John P. Sloane | 1946-2000 |

This edition is dedicated to the memory of our friend and colleague who pioneered the quality assurance of breast pathology in the UK and throughout Europe

N. Perry
Quality Assurance Reference Centre
London Region Breast Screening Programme
St Bartholomew's Hospital
90 Bartholomew Close
London EC1A 7BE
United Kingdom

M. Broeders
Department of Epidemiology and
Biostatistics / EUREF Office 451
University Medical Centre Nijmegen
PO Box 9101
6500 HB Nijmegen
The Netherlands

C. de Wolf
Institute of Social and Preventive Medicine (IMSP)
University of Geneva
55 Bd de la Cluse
1205 Geneva
Switzerland

S. Törnberg
Cancer Screening Unit
Oncologic Centre
Karolinska Hospital
17176 Stockholm
Sweden

J. Schouten
EUREF Office 451
University Medical Centre Nijmegen
PO Box 9101
6500 HB Nijmegen
The Netherlands

Contributors

N. Ascunce, Gobierno de Navarra, Programme Cancer de Mamma, Pamplona, Spain

R. Blamey, Professorial Unit of Surgery, Nottingham City Hospital, United Kingdom

M. Blichert-Toft, Department of Surgery, Rigshospitalet, Denmark

R. Bordon, Breast Unit, St. Anna Hospital, Turin, Italy

M. Broeders, Department of Epidemiology and Biostatistics / EUREF Office, University Medical Centre Nijmegen, The Netherlands

J. Caseldine, NHS Breast Screening Programme, Sheffield, United Kingdom

L. Cataliotti, Instituto di Clinica Chirurgia, University of Florence, Italy

M. Codd, Department of Epidemiology, Mater Hospital, Dublin, Ireland

V. Distante, Instituto di Clinica Chirurgia, University of Florence, Italy

D. Giorgi, Unit of Epidemiology, CSPO, Florence, Italy

T. Gorey, Department of Surgery, Mater Hospital, Dublin, Ireland

J. Hendriks, National Expert and Training Centre for Breast Cancer Screening, Nijmegen, The Netherlands

R. Holland, National Expert and Training Centre for Breast Cancer Screening, Nijmegen, The Netherlands

L. Holmberg, Oncologic centre, Uppsala, Sweden

A. Linos, Department of Hygiene and Epidemiology, University Medical School, Athens, Greece

D. Linos, Department of Surgery, Hospital Hygeia, 1st Surgical Clinic, Athens, Greece

M. Mano, Breast Unit, St. Anna Hospital, Turin, Italy

R. Mansel, University Department of Surgery, University of Wales, Cardiff, United Kingdom

W. Mattheiem, Institute Jules-Bordet, Brussels, Belgium

L. Nyström, Department of Public Health and Clinical Medicine Epidemiology, University of Umeå, Sweden

N. O'Higgins, Department of Surgery, University College Dublin, St. Vincent's Hospital, Ireland

N. Perry, London Region Breast Screening Programme, St. Bartholomew's Hospital, London, United Kingdom

A. Ponti, CPO Piemonte, Turin, Italy

H. Rijken, National Expert and Training Centre for Breast Cancer Screening, Nijmegen, The Netherlands

E. Riza, Department of Hygiene and Epidemiology, University Medical School, Athens, Greece

P. Roberts, Department of Surgery, University of Helsinki, Finland

F. Rochard, Institute Gustave Roussy, France

V. Rodrigues, Programa de Cancro de Mama, Liga Portuguesa Contra o Cancro, Coimbra, Portugal

M. Rosselli del Turco, Breast Unit, CSPO, Florence, Italy

E. Rutgers, Department of Surgery, Netherlands Cancer Institute, The Netherlands

R. Sainsbury, University College Hospital - NHS Trust, 9th floor, St. Martin's House, 140 Tottenham Court Road, London W1P 9LM, UK

K. Schulz, Universitaets-Frauenklinik, Marburg, Germany

N. Segnan, CPO Piemonte, Turin, Italy

M. da Silva, Centro de Coimbra do Instituto Portugues de Oncologia de Francisco Gentil, Portugal

M. Smola, Universitaetsklinik fur Chirurgie, Karl Franzens Universitaet, Austria

J. Sloane†, Department of Pathology, University of Liverpool, Liverpool, United Kingdom

M. Thijssen, National Expert and Training Centre for Breast Cancer Screening, Nijmegen, The Netherlands

S. Törnberg, Cancer Screening Unit, Oncologic Centre, Karolinska Hospital, Stockholm, Sweden

C. de Wolf, Institute of Social and Preventive Medicine (IMSP), University of Geneva, 55 Bd de la Cluse, 1205 Geneva, Switzerland

S. van Woudenberg, National Expert and Training Centre for Breast Cancer Screening, Nijmegen, The Netherlands

K. Young, National Coordinating Centre for Physics of Mammography, Guildford, United Kingdom

Table of contents

4. Radiographical guidelines

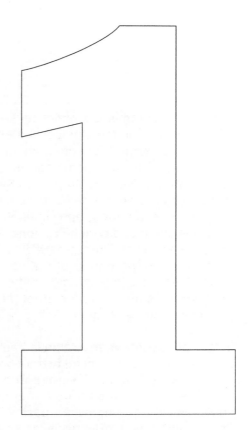

Introduction

Author
N. Perry

Breast cancer remains a major cause of mortality and morbidity, and of significant concern to many women in the Member States. Mammography is a widely used imaging procedure, whether performed for screening or diagnostic purposes. The exact number performed throughout Europe each year is unknown, but probably in excess of ten million examinations. The UK, Dutch and Swedish screening programmes alone perform nearly three million mammograms annually, and in those countries with organised screening programmes mammography is likely to be the third commonest radiographic procedure following chest and peripheral bone X-rays. The major benefits of breast screening are the early detection of breast cancer and the subsequent reduction in mortality from the disease. The potential harm caused by mammography includes the creation of unnecessary anxiety and morbidity, inappropriate economic cost and the use of ionising radiation. It is for this reason that the strongest possible emphasis on quality control and quality assurance is required.

In the last twenty years we have had ample evidence that mammographic screening can successfully reduce mortality from breast cancer. These benefits are sufficiently clear cut and cost-effective for several European Member States - Sweden, the Netherlands, UK and Finland - to embark upon national population based screening programmes. The Luxembourg Programme as part of the Europe Against Cancer funded Breast Cancer Screening Network effectively also has national coverage. France and Ireland have set up and are about to implement national programmes. Many other countries have high quality regionally based screening.

Even with a high level of professional skill and a comprehensive QA system, no screening programme can be truly successful without a long term political commitment. Breast screening is a major public health management issue which requires a far reaching political responsibility in order to be effective. This will entail the organisation of a suitable infrastructure, setting of screening policy, coordination of professional groups and economic programme evaluation.

Critics of breast screening question cost-effectiveness and the overall benefit conferred to women. Critical analysis and experience demonstrate that there is indeed a fine balance between desirable and undesirable effects even in organised high quality programmes. Sensitivity and specificity need to be optimal in order to obtain the maximum benefit from breast screening. This can only be achieved as skill and a comprehensive quality assurance system is applied to the entire process, involving each individual part of the programme. Use of sub-optimal equipment by poorly trained and unskilled staff will significantly reduce the major benefits of screening and result in ineffective and costly mammography services. Under these circumstances, the critics of screening are correct and it is our responsibility to discourage and if possible prevent screening of inadequate quality.

The key operational objectives for a successful population screening programme have not altered and should be re-emphasised:
1. To identify and invite eligible women for mammography screening.
2. To maximise compliance in the eligible population.
3. To ensure that mammography of the highest possible standard is performed and that films are read by personnel with proper training and proven skills in this area.
4. To maximise the acceptability of the service.
5. To provide prompt and effective further investigations and treatment where indicated.
6. To minimise the adverse effects of screening while optimising cancer detection.

7. To monitor outcomes and continuously evaluate the entire screening process.
8. To perform regular audit of programme activities and to provide appropriate feedback to staff.
9. To provide a cost-effective service.
10. To ensure that all staff undergo initial training with regular updating and continuing professional development.

To achieve these objectives requires a multi-faceted and multidisciplinary approach, a weak link anywhere will diminish the overall effectiveness of the programme. This is the reason why guidelines such as these are essential for all stages of the screening and diagnostic process and for all professional disciplines involved. They should provide the basis of local quality assurance manuals, and practice protocols which must exist in any programme. They should always be used in conjunction with any existing professionally agreed guidelines.

These European guidelines are based upon experience gained through the national screening programmes, the Europe Against Cancer funded European Network for Breast Cancer Screening which commenced in 1988 and EUREF (see annex VIII). There is much important information contained within which can be applied at all levels and will also be useful for those active in the diagnosis of breast disease within locally based mammographic facilities. Genuine improvement may be achieved purely by following the technical advice given. It is sometimes easier to be more specific in national guidelines that pertain to one particular healthcare system, than across Europe where professional and political attitudes and healthcare systems are more diverse. These issues have been taken into account in the setting of some targets, however varying practice must never be allowed to compromise the quality and outcomes of a programme.

It is the belief of many that screening programmes can also achieve significant gains for women outside the screened population, despite the fact that the majority of all breast cancers in the population will be detected symptomatically. The reason for such optimism is that the skill, expertise, knowledge and multidisciplinary team working fostered by organised screening will reap huge rewards in the streamlining of effective diagnosis and treatment of all breast cancers passing through an experienced unit. It would be unjustifiable not to fully utilise these skills to benefit symptomatic breast services where good image quality, correct interpretation and skilled assessment carry just as much importance as in screening. To this end we have included the EUSOMA document on quality assurance in the diagnosis of breast disease as annex.

This third edition has been revised and expanded to reflect further experiences in the four years since the previous edition was published. There are additions of fuller sections for radiologists and radiographers, with sections on training requirements and data collection. The surgical aspects of multidisciplinary team work, and involvement in the diagnosis and management of small screen detected cancers are central to the effectiveness of screening and so the previously published guidelines for surgeons have been incorporated. Annexes have been rearranged to reflect current status and activity.

What future developments might be expected by the time of the next edition? The most likely would seem to be related to digital technology. Digital acquisition of mammographic images either in a full field system or in a more localised field for assessment and sampling is certain to become more widely used. This leads on to other exciting possibilities regarding the use of computer aided detection and tele-radiology. These may become significant issues as the need for breast imaging radiologists becomes even more acute with the ever expanding utilisation of screening, and the steeply rising population in the screening age group (the post-war baby boom). Speed of acquisition of images and potential archiving advantages of digital mammography are likely to become important factors. Increasing attention will be paid to the accuracy of pre-operative diagnosis in order to further reduce the numbers of unnecessary benign surgical biopsies, and to maximise the effectiveness of one stage surgery for breast cancer. There are likely to be advances in new techniques for percutaneous sampling, and ultrasound technology using contrast. The place of MRI in breast diagnosis will become more precisely understood, as will the use of sentinel node biopsy to avoid unnecessary axillary dissection. It remains to be seen how many of these techniques become sufficiently established and available, cost-effective and relevant to screening, in order to be suitable for inclusion in the next edition of the guidelines.

Quality is a word subject to frequent over-use, particularly where commercial considerations are involved, in order to impart or imply confidence in a system which may be ill founded. This cannot be tolerated in breast cancer screening which requires a long term commitment and will only work effectively with a genuine and constant high level of quality. We must strive to achieve a system free from variable standards and performance levels. There needs to be a tangible benchmark that quality is real and is maintained at a sufficient level to satisfy external inspection. Such evidence should be available for the public, politicians and funding organisations alike. Voluntary codes of practice and self regulation are unlikely to be sufficiently effective.

Whereas the previous edition recommended the certification of knowledge acquired through training, it is now the general belief that certification of overall system quality by suitable and approved organisations will provide the only real and meaningful confidence. Accordingly the EUREF Certification Protocol, describing the certification process of breast screening and diagnostic institutions at different levels, is included in the annexes. The EUREF organisation has commenced its certification programme in 2000. The strongly worded EURATOM Council Directive (97/43) supports this aim. This document concerns health protection of individuals against the dangers of ionising radiation in relation to medical exposure, mentions screening specifically and became European law as of 13th May 2000.

Research to achieve major new advances in diagnosis and treatment of breast cancer is essential and requires further support. Breast cancer screening is available and effective. There is an obligation to ensure achievable quality is optimised in order to obtain the maximum benefit from this already proven technique.

The contributors to this latest edition have dedicated much of their careers to such issues. I thank them for their contributions and have great pleasure in introducing these guidelines to you. I have no doubt that this document is of major public health importance and will further the continuous task of striving to improve the outlook for women with early detectable breast cancer.

Table 3: Breast cancer occurrence, rates/100,000 women per year

Age group	Breast cancer incidence* Number	/100,000	Breast cancer mortality* Number	/100,000
50-54				
55-59				
60-64				
World age-standardised rate* in the year	NA		NA	

* cf Glossary of terms
NA = not applicable

Table 4 refers to a variety of methods potentially available to publicise the screening programme. Depending on the target population and the local geographical, municipal and cultural conditions, the need for and intensity of programme promotion may vary. Please indicate the intensity of the activities in your screening programme, using the classification 'no', 'low', 'medium' or 'high'.

Table 4: Programme promotion

Mode of promotion	Intensity of activity (no/low/medium/high)
Press	
TV	
Radio	
Physician/GP	
Church	
Schools	
Municipal authorities	
Social clubs	
Other:	

Table 5 A potential determinant of participation in a breast screening programme is whether the participating woman is required to pay for the screening examination. When a consultation with a family practitioner is required to gain access to the screening examination, the costs of this consultation should be included in the fee paid. In some screening programmes, the fee for the screening examination will be paid, partly or completely, by a third party. Third party payment may be either through vouchers available to the woman before screening or through a system in which the woman pays in advance and gets reimbursed after the screening. Alternatively, a third party may pay the fee directly to the screening unit or organisation.

Table 5: Fees paid for the screening examination

Fees paid by the woman herself (in Euros):
• For the screening examination
• To receive the results

Third party payment (% of costs covered):
• Through vouchers
• Through reimbursement system
• Directly to screening unit*

* cf Glossary of terms

Table 6 Many factors can be identified which encourage or impede the setting up of a breast screening programme. Such potential factors are: cost, fear, lack of interest, integration into the existing health care system, data protection legislation. These can also include reasons for not responding to the invitation to be screened, and women's attitudes about and knowledge of screening guidelines.

Table 6: Potential conditions for/against screening

Please specify any conditions that may have worked for or against screening in your screening programme:

2.3 Invitation scheme

The aim of this paragraph is to describe the invitation scheme used by the screening programme, i.e. the methodology used to identify and invite members of the target population. A number of data sources can be used. For each source, information on its accuracy is requested.

Table 7 lists the sources of demographic data potentially used and the contribution of each to the identification of the target population in preparation for the first screening round. It is recognised that relative contributions of these sources will vary and may be difficult to estimate.

Table 7: Sources and accuracy of target population data (first round)

Data source	Target population* identified (%)	Best estimate of register accuracy (%)	Computer (C)/ Manual (M)
Population register			
Electoral register			
Other registers			
Self-registration*			
Other:			

* cf Glossary of terms

Table 8 After the creation of a screening register which identifies the target population at the start of the screening programme with maximal accuracy, every effort should be made to ensure that this information remains up-to-date. Ideally, a permanent link with a population register should be established, offering the possibility of daily updates of the screening register. In this way, women who move into or out of the screening area or who have died, can be identified and included or excluded from the invitation scheme. Potential access to other sources allowing for adjustments of the screening register are also listed. Please also indicate the frequency with which this information is used to update the screening register.

Table 8: Maintenance of the screening register

Estimate of screening register completeness (%)	
Estimate of screening register accuracy (%)	
Sources of screening register updates (yes/no): • Census data • Cancer registration • Death registration • Social insurance/tax records • Data on population migration • Returned invitations • Other:	
Frequency with which screening register is updated	

Table 9 Depending on the programme several types of call systems may be used. Invitations may be by personalised letter, by personal oral invitation or by open non-personal invitation, or by a combination of all three. Women who do not respond to the initial invitation may be issued a reminder, again by any available means listed below. The time interval (column 4 and 7) between invitation and reminder usually varies by programme. Some programmes may issue more than one reminder, or reminders by multiple methods. It may not be possible to ascertain the success of individual types of reminders.

Table 9: Mode of invitation

Mode of invitation	Initial screening*			Subsequent screening*		
	Invitation (yes/no)	Reminder (yes/no)	Interval* (weeks)	Invitation (yes/no)	Reminder (yes/no)	Interval* (weeks)
Personal letter • By mail • Other • Fixed date						
Personal oral invitation • By screening unit* • Other • Fixed date						
Non-personal invitation • Letter • Public announcement						

* cf Glossary of terms

Table 10 In the context of these epidemiological guidelines, the target population for the breast screening programme includes all persons eligible to attend screening on the basis of age and geographic location. However, each programme may apply additional inclusion/exclusion criteria to identify the 'eligible population' for screening. In addition, screening programmes may apply their own criteria to exclude certain women from screening outcomes. Potential exclusions from both the target population and screening outcomes for initial and subsequent screening examinations are listed in table 10. The ease with which such individuals can be identified and excluded from the target population will vary by programme; for some programmes it may not be possible to identify any category of potential exclusion prior to invitation.

Table 10: Potential adjustments

	Initial screening*		Subsequent screening*	
Target population* (n)				
Eligible population* (n)				
Reason for exclusion	**Excluded from**		**Excluded from**	
	Target (yes/no, n)	Outcomes (yes/no, n)	Target (yes/no, n)	Outcomes (yes/no, n)
Previous breast cancer				
Previous mastectomy • Unilateral • Bilateral				
Recent mammogram*				
Symptomatic women*				
Incapacitated • Physical • Mental • Other				
Death				
Other:				

* cf Glossary of terms
n = number

2.4 Screening process and further assessment

The aim of this paragraph is to describe the entire screening and assessment process, from mammographic detection of breast abnormalities through further investigation of those abnormalities, to diagnosis or otherwise of a malignant lesion.

Table 11 describes the screening facilities available and whether they are dedicated completely to breast cancer screening. It also requires information on the availability of assessment centres, where women might go for further assessment of a perceived abnormality detected at the screening examination.

Table 11: Screening facilities

Screening facilities	Number	Dedicated*
Mammography machines		
Static units		
Semi-mobile units		
Mobile units		
Other units		
Assessment centres		

* cf Glossary of terms

In **table 12** further details on the screening policy of the programme are requested such as: the screening test used (whether single or two-view mammography, with or without clinical examination), the interval between screening examinations and the assessment facilities for invasive investigations (centralised or not). If the majority of screening mammograms are double read, please also specify the policy to resolve discrepancies between the interpretations of the two readers, e.g. the woman is always recalled, discussion between readers, review by third reader, review by consensus panel or committee. In case your screening programme changed its policy after the introduction, please complete table 12 a second time to reflect any changes made.

Table 12: Screening policy*

Screening test* • Initial screening* • Subsequent screening*
Screening interval* (months)
Double reading (%)
Policy to resolve discrepancies
Centralised assessment (yes/no)

* cf Glossary of terms

Tables 13 and 14 describe the outcomes of screening examinations, as well as the additional investigations which may be undertaken prior to, and including surgery. The order of investigations as listed does not necessarily imply that each participant will go through all stages before surgical excision and final diagnosis. All tables should be reported separately for the three groups of women, as described in the introduction:
• initial screening, i.e. the first screening examination of individual women within the screening programme, regardless of the organisational screening round (INITIAL)
• subsequent screening at the regular interval, in accordance with the routine interval defined by the screening policy (SUBS-R)
• subsequent screening at irregular intervals, those who miss an invitation to routine screening and return in a subsequent organisational screening round (SUBS-IRR)

For all investigations listed the numbers should reflect women, not breasts. The age category in which the result of an individual woman should be recorded is determined as the age of the woman at the time of the screening examination for a particular screening round. For non-participants, age should be determined as the age of the woman at the time of invitation (not the age at reminder). A woman's results should thus be recorded in the same age category throughout a particular screening episode.

Table 13 lists the number of women that are targeted, eligible, invited and finally screened. The result of the screening examination can be recorded in various categories, that may not all be available in the screening programme, e.g. a screening programme may not have the option of intermediate mammography directly following the screening examination. Further assessment includes non-invasive and invasive investigations for medical reasons.

Table 13: Screening outcomes (INITIAL/SUBS-R/SUBS-IRR)

	Age group 50-54	55-59	60-64	Total
Target population*				
Eligible population*				
Women invited*				
Women screened*				
Participation rate (%)*				

Result of screening test:
• Negative
• Intermediate mammogram following screening*
• Repeat screening test*
  - recommended
  - performed
• Further assessment*
  - recommended
  - performed
• Unknown/not available				

* cf Glossary of terms

Table 14 describes the outcomes of non-invasive and invasive investigations following the screening examination. These investigations can be done at the time of screening when facilities are available in the screening unit or they can be performed on recall, i.e. the woman will have to come back to the screening unit for further investigation. As a result of non-invasive assessment, further clarification of the perceived abnormality may be required using invasive investigations. It should be noted however, that a woman may also undergo further assessment by invasive investigations directly following the screening examination.

Table 14: Screening outcomes: further investigations (INITIAL/SUBS-R/SUBS-IRR)

Investigations after screening	Age group			
	50-54	55-59	60-64	Total
Repeat screening test*				
• At screening				
• On recall*				
Additional imaging*				
• At screening				
• On recall*				
Additional imaging rate* (%)				
Recall rate* (%)				
Types of additional imaging*				
• Repeat views (medical)				
• Cranio-caudal view				
• Other views				
• Ultrasound				
• MRI				
Invasive investigations				
• Recommended				
• Performed				
- at screening				
- on recall*				
Cytology*				
• Recommended				
• Performed				
Core biopsy*				
• Recommended				
• Performed				
Open biopsy*				
• Recommended				
• Performed				

* cf Glossary of terms

Table 15 classifies the results of the overall screening process in four categories, partly overlapping with the results of the screening test in table 13.

An overall breast cancer detection rate represents the performance of a screening programme but also reflects the age structure of the population being screened. To provide a more sensitive measure of performance, table 15 also allows for the calculation of age-specific detection ratios per 5-year age groups. The incidence rate for breast cancer in the denominator of the formula should reflect the underlying (expected) incidence rate in the absence of screening. It should be noted that the expected rates will increase marginally with each screening year because of the annual increase in the estimated background incidence.

$$\textbf{Age-specific detection ratio} = \frac{\text{Cancer detection rate in a 5-year age group}}{\substack{\text{Underlying expected breast cancer incidence in} \\ \text{that age group in the absence of screening}}}$$

Table 15: Result of screening process after assessment (INITIAL/SUBS-R/SUBS-IRR)

	Age group			
	50-54	55-59	60-64	Total
Result of screening process:				
• Negative				
• Intermediate mammogram following assessment*				
• Breast cancers detected:				
- DCIS				
- invasive cancers				
• Unknown/not available				
Breast cancers detected:				
• At routine screen				
• At intermediate mammography*				
Breast cancer detection rate*				
Breast cancer incidence rate*				
Age-specific detection ratio*				

* cf Glossary of terms

Table 16 summarises the results of screening in terms of positive predictive values (PPV) of specific interventions which take place in the course of mammographic screening and in further assessment of abnormal lesions. Results can be expected to vary between initial and subsequent screening examinations. PPV is expressed as a proportion. Please refer to the Glossary of terms (paragraph 2.10) for definition of the individual PPVs listed in table 16.

Table 16: Positive predictive value of specific interventions in screening for breast cancer, age group 50-64 (INITIAL/SUBS-R/SUBS-IRR)

Outcome of the intervention		Breast cancer detected		
		Yes	No	PPV*
Screening test*	Positive			
	Negative			
Additional imaging*	Positive			
	Negative			
Recall*	Positive			
	Negative			
Cytology*	Positive			
	Negative			
Recommendation * for open biopsy	Positive			
	Negative			

* cf Glossary of terms

2.5 Disease stage of screen-detected cancers

The aim of this paragraph is to describe the disease stage of screen-detected cancer cases. More detailed guidance on the pathological service in a breast screening programme can be found in the pathology chapters. A prerequisite for a reduction in breast cancer mortality is a more favourable stage distribution in screen-detected cancers compared with clinically diagnosed cancers. Tumour size and axillary lymph node involvement for invasive cancers are of central importance here, and are assessed preferably after surgery (pT and pN). Age categories in **tables 17 and 18** refer to the age of a woman at the preceding screening examination.

The categorisation of size according to pathological diameter is based on the TNM-classification (UICC, 1997) for reasons of comparison. It is recommended however to also register the size of the tumour on a continuous scale. This will facilitate recategorisation in the event that consensus is reached on a different prognostic threshold (e.g. 15 mm).

Primary tumour (T) is classified as follows:
pTx   primary tumour cannot be assessed
pT0   no evidence of primary tumour
pTis   ductal carcinoma in situ
pT1ab tumour ≤ 10 mm in greatest dimension
pT1c   tumour ≤ 20 mm in greatest dimension
pT2   tumour ≤ 50 mm in greatest dimension
pT3   tumour > 50 mm in greatest dimension
pT4   tumour of any size with direct extension to chest wall or skin

Regional lymph node involvement (N) is classified as follows:
Nx   regional lymph nodes cannot be assessed
N0   no regional lymph node metastasis
N1   metastasis to movable ipsilateral axillary lymph node(s)
N2   metastasis to ipsilateral axillary lymph node(s) fixed to one another or to other structures
N3   metastasis to ipsilateral internal mammary lymph node(s)

Distant metastasis (M) is classified as follows:
Mx   presence of distant metastasis cannot be assessed
M0   no distant metastasis
M1   distant metastasis (includes metastasis to ipsilateral supraclavicular lymph node(s)

Stage grouping

Stage 0	Tis	N0	M0
Stage I	T1	N0	M0
Stage IIA	T0	N1	M0
	T1	N1	M0
	T2	N0	M0
Stage IIB	T2	N1	M0
	T3	N0	M0
Stage IIIA	T0	N2	M0
	T1	N2	M0
	T2	N2	M0
	T3	N1	M0
	T3	N2	M0
Stage IIIB	T4	any N	M0
	any T	N3	M0
Stage IV	any T	any N	M1

Table 17: Size and nodal status of screen-detected cancers (INITIAL/SUBS-R/ SUBS-IRR)

| | Age group | | | |
	50-54	55-59	60-64	Total
pTis				
• N–				
• N+				
• Nx				
pT1ab				
• N–				
• N+				
• Nx				
pT1c				
• N–				
• N+				
• Nx				
pT2				
• N–				
• N+				
• Nx				
pT3				
• N–				
• N+				
• Nx				
pT4				
• N–				
• N+				
• Nx				
pTx				
• N–				
• N+				
• Nx				

N– = axillary node negative (N0)

N+ = axillary node positive (any node positive; N1-3)

Nx = nodal status cannot be assessed (e.g. previously removed, not done)

Table 18: Disease stage of screen-detected cancers according to the TNM-classification (INITIAL/SUBS-R/SUBS-IRR)

	Age group			
	50-54	55-59	60-64	Total
Stage 0 • TisN0M0				
Stage I • T1N0M0				
Stage IIA • T0N1M0 • T1N1M0 • T2N0M0				
Stage IIB • T2N1M0 • T3N0M0				
Stage IIIA • T0N2M0 • T1N2M0 • T2N2M0 • T3N1M0 • T3N2M0				
Stage IIIB • T4anyNM0 • AnyTN3M0				
Stage IV • AnyTanyNM1				
Unknown				

2.6 Treatment of screen-detected cancers

It is recognised that collecting data on treatment on a regular basis may be a difficult and time consuming activity, especially in those screening programmes where treatment is not considered to be part of the screening process. On the other hand, it should be realised that the effect of screening in the long term will be heavily influenced by the way screen-detected cases are treated. A high-quality screening programme can only lead to a long-term mortality reduction if the treatment of women detected at screening is of equally high quality. Thus it is considered of the utmost importance to collect this type of data. More detailed guidance on the management of screen-detected lesions and appropriate quality indicators can be found in the surgical chapters in this document.

All women with breast cancer detected at screening, with or without signs of distant metastases, will be offered some form of primary treatment. For ductal carcinoma in situ (DCIS) and invasive cancers several types of treatment are categorised in **tables 19, 20 and 21**. Women with axillary lymph node metastases are assumed to receive adjuvant systemic therapy in the majority of cases. The treatment options according to disease stage of breast cancer diagnosed outside screening (interval cancer as well as other 'control' cancers) can be optionally registered in **table 22**.

Table 19: Primary treatment* of screen-detected *ductal carcinoma in situ*

| | Age group | | | |
	50-54	55-59	60-64	Total
Breast conserving surgery[1]				
• Axillary dissection performed				
• With radiotherapy				
• Without radiotherapy				
• Radiotherapy unknown				
Mastectomy				
• Axillary dissection performed				
Treatment refusal/unknown				

[1] less than mastectomy
* cf Glossary of terms

Table 20: Primary treatment* of screen-detected *invasive* breast cancers

| | Age group | | | |
	50-54	55-59	60-64	Total
Breast conserving surgery[1]				
• Axillary dissection performed				
• With radiotherapy				
• Without radiotherapy				
• Radiotherapy unknown				
• Adjuvant therapy*				
Mastectomy				
• Axillary dissection performed				
• With radiotherapy				
• Without radiotherapy				
• Radiotherapy unknown				
• Adjuvant therapy*				

	Age group			
	50-54	55-59	60-64	Total
Chemotherapy				
• With radiotherapy				
• Without radiotherapy				
• Radiotherapy unknown				
• Adjuvant therapy*				
Radiotherapy				
• Adjuvant therapy*				
Treatment refusal/unknown				

[1] less than mastectomy
* cf Glossary of terms

Table 21: Primary treatment* of screen-detected breast cancers according to stage at diagnosis

	Stage at diagnosis							
	0	I	IIA	IIB	IIIA	IIIB	IV	Unk[2]
Breast conserving surgery[1]								
• Axillary dissection performed								
• With radiotherapy								
• Without radiotherapy								
• Radiotherapy unknown								
• Adjuvant therapy*								
Mastectomy								
• Axillary dissection performed								
• With radiotherapy								
• Without radiotherapy								
• Radiotherapy unknown								
• Adjuvant therapy*								
Chemotherapy								
• With radiotherapy								
• Without radiotherapy								
• Radiotherapy unknown								
• Adjuvant therapy*								
Radiotherapy								
• Adjuvant therapy*								
Treatment refusal/unknown								

[1] less than mastectomy   [2] unk = unknown   * cf Glossary of terms

Table 22: Primary treatment* of breast cancers diagnosed *outside* screening according to stage at diagnosis (OPTIONAL)

	Stage at diagnosis							
	0	I	IIA	IIB	IIIA	IIIB	IV	Unk[2]
Breast conserving surgery[1]								
• Axillary dissection performed								
• With radiotherapy								
• Without radiotherapy								
• Radiotherapy unknown								
• Adjuvant therapy*								
Mastectomy								
• Axillary dissection performed								
• With radiotherapy								
• Without radiotherapy								
• Radiotherapy unknown								
• Adjuvant therapy*								
Chemotherapy								
• With radiotherapy								
• Without radiotherapy								
• Radiotherapy unknown								
• Adjuvant therapy*								
Radiotherapy								
• Adjuvant therapy*								
Treatment refusal/unknown								

[1] less than mastectomy
[2] unk = unknown
* cf Glossary of terms

Table 23 reflects the distribution of the number of days between the day of screening and the day of surgery for those women undergoing surgery as a result of the screening examination. For those women not undergoing surgery, the interval between the day of screening and the day of final assessment should be registered.

In case a cancer is detected at intermediate mammography, which is by definition a screen-detected cancer, the day of screening should be replaced by the day that the intermediate mammogram was performed.

Table 23: Number of days between screening and surgery or screening and final assessment (age group 50 - 64 years) for screen-detected cancers

			Quantiles		
	5%	25%	50%	75%	95%
Day of screening - day of surgery					
Day of screening - day of final assessment					

2.7 Follow up of the target population and ascertainment of interval cancers[1]

Introduction

The aim of this paragraph is to describe objectives and document the processes of follow up of the target population of a mammographic screening programme.

The purpose of monitoring interval cancers is two fold. On the one hand, it serves quality assurance and training (see radiology chapter). On the other hand, it allows for the calculation of parameters providing an early estimate of the impact of the screening programme in modifying the appearance of the disease, and thereby its effects, in the population. Therefore, data collection and reporting should be directed to all cancers appearing in the target population. Completeness of data collection and the use of different inclusion and exclusion criteria may limit the comparability of interval cancer rates in different populations. Tables and parameters suggested in this section aim at reducing these sources of variation and assist in the estimation of the effect of screening within each programme. Background incidence, breast awareness, the availability of timely diagnosis and the diffusion of spontaneous screening can also affect comparisons. For this reason it is recommended that numerical targets, not provided here, be set at a national or regional level.

Comprehensive follow up of a target population necessitates ascertainment and reporting of all breast cancers in all members of the target population. Such a target population consists of three groups:
a. those women who were invited for screening and who attended
b. those women who were invited for screening but who did not attend
c. those women who were not invited for screening

Group c includes women not yet invited for screening at the time of follow up as well as those women of the target population who were never invited because of inadequate or

---

[1] This paragraph is based on the work of the interval cancer project group, represented by M Codd, A Ponti, V Rodrigues and S Törnberg (supported in part by a grant from the 'Europe Against Cancer' Programme, 98/CAN/40211).

---

incomplete population registers. The size and complexity of this group may differ between health care environments and may be determined in part by the frequency of update of population registers.

Methods of follow up for cancer occurrence

Methods of follow up for cancer occurrence may differ by country, by region or by screening programme, depending on the availability and accessibility of data and data sources. **Table 24** outlines the methods by which the target population may be followed to ascertain breast cancer occurrence, for each of the groups as defined above. It is sufficient to mark the boxes with a ✓.

Table 24: Methods of follow up for cancer occurrence

Data source	Participants	Non-participants	Persons not invited
Screening programme register			
Cancer / pathology register			
Breast care / clinical records			
Death register / certificate review			
Other, specify:			

Categories of cancer in the target population

Combining data on cancer occurrence from whatever source, with information on individual screening histories, including date of invitation, response to invitation, attendance for and outcome of screening with/without further assessment, permits classification of cancers which occur in members of the target population into the following categories:

a. **Screen-detected cancer:**
   A primary breast cancer which is identified by the screening test, with/without further assessment, in a member of the target population, who was invited for and attended for screening.

b. **Interval cancer:**
   A primary breast cancer which is diagnosed in a woman who had a screening test, with/without further assessment, which was negative for malignancy, either:
   • before the next invitation to screening, or
   • within a time period equal to a screening interval in case the woman has reached the upper age limit for screening.

c. **Cancer in non-participant:**
   A primary breast cancer which occurs in a member of the target population who was invited for screening but did not attend.

d. **Cancer in women not invited:**
   A primary breast cancer which occurs in a member of the target population who was not, or not yet, invited for screening.

Typically, a mammographic screening programme is organised into 'rounds' of screening, i.e. first, second, etc. at a defined interval, e.g. 24 months, depending on the programme's screening policy. Follow up begins at the start of a screening round and extends to the time of the next routine screening examination for those who attend screening as scheduled. For those who do not attend regularly, and for those women who, during the follow up period, exceed the upper age limit for screening, follow up should be continued for a period at least commensurate with the usual screening interval. This applies to all categories of women, i.e. participants, non-participants and those not invited for screening, in so far as this is possible.

In follow up of the target population it is relevant to examine *separately* those cancers (of all categories) identified during, or occurring after, the first round of screening, and those identified during, or occurring after, a subsequent round of screening. This is because the first round of screening is comprised entirely of women being screened for the first time (initial screenees); subsequent rounds of screening are comprised of women being screened for the first time, as well as those who have previously been screened.

Table 25 documents the number of breast cancers in the target population for first and second rounds of screening, and for initial and subsequent screening examinations. Data for additional, subsequent, rounds of screening should be recorded as for the second round.

Table 25: Breast cancers in the target population by screening round and by initial/ subsequent screening*

	First round	Second/Subsequent round(s)	
Screening period (dates) (mth/yr – mth/yr)			
Follow up period (dates) (mth/yr – mth/yr)			
	Initial (n)	Initial (n)	Subsequent (n)
Screen-detected cancer Interval cancer* Cancer non-participants Cancer not invited			
TOTAL			

* cf Glossary of terms

Date of diagnosis of breast cancers in the target population
An important consideration in classifying breast cancers which occur in the target population is the date used as the date of diagnosis. The category to which a cancer will

be assigned may depend on which one of several possible dates of diagnosis is used. For the cancers reported in table 25, it is suggested that the 'date used' be recorded, primarily for the purpose of quality assurance in the ascertainment and classification of cancers. **Table 26** provides the opportunity to do this.

Table 26: Date of diagnosis of breast cancers in the target population

Source for date of diagnosis	SD	IC	NP	NI
Date of clinical examination				
Date of screening mammogram				
Date of diagnostic mammogram				
Date of cytology				
Date of surgery				
Date of pathology				
Date of death				
Other, specify:				

SD = screen-detected cancer
IC = interval cancer
NP = cancer in non-participant
NI = cancer in not invited

Relationship of breast cancers in the target population to selected programme performance indicators

Examination of the relationship between breast cancer occurrence in the target population and programme performance indicators is an important component of the evaluation of a mammographic screening programme.

Table 27 provides the opportunity to record breast cancer occurrence along with selected programme performance indicators e.g. participation rate, additional imaging rate, recall rate, assessment rate, benign biopsy rate. Of particular interest is the relation of an indicator of sensitivity of the screening programme, such as the interval cancer rate, with indicators of specificity, such as additional imaging rate, recall rate, assessment rate and benign biopsy rate (see Glossary of terms for definitions).

Table 27: Relationship of breast cancers in the target population to selected programme performance indicators

Performance indicator	First round Initial*	Second round	
		Initial*	Subsequent*
Women invited* (n)			
Women screened* (n)			
Participation rate* (%)			
Additional imaging rate at time of screening* (%)			
Recall rate* (%)			
Intermediate mammography rate* (%)			
Further assessment* rate (%)			
Benign biopsies /10,000 screened			
Screen-detected cancers (n)			
Benign to malignant biopsy ratio*			
Breast cancer detection rate* • In situ / 10,000 screened • Invasive / 10,000 screened			
Interval cancers (n)			
Interval cancer rate • 0-11 months / 10,000 screened • 12-23 months / 10,000 screened • 24+ months / 10,000 screened			
Cancers in non-participants (n)			
Cancers in not invited (n)			
Cancer in non-screened population / 10,000 population not screened			
Total cancers in target population (n)			
Cancer / 10,000 target population			

* cf Glossary of terms
n = number

International comparisons of these relationships are currently under way to define the direction of the relationships and programme factors most strongly associated with the occurrence of interval cancers.

Relationship of breast cancers in the target population to tumour size and stage at diagnosis

Tumour size and stage at diagnosis of breast cancer differ according to the category of cancer, i.e. whether screen-detected, interval or non-participant cancer. While such detailed data may not be available from all data sources, it is recommended that these data are collected on all categories of cancer in so far as it is possible. This would permit comparison between the categories of cancer with respect to tumour size and stage at diagnosis as outlined in **table 28**. The classification used is defined in paragraph 2.6 of this chapter.

Table 28: Relationship of breast cancers in the target population to tumour size and stage at diagnosis

Size of primary tumour	SD	IC	NP	NI
pTis				
pT1a				
pT1b				
pT1c				
pT2				
pT3				
pT4				
pTx				
TOTAL				

SD = screen-detected cancer
IC = interval cancer
NP = cancer in non-participant
NI = cancer in not invited

Table 28, continued

Stage at diagnosis	SD	IC	NP	NI
Stage 0				
Stage I				
Stage II				
Stage III				
Stage IV				
Stage unknown				
TOTAL				

SD = screen-detected cancer
IC = interval cancer
NP = cancer in non-participant
NI = cancer in not invited

Classification of interval cancers

This section concentrates specifically on interval cancers of a mammographic screening programme. Interval cancers are a heterogeneous group of cancers that may be classified into subgroups when reviewed radiologically, as outlined in the radiology chapter. This information is the key to quality assurance in radiology and a valuable resource for training.

Interval cancers by type in defined time periods following screening

While the aspiration in a screening programme is to have a fixed interval between screening examinations, e.g. 24 months, in practice it may not be possible to have the exact interval for every woman. This 'round slippage' may be due to several factors, including administrative factors, changes to scheduled invitations, etc. In a screening programme with a screening interval of 24 months, it is customary to group together those interval cancers which occur in the first 12 months after a negative screening examination, those which occur in the second 12 months after a negative screening examination and those which occur after 24 months. This highlights the need to define the date of diagnosis of the interval cancer.

Table 29 provides the opportunity to record interval cancers by type in defined time periods following screening, separately for initial and subsequent screening examinations. This table may be reproduced if desired to examine interval cancers by type in defined time periods following first and subsequent screening rounds.

Table 29: Classification of interval cancers by type in defined time periods following initial and subsequent screening examinations

Type of interval cancer	Time since negative screening examination (mths)		
	0-11	12-23	24+
Initial screening*			
• True interval			
• Radiologically occult			
• Minimal signs			
• False negative			
• Unclassifiable			
TOTAL (n)			
Subsequent screening*			
• True interval			
• Radiologically occult			
• Minimal signs			
• False negative			
• Unclassifiable			
TOTAL (n)			

* cf Glossary of terms

Interval cancers by type and age group in defined periods following screening
The type of interval cancer that occurs may also be related to age.

Table 30 provides the opportunity to record interval cancers by type and age group in five year age intervals at defined time periods following screening, i.e. 0-11 months, 12-23 months and 24+ months. This table can be reproduced for initial and subsequent screening examinations or for first and subsequent rounds of screening as desired.

Table 30: Interval cancer occurrence by type and age group at defined time periods following screening

Type of interval cancer	Age at diagnosis (years)			
	50-54	55-59	60-64	65+
0-11 months				
• True interval				
• Radiologically occult				
• Minimal signs				
• False negative				
• Unclassifiable				
TOTAL (n)				

Table 30, continued

Type of interval cancer	Age at diagnosis (years)			
	50-54	55-59	60-64	65+
12-23 months				
• True interval				
• Radiologically occult				
• Minimal signs				
• False negative				
• Unclassifiable				
TOTAL (n)				
24+ months				
• True interval				
• Radiologically occult				
• Minimal signs				
• False negative				
• Unclassifiable				
TOTAL (n)				

Interval cases for estimating sensitivity of the screening programme and its impact

Sensitivity of the screening test is defined as the ability of identifying a case during its detectable phase. However, the impact of screening depends not only on the sensitivity of the screening test but also on the length of the screening interval. Therefore it is recommended that the following more general expression is computed:

$$\text{Sensitivity of the screening programme} = \frac{\text{screen-detected cases}}{\text{screen-detected cases} + \text{all interval cancer cases}}$$

This proportion includes interval cancer cases whose preclinical detectable phase was not initiated at the time of the screening test, and therefore reflects sensitivity of the screening test, lead time, and length of the screening interval. This easy to calculate measure is useful in assessing the overall impact of a screening programme in detecting cancers in the screened population and does not require radiological classification of interval cancers. It is strongly suggested that size or stage categories are taken into account, as the benefit of the screening programme diminishes if interval cancers tend to be advanced. Survival of ductal carcinoma in situ and of invasive cancers up to 10 mm in size has been shown to be very good, irrespective of grade and (for invasive cancers) nodal status. Therefore, interval cancers diagnosed at these stages, as opposed to dectecting the same lesions at screening, is likely to affect breast cancer mortality only marginally. The proportion of cases with unknown pathological size (pTx) should also be carefully noted. Although these cases would not be included in stage-specific calculations, it is obvious that results would be meaningless if cases with pTx are numerous.

Calculation of screening programme sensitivity, as defined above, excludes potentially detectable cases being diagnosed after the screening interval or at the subsequent screening examination. Since the probability of diagnosing a case during the screening interval varies according to local diagnostic delay and the occurrence of spontaneous screening, comparisons across programmes should be made with caution. However, the proportion calculated for 'advanced cases' (pT2 or more) only is less likely to be affected by these factors.

It is important to calculate sensitivity of the screening programme separately for initial and subsequent screening examinations (**table 31**) as the rate and stage distribution of screen-detected cancers are quite different. If numbers allow, the table should also be computed for 5-year age categories.

Table 31: Ratio of the number of interval cancers to total number of cancers detected in screened women

| Size at diagnosis | Initial screening | | | | | | Subsequent screening | | | | | |
| | Screen-detected cancers | | Interval cancers | | Total | | Screen-detected cancers | | Interval cancers | | Total | |
	N	(%)	N	(%)	N	(%)	N	(%)	N	(%)	N	(%)
pTis												
pT1ab												
pT1c												
pT2+												
pTx												
TOTAL		100		100		100		100		100		100

The occurrence of interval cancers can also be related to the background population incidence of cancer in the absence of screening (**table 32**). Several limitations arise in this respect:

a. The population incidence of breast cancer is altered by screening. While population incidence of breast cancer in the absence of screening can be used in the early stages of a screening programme, the longer a screening programme proceeds, the more difficult it becomes to determine what the incidence of breast cancer would be in the absence of screening.

b. Thus far, the focus of this paragraph has been entirely on the 'individual interval', i.e. the interval between the date of the screening mammogram and development of the interval cancer. In the evolution of a screening programme, individual intervals begin and end at different times. It is therefore of some concern to select the appropriate background incidence rate and detection rate for a time period which compares appropriately to the time period covered by the combined individual data for a particular round of screening or period of interest.

If background incidence does not include in situ cancers, these should also be excluded from interval cancers for the calculation of this outcome measure. If numbers allow, the table should also be computed for 5-year age categories. In calculating the observed rates of interval cancers, the denominator should be the number of 'negative' screening tests (with/without further assessment). If available, the number of 'woman-years of follow up' after a negative test should be used instead, taking into account women 'lost to follow up'.

Table 32: Relationship of observed interval cancer rate, by time since last negative screening examination, to background incidence rate

Time since last negative screening examination	Initial screening examinations			Subsequent screening examinations		
	Background incidence/ 10,000 (E) Year ____	Interval cancers 10,000 (O) Year____	O/E	Background incidence/ 10,000 (E) Year ____	Interval cancers 10,000 (O) Year ____	O/E
0-11 mths						
12-23 mths						
24+ mths						
TOTAL All ICs						

IC = interval cancer

Summary
Completion of the tables in this paragraph requires considerable attention to, and resources for, data collection, links to cancer registration and other data sources, and extensive quality assurance in data management. It is recognised that these exercises differ between programmes, thus limiting the extent to which results can be compared between programmes. The tables suggested in this section are, therefore, intended to assist each programme to assess its own data collection exercises as well as its performance in relation to breast cancer occurrence in the target population. They may also act as a prompt to improve data collection and quality assurance measures.

2.8 Evaluation and interpretation of screening outcomes

Screening outcomes become available throughout the screening process and afterwards. It is important to define the audience for the evaluation results, since the responsibilities and expertise of the decision-makers will affect what questions should be asked. In general, a distinction can be made between evaluating the performance of the screening programme and its impact on health indicators such as mortality. Monitoring performance indicators is an organisational responsibility to be carried out by the project leader or relevant professional and administrative disciplines. Evaluating the impact on mortality and cost-effectiveness of a screening programme requires the application of complex epidemiological and statistical methodologies.

2.8.1 Performance indicators

Performance evaluation, as suggested by Habicht et al (1999), can be applied to the provision of the service, its utilisation and coverage. The screening programme should be available and accessible to the target population and of high quality. Women in the target population should accept the invitation for screening and attend at regular intervals which will result in a certain population coverage. Coverage is a particularly useful performance measure, representing the interface between service delivery (the managerial process) and the population (the epidemiological picture).

Performance indicators reflect the provision and quality of the activities constituting the screening process without contributing directly to reduction in mortality. It is essential however that data elements are recorded and that indicators are produced and monitored at regular intervals. This is the basis of quality assurance actitivities within and between specialties.

There is an infinite number of possible process indicators reflecting specific parts of the screening programme. This outline is confined to those which pertain to the screening process and its sequelae.

The performance indicators to be evaluated include:
• Participation rate
• Technical repeat rate
• Recall rate
• Additional imaging rate at the time of screening
• Rate of invasive investigations (cytology, core biopsy, open biopsy)
• Proportion of malignant lesions with a pre-treatment diagnosis of malignancy
• Proportion of image-guided FNAC procedures with an insufficient result
• Positive predictive value of screening test, additional imaging, cytology and recommendation for open biopsy
• Benign to malignant biopsy ratio
• Specificity of the screening test
• Surgical procedures performed
• Interval between screening test and final assessment/surgery
• Proportion of women reinvited within the specified screening interval

Table 33 lists those performance indicators for which acceptable and desirable levels could reasonably be specified in a European context. Each screening programme could decide to expand this table to include other performance indicators.

Table 33: Indicators by which the performance of a breast screening programme is assessed

Performance indicator	Acceptable level	Desirable level	Screening programme 50-64
Participation rate*	> 70%	> 75%	
Technical repeat rate*	< 3%	< 1%	
Recall rate* • Initial screening • Subsequent-regular screening	< 7% < 5%	< 5% < 3%	
Additional imaging rate at the time of screening*	< 5%	< 1%	
Pre-treatment diagnosis in malignant lesions (%)	> 70%	> 90%	
Image-guided FNAC procedures with insufficient result (%)	< 25%	< 15%	
Benign to malignant biopsy ratio* • Initial screening • Subsequent-regular screening	≤ 1:1 ≤ 1:1	≤ 0.5:1 ≤ 0.2:1	
Women reinvited within the specified screening interval (%)	> 95%	100%	

* cf Glossary of terms
FNAC = fine needle aspiration cytology

2.8.2 Impact indicators

Achievement of the objective of screening for breast cancer, i.e. mortality reduction, is inevitably long-term. Ascertainment of impact on mortality demands (a) that follow up of the screened cohorts continues over extended periods of time, (b) that data on vital status and disease-free interval be vigorously sought and recorded despite the problems of follow up, and (c) that adequate links exist between programme data and other relevant data sources, e.g. medical records, pathology registers, death certificate information. Models for evaluating the impact of screening on mortality have not yet been fully developed. Given that this area of analysis is still evolving, a frequently used alternative is to identify and monitor early surrogate measures which can possibly predict outcome (for relevant publications see paragraph 2.9).

Analysis of breast cancer mortality
The objective of a breast cancer screening programme is to detect the tumour as early as possible to facilitate effective treatment and thereby reduce the mortality due to the disease. Continuous evaluation of the programme is necessary to ensure that it is as effective as expected.

That a breast cancer screening programme can reduce the breast cancer mortality in the age group 40-74 years has been proved in several randomised controlled trials and in the overview of the Swedish randomised trials. The level of reduction has varied from a few percent up to 40% (HIP trial). The reason for this variation has not been analysed but can be due to the type of intervention i.e. mammography alone (Swedish trials) or including palpation (HIP, Edinburgh and Canadian trial). It can also be affected by the duration of the intervention i.e. the time period from the start of the screening programme until the control group was also invited to screening, awareness of the disease, screening outside the programme, and the quality of screening. While it may be tempting to predict that a programme can achieve a reduction in mortality in the range of the higher estimates quoted above, recent data examining non-randomised general population screening suggest that the impact in these settings is lower.

To evaluate whether a service screening programme is as effective as the randomised trials is important but not easy as a non-randomised study design must be applied. So far, two main approaches have been used in the evaluation of the service screening programmes. The most commonly used implies study of the age-specific trends in the breast cancer mortality comparing the development before and after introduction of the programme. The other approach is based on a comparison of trends between areas with and without a programme. Both methods have been questioned from a methodological point of view and there is a lack of development of methods for the statistical analysis of the trends as well as comparison of trends.

To estimate the effect of the screening programme based on the trend in the breast cancer mortality raises several questions e.g. How long a time period before introduction of screening should be included as a reference period? How many years after introduction of the programme do we have to wait before we can expect an effect (study period)? The situation can be further complicated by the introduction of the programme, e.g. by the phased introduction of screening in specific geographic areas and age groups.
To estimate the effect of the screening programme based on a comparison of the trend in the breast cancer mortality in areas with and without a programme also raises questions besides those mentioned above. The most complicated is how the control area should be selected? What aspects should be prioritised with respect to comparability of the areas – risk factor pattern for breast cancer (often unknown), treatment programmes for breast cancer, accessibility to health care, etc.

Apart from the trend studies described above, methods using novel mortality measures or simulation and other modelling techniques to describe the impact of screening on mortality are under development. In addition, efforts should also be made to enable evaluation of longitudinal, individual data directly linking a woman's screening history to her cause of death.

The disadvantage of using breast cancer mortality as the endpoint in evaluation of a screening programme is that it takes many years before an effect can be expected. It takes years until the study population is screened for the first round and many more years until it is possible to see an effect of the intervention. It is recommended to try to estimate the proportion of the study population exposed to the intervention from the start of the screening programme to be able to estimate when it is realistic to expect an effect.

Analysis of surrogate indicators

An attractive alternative to analysing breast cancer mortality is to identify early surrogate indicators and follow their development over time. Several characteristics have been indicated to predict a reduction in the breast cancer mortality e.g.
- Interval cancer rate*
- Breast cancer detection rate*
- Stage at diagnosis of screen-detected cancers
- Proportion of screen-detected invasive cancers ≤ 10 mm
- Proportion of screen-detected cancers that are invasive
- Proportion of screen-detected cancers with lymph node metastases

* cf Glossary of terms

After ascertainment, confirmation and classification of interval cancer cases identified, the following additional measures can be calculated, as outlined in paragraph 2.7:
- Number of interval cancers per 10,000 women screened negative by time since last screening examination
- The interval cancer rate in a defined period after screening expressed as a proportion of the background (expected) breast cancer incidence rate in the absence of screening. Please note that proportions for e.g. the first and second year after screening should not be considered cumulative.
- Age-specific interval cancer rates
- Round-specific interval cancer rates
- Association of interval cancer rates with other performance indicators of screening such as participation rate, recall/additional imaging rate and positive predictive value of screening mammography and of each investigation undertaken as further assessment of screen-detected lesions
- Sensitivity and impact of the screening programme

Table 34 lists those early surrogate indicators for which acceptable and desirable levels could reasonably be specified in a European context. Each screening programme could decide to expand this table to include other surrogate indicators.

Table 34: Early surrogate indicators by which the impact of a breast screening programme is assessed

Surrogate indicator	Acceptable level	Desirable level	Screening programme 50-64
Interval cancer rate* / Background incidence rate* (%)			
• 0-11 months	30%	< 30%	
• 12-23 months	50%	< 50%	
Breast cancer detection rate*			
• Initial screening	3xIR	> 3xIR	
• Subsequent-regular screening	1.5xIR	> 1.5xIR	
Stage II+/Total cancers screen-detected (%)			
• Initial screening	25%	< 25%	
• Subsequent-regular screening	20%	< 20%	
Invasive cancers ≤ 10 mm/ Total invasive cancers screen-detected (%)			
• Initial screening	≥ 20%	≥ 25%	
• Subsequent-regular screening	≥ 25%	≥ 30%	
Invasive cancers/ Total cancers screen-detected (%)	90%	80-90%	
Node-negative cancers/ Total cancers screen-detected (%)			
• Initial screening	70%	> 70%	
• Subsequent-regular screening	75%	> 75%	

* cf Glossary of terms

2.8.3 Cost-effectiveness

Prior to inception, a screening programme should carry out cost-effectiveness analyses to demonstrate the cost of achieving its proposed objectives. A computer simulation package (MISCAN) has been developed by the Erasmus University in Rotterdam (The Netherlands) for analysing and reproducing the observed results of screening projects and for predicting the future effects of alternative screening programmes. In the present MISCAN model, breast cancer has four invasive, screen-detectable, pre-clinical states (<0.5 cm, 0.5-1 cm, 1-2 cm and >2cm) and one non-invasive state, ductal carcinoma in situ. By generating individual life histories a dynamic population is simulated, representing the demography, mortality of all causes and incidence and mortality from breast cancer. In the disease part of the programme the relevant stages of breast cancer are discerned and the natural history is simulated as a progression through these stages. Key parameters in the model of the performance of screening are mean duration of screen-detectable preclinical disease, sensitivity and improvement of prognosis for screen-detected cancers. The MISCAN model has been tested in several screening programmes throughout Europe. Other cost-effectiveness analyses, based on Markov and Monte Carlo computer models, have also been employed in studying the cost-effectiveness of breast cancer screening, in particular of women aged 40 to 49 years (for literature references see paragraph 2.9).

2.9 Bibliography

Randomised controlled trials
Alexander FE, Anderson TJ, Brown HK, et al. 14 years of follow-up from the Edinburgh randomised trial of breast cancer screening. Lancet 1999;353:1903-8

Andersson I, Aspegren K, Janzon L, et al. Mammographic screening and mortality from breast cancer: the Malmo mammographic screening trial. BMJ 1988;297:943-8.

Bjurstam N, Bjorneld L, Duffy SW, et al. The Gothenburg breast screening trial: first results on mortality, incidence, and mode of detection for women ages 39-49 years at randomization. Cancer 1997;80:2091-99.

Frisell J, Eklund G, Hellstrom L, et al. Randomised trial of mammography screening - preliminary report on mortality in the Stockholm trial. Breast Cancer Res Treat 1991;18:49-56.

Kerlikowske K, Grady D, Rubin SM, et al. Efficacy of screening mammography. A meta-analysis. JAMA 1995;273:149-54.

Nyström L, Rutqvist LE, Wall S, et al. Breast cancer screening with mammograpy; overview of Swedish randomised trials. Lancet 1993;341:973-8.

Shapiro S, Strax P, Venet L. Periodic breast cancer screening in reducing mortality from breast cancer. JAMA 1971;215:1777-85.

Tabar L, Fagerberg G, Duffy SW, et al. The Swedish two county trial of mammographic screening for breast cancer: recent results and calculation of benefit. J Epidemiol Community Health 1989;43:107-14.

Demonstration projects
Collette HJA, Day NE, Rombach LL, et al. Evaluation of screening for breast cancer in a non-randomised study (the DOM Project) by means of a case-control study. Lancet 1984;1:1224-6.

Morrison AS, Brisson J, Khalid N. Breast cancer incidence and mortality in the Breast Cancer Detection and Demonstration Project. JNCI 1988;80:1540-7.

Palli D, Rosselli del Turco M, Buiatti E, et al. A case-control study of the efficacy of a non-randomised breast cancer screening program in Florence (Italy). Int J Cancer 1986;38:501-4.

UK Trial of Early Detection of Breast Cancer Group. 16-year mortality from breast cancer in the UK Trial of Early Detection of Breast Cancer. Lancet 1999;353:1909-14.

Verbeek ALM, Hendriks JHCL, Holland R, et al. Mammographic screening and breast cancer mortality: age-specific effects in Nijmegen project, 1975-1982. Lancet 1985;1:865-6.

National programmes
Hakama M, Pukkala E, Heikkilä M, et al. Effectiveness of the public health policy for breast cancer screening in Finland: population-based cohort study. BMJ 1997;314:864-7.

Lenner P, Jonsson H. Excess mortality from breast cancer in relation to mammography screening in northern Sweden. J Med Screen 1997;4:6-9.

Quinn M, Allen E, on behalf of the United Kingdom Association of Cancer Registries. Changes in incidence and mortality from breast cancer in England and Wales since introduction of screening. BMJ 1995;311:1391-5.

Van den Akker-van Marle E, de Koning H, Boer R, et al. Reduction in breast cancer mortality due to the introduction of mass screening in The Netherlands: comparison with the United Kingdom. J Med Screen 1999; 6:30-4.

Evaluation
Day N, Williams DRR, Khaw KT. Breast cancer screening programmes: the development of a monitoring and evaluation system. Br J Cancer 1989;59:954-58.

Habicht JP, Victoria CG, Vaughan JP. Evaluation designs for adequacy, plausibility and probability of public health programme performance and impact. Int J Epidemiol 1999;28:10-8.

Hakama M, Pukkala E, Södermann B, et al. Implementation of screening as a public health policy: issues in design and evaluation. J Med Screen 1999;6:209-16.

Törnberg S, Carstensen J, Hakulinen T, et al. Evaluation of the effect on breast cancer mortality of population-based mammography screening programmes. J Med Screen 1994;1:184-7.

Interval cancers

Burrell HC, Sibbering DM, Wilson ARM, et al. Screening interval breast cancers: mammographic features and prognostic factors. Radiology 1996;199:811-7.

Day N, McCann J, Camilleri-Ferrante C, et al. Monitoring interval cancers in breast screening programmes: the East Anglian experience. J Med Screen 1995;2:180-5.

Everington D, Gilbert FJ, Tyack C, et al. The Scottish breast screening programme's experience of monitoring interval cancers. J Med Screen 1999;6:21-7.

Exbrayat C, Garnier A, Colonna M, et al. Analysis and classification of interval cancers in a French breast screening programme (département of Isère). Eur J Cancer Prev 1999;8:255-60.

Faux AM, Richardson DC, Lawrence GM, et al. Interval cancers in the NHS Breast Screening Programme: does the current definition exclude too many? J Med Screen 1997;4:169-73.

Fracheboud J, de Koning HJ, Beemsterboer PMM, et al. Interval cancers in the Dutch breast screening programme. Br J Cancer 1999;81:912-7.

Klemi PJ, Toikkanen S, Räsänen O, et al. Mammography screening interval and the frequency of interval cancers in a population-based screening. Br J Cancer 1997;75:762-66.

Moberg K, Grundström H, Törnberg S, et al. Two models for radiological reviewing of interval cancers. J Med Screen 1999;6:35-39.

Schouten LJ, de Rijke JM, Schlangen JT, et al. Evaluation of the effect of breast cancer screening by record linkage with the cancer registry, the Netherlands. J Med Screen 1998;5:37-41.

Vitak B, Stål O, Månson JC, et al. Interval cancers and cancers in non-attenders in the Östergötland Mammographic Screening Programme. Duration between screening and diagnosis, S-phase fraction and distant recurrence. Eur J Cancer 1997;33:1453-60.

Woodman CBJ, Threlfall AG, Boggis CRM, et al. Is the three year breast screening interval too long? Occurrence of interval cancers in NHS breast screening programme's north western region. BMJ 1995;310:224-6.

Performance indicators

Blanks RG, Day NE, Moss SM. Monitoring the performance of breast screening programmes: use of indirect standardisation in evaluating the invasive cancer detection rate. J Med Screen 1996;3:79-81.

Bleyen L, van Landeghem P, Pelfrene E, et al. Screening for breast cancer in Ghent, Belgium: First results of a programme involving the existing health services. Eur J Cancer 1998;34.1410-4.

Giordano L, Giorgi D, Fasolo G, et al. Breast cancer screening: characteristics and results of the Italian programmes in the Italian group for planning and evaluating breast cancer screening programmes (GISMa). Tumori 1996;82:31-7.

Lacour A, Mamelle N, Arnold F, et al. Mass screening programs for breast cancer in France – average values of assessment criteria. Cancer Detection Prevention 1997;21:221-30.

McCann J, Wait S, Séradour B, et al. A comparison of the performance and impact of breast cancer screening programmes in East Anglia, UK and Bouches Du Rhone, France. Eur J Cancer 1997;33.429-35.

McCann J, Stockton D, Day N. Breast cancer in East Anglia: the impact of the breast screening programme on stage at diagnosis. J Med Screen 1998;5:42-8.

Ong GJ, Austoker J, Michell M. Early rescreen/recall in the UK National Health Service breast screening programme: epidemiological data. J Med Screen 1998;5:146-55.

Paci E, Ciatto S, Buiatti E, et al. Early indicators of efficacy of breast cancer screening programmes; results of the Florence district programme. Int J Cancer 1990;46:198-202.

Van den Akker-van Marle ME, Reep-van den Bergh CMM, Boer R, et al. Breast cancer screening in Navarra: Interpretation of a high detection rate at the first screening round and a low rate at the second round. Int J Cancer 1997;73:464-9.

Cost-effectiveness

Beemsterboer PMM, Warmerdam PG, Boer R, et al. Screening for breast cancer in Catalonia, which policy is preferred? Eur J Public Health 1993;8:214-46.

Beemsterboer PMM, de Koning HJ, Warmerdam PG, et al. Prediction of the effects and costs of breast cancer screening in Germany. Int J Cancer 1994;58:623-28.

Habbema JD, van Oortmarssen GJ, Lubbe JT, et al. The MISCAN simulation program for the evaluation of screening for disease. Comput Methods Programs Biomed 1985;20:79-93.

Rosenquist CJ, Lindfors KK. Screening mammography in women aged 40-49 years: analysis of cost-effectiveness. Radiology 1994;191:647-50.

Salzmann P, Kerlikowske K, Phillips K. Cost-effectiveness of extending screening mammography guidelines to include women 40 to 49 years of age. Ann Intern Med 1997;127:955-65.

2.10 Glossary of terms

Additional imaging: after evaluation of the screening mammogram, additional imaging may be required for medical reasons. This may take the form of repeat mammography, specialised views (e.g. magnification, extended craniocaudal, paddle views), ultrasound or magnetic resonance imaging (MRI). Additional radiology includes additional views taken at the time of the screening mammogram, as well as those carried out on recall. It does not include repeat mammograms for technical reasons. It also does not include intermediate mammograms. On the basis of additional imaging, a woman may be dismissed, or may be recommended to have cytology or biopsy. Please note the difference between additional imaging and an intermediate mammogram.

Additional imaging rate: the number of women who have an additional imaging investigation as a proportion of all women who have a screening test. This includes additional images taken at the time of the screening test, as well as imaging for which women are recalled. The additional imaging rate does not include repeat mammography for technical reasons. It also does not include intermediate mammograms. Within the group with additional imaging, the rates of individual imaging procedures may be derived.

Adjuvant therapy: women with axillary lymph node metastases are assumed to receive adjuvant systemic therapy (chemotherapy and/or hormonal therapy) in the majority of cases.

Age-specific detection ratio: the breast cancer detection rate in a specified age group divided by the underlying (expected) incidence of breast cancer in that same age group in the absence of screening.

Benign to malignant biopsy ratio: the ratio of pathologically-proven benign lesions to malignant lesions surgically removed in any round of screening. This ratio may vary between initial and subsequent screening examinations.

Background incidence rate: the breast cancer incidence rate that would be expected in the screened population in the absence of screening.

Breast cancer: a pathologically-proven malignant lesion which is classified as ductal carcinoma in situ or invasive breast cancer.

Breast cancer detection rate: the number of pathologically-proven malignant lesions of the breast (both in situ and invasive) detected in a screening round per 1000 women screened in that round. This rate will differ for initial versus subsequent screening examinations. Cancers detected at intermediate mammography should be regarded as screen-detected cancers and thus be included in the cancer detection rate. Recurrent breast cancers, detected for the first time at mammographic screening, should also be regarded as screen-detected cancers since they will be identified and diagnosed in the same way as a primary breast cancer. Cancer metastases diagnosed in the breast as a consequence of a primary cancer outside the breast should not be included in the cancer detection rate.

Breast cancer incidence rate: the rate at which new cases of breast cancer occur in a population. The *numerator* is the number of newly diagnosed cases of breast cancer that occur in a defined time period. The *denominator* is the population at risk of being diagnosed with breast cancer during this defined period, sometimes expressed in person-time.

Breast cancer mortality rate: the rate at which deaths of breast cancer occur in a population. The *numerator* is the number of breast cancer deaths that occur in a defined time period. The *denominator* is the population at risk of dying from breast cancer during this defined period, sometimes expressed in person-time.

Breast cancer register: when a country or region does not have or can not access a pathology register and/or cancer register, a screening programme may take it upon itself to create a 'breast cancer register' specifically for the programme.

Core biopsy: closed biopsy of a breast lesion providing a histological specimen of breast tissue for diagnostic purposes.

Cytology: technique used to extract cells from breast lesions for cytological examination. Cytology can distinguish between cystic and solid breast lesions. Material from solid lesions can be examined cytologically for evidence of malignancy. Cytology may be performed with or without radiological (stereotactic) control. The latter may be referred to as Stereotactic Biopsy (STB) to distinguish it from cytology performed clinically, as in an outpatient clinic where a surgeon may aspirate a palpable breast lump for fluid or cells, or using ultrasound guidance.

Dedicated screening facility: a facility that is used solely for screening examinations and/or further assessment of women where a perceived abnormality was detected at the screening examination.

Dynamic cohort: a cohort that gains and loses members. The composition of the cohort is continuously changing allowing for the addition of new members for screening and follow up, and cessation of screening for those who become older than the maximum screening age. In order for estimates of screening efficacy to be accurately derived it is essential to know the denominator of the dynamic cohort at all times.

Eligible population: the adjusted target population, i.e. the target population minus those women that are to be excluded according to screening policy on the basis of eligibility criteria other than age, gender and geographic location.

Fixed cohort: a cohort for which membership is determined by being present at some defining event. Thus, there are no entries during the study period, including the follow up period. In a screening programme this means that a specific birth cohort is selected for screening and follow up. Women entering the age category in subsequent years of the screening programme are not included in the study cohort.

Further assessment: additional diagnostic techniques (either non-invasive or invasive) that are performed for medical reasons in order to clarify the nature of a perceived abnormality detected at the screening examination. Further assessment can take place at the time of the screening test or on recall.

Initial screening: first screening examination of individual women within the screening programme, regardless of the organisational screening round in which women are screened.

Intermediate mammogram following screening: if, as a result of the screening test, a mammogram is required out of sequence with the screening interval (say at 6 or 12 months), this is referred to as an intermediate mammogram following screening. Cancers detected at intermediate mammography should be regarded as screen-detected cancers (not interval cancers). However they also represent a delayed diagnosis and should be subject to separate analysis and review.

Intermediate mammogram following further assessment:
if, as a result of the screening test and further assessment, a mammogram is required out of sequence with the screening interval (say at 6 or 12 months), this is referred to as an intermediate mammogram following further assessment. Cancers detected at intermediate mammography following further assessment should be regarded as screen-detected cancers (not interval cancers). However they also represent a delayed diagnosis and should be subject to separate analysis and review. In the radiology chapter the term 'early recall' is used to refer to an intermediate mammogram following further assessment.

Interval cancer:
a primary breast cancer which is diagnosed in a woman who had a screening test, with/without further assessment, which was negative for malignancy, either:
• before the next invitation to screening, or
• within a time period equal to a screening interval for a woman who has reached the upper age limit for screening.

Interval cancer rate:
the number of interval cancers diagnosed within a defined time period since the last negative screening examination per 10,000 women screened negative. The rate of interval cancers can also be expressed as a proportion of the background (expected) breast cancer incidence rate in the screened group.

Open biopsy:
refers to surgical removal of (part of) a breast lesion.

Open biopsy rate:
the number of women undergoing open biopsy as a proportion of all women who have a screening examination. This rate may differ for initial versus subsequent screening examinations.

Opportunistic screening:
refers to screening that takes place outside an organised or population-based screening programme. This type of screening may be the result of e.g. a recommendation made during a routine medical consultation, consultation for an unrelated condition, on the basis of a possible increased risk of developing breast cancer (family history or other known risk factor).

Participation rate:
the number of women who have a screening test as a proportion of all women who are invited to attend for screening.

Primary treatment:
all women with breast cancer, with or without signs of distant metastases, will be offered some form of primary treatment,

e.g. breast conserving surgery, mastectomy, chemotherapy, radiotherapy.

Population-based: pertains to a population defined by geographical boundaries. For a screening programme to be population-based every member of the target population who is eligible to attend on the basis of predecided criteria must be known to the programme. This emphasises the need for accurate information on the population at risk, constituting the denominator of most rates.

Positive predictive value (PPV): refers to the ratio of lesions which are truly positive to those test positive. It is intimately effected by the prevalence of the condition under study. Thus, with a prevalence of < 1%, as with breast cancer, one can expect a low positive predictive and a very high negative predictive value for screening mammography.

PPV of additional imaging: the number of cancers detected as a proportion of the women with positive results in additional imaging (i.e. suspicion of malignancy). The denominator should include additional views performed for medical reasons at the time of the screening examination or on recall. Additional views taken for technical reasons should be excluded. Intermediate mammograms should also be excluded. In practice, the denominator corresponds to those women who, after additional imaging, undergo invasive tests for diagnostic confirmation.

PPV of cytology: the number of cancers detected as a proportion of the women with positive cytology (i.e. suspicion of malignancy). In practice, the denominator corresponds to those women who undergo biopsy after cytology.

PPV of recall: the number of cancers detected as a proportion of the women who were physically recalled for further assessment (but excluding those for technical recall).

PPV of recommendation for open biopsy: the number of cancers detected as a proportion of the women who were recommended for open biopsy. Since biopsy is the 'gold standard', i.e. the test used for diagnostic confirmation, there is no such thing as a PPV of open biopsy.

PPV of screening test: the number of cancers detected as a proportion of the women with a positive screening test. In practice, the denominator corresponds to women undergoing further assessment either at the time of screening or on recall. Further assessment does not include additional mammograms for technical reasons (repeat screening tests).

Recall:	refers to women who have to come back to the screening unit, i.e. who are physically recalled, as a consequence of the screening examination for:
a) a repeat mammogram because of a technical inadequacy of the screening mammogram (technical recall); or
b) clarification of a perceived abnormality detected at the screening examination, by performance of an additional procedure (recall for further assessment).
This group is different from those who may have additional investigations performed at the time of the screening examination, but who were not physically recalled for that extra procedure.

Recall rate:	the number of women recalled for further assessment as a proportion of all women who had a screening examination.

Recent mammogram:	a mammogram performed at a shorter time interval than the regular screening interval. Women who had a recent mammogram (either diagnostic or screening) may potentially be excluded from the target population and/or the results dependent on screening policy.

Repeat screening test:	refers to the need to repeat a screening test for technical reasons, either at the time of the screening examination or on recall. The most common reasons for a repeat screening test are:
a) processing error;
b) inadequate positioning of the breast; or
c) machine or operator errors.
Technical recalls will be reduced considerably, though not necessarily completely eliminated, by onsite processing taking place before a woman is dismissed.

Screening interval:	the fixed interval between routine screens decided upon in each screening programme dependent on screening policy.

Screening policy:	the specific policy of a screening programme which dictates the targeted age and gender group, the geographic area to target, the screening interval (usually two or three years), etcetera.

Screening test: the test that is applied to all women in the programme. This may be a single or two-view mammogram with or without clinical examination. The screening test does not include additional imaging tests carried out at the time of the initial screening examination.

Screening unit: a screening unit refers to the facilities where screening examinations take place. It does not refer to the exact number of e.g. mammography machines within the unit.

Self-registration: women not invited for screening may present themselves and be included in the screening roster. It is the responsibility of the screening staff to decide whether self-registered women qualify to become members of the screening roster or not. It would be expected that only women who are members of the target population and thus eligible to attend would be allowed to self-refer.

Sensitivity: is the proportion of truly diseased persons in the screened population who are identified as diseased by the screening test. The more general expression for 'sensitivity of the screening programme' refers to the ratio of breast cancers correctly identified at the screening examination to breast cancers identified and not identified at the screening examination (i.e. true positives/true positives + false negatives). It is clear that to establish the sensitivity of the screening test in a particular programme there must be a flawless system for identification and classification of all interval cancers (false negatives).

Sources of demographic data: demographic data for the purpose of issuing invitations to screening may come from a population register, an electoral register, other registers, population survey, or census data.

Specificity: is the proportion of truly non-diseased persons in the screened population who are identified as non-diseased by the screening test. Here it refers to the ratio of truly negative screening examinations to those that are truly negative and falsely positive (i.e. true negatives/true negatives + false positive). To derive an absolutely accurate estimate of specificity would require that each person dismissed as having a negative screening test is followed for ascertainment of subsequent negativity, and that those who are recalled for additional investigation following the screening test are regarded as potentially all having a malignancy. The false positives are those who have a histologically-proven benign lesion.

A note of caution is warranted here, however, in that, not infrequently, it is known beforehand, on the basis of radiological investigation, that the offending lesion is benign. The reason for surgery on a benign lesion may be surgeon or patient preference for excision. In practice ascertainment of specificity is frequently made on the basis of the results of initial mammograms.

Subsequent screening: all screening examinations of individual women within the screening programme following an initial screening examination, regardless of the organisational screening round in which women are screened. There are two types of subsequent screening examination:
- subsequent screening at the regular screening interval, i.e. in accordance with the routine interval defined by the screening policy (SUBS-R);
- subsequent screening at irregular intervals, i.e. those who miss an invitation to routine screening and return in a subsequent organisational screening round (SUBS-IRR).

Symptomatic women: women reporting breast complaints or symptoms at the screening examination may potentially be excluded from the target population and/or results according to screening policy.

Target population: the group of persons for whom the intervention is planned. In screening for breast cancer, it refers to all women eligible to attend for screening on the basis of age and geographic location (dictated by screening policy). This includes special groups such as institutionalised or minority groups.

Women invited: all women invited in the period to which data refer, even if they have yet to receive a reminder.

Women screened: all women screened in the period to which data refer, even if results of mammograms are not yet available.

World age-standardised rate: using 'direct' standardisation, this is the rate which would have occurred if the observed age-specific rates had operated in the standard world population:

Standard world population used for the computation of age-standardised mortality and incidence rates[1]:

Age (yrs)	World
0	2 400
1	9 600
5	10 000
10	9 000
15	9 000
20	8 000
25	8 000
30	6 000
35	6 000
40	6 000
45	6 000
50	5 000
55	4 000
60	4 000
65	3 000
70	2 000
75	1 000
80	500
85 +	500
TOTAL	100 000

[1] Smith PG (1992) Comparison between registries: age-standardized rates. In: Parkin DM, Muir CS, Whelan SL, Gao Y-T, Ferlay J, Powell J (eds) Cancer Incidence in Five Continents, Volume VI. IARC Scientific Publications No 120, Lyon, p 865-870

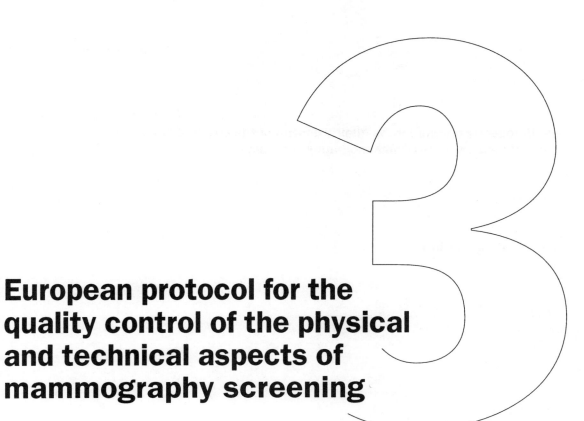

European protocol for the quality control of the physical and technical aspects of mammography screening

Authors

S. van Woudenberg

M. Thijssen

K. Young

The European protocol for the quality control of the physical and technical aspects of mammography screening

Third edition

Collaborating institutes
QUARAD
LUCK
ARCADES
LRCB
EMIFMA
NCCPM
PM

Contributors
M. Fitzgerald, London, UK
P. Heid, Marseille, FR
R. van Loon, Brussels, BE
H. Mol, Brussels, BE
D. Dierckx, Brussels, BE
F. Verdun, Lausanne, CH
M. Säbel, Erlangen, DE
D. Dance, London, UK
A. Ferro de Carvalho, Lisbon, PT
A. Flioni Vyza, Athens, GR
M. Gambaccini, Ferrara, IT
C. Maccia, Cachan, FR
W. Leitz, Stockholm, SE
E. Vaño, Madrid, ES
J. Shekdhar, London, UK
T. Deprez, Leuven, BE
H. Bosmans, Leuven, BE
A. Carton, Leuven, BE
N. Gerardy, Brussels, BE
J. Lindeijer, Nijmegen, NL
R. Bijkerk, Nijmegen, NL
B. Moores, Liverpool, UK
H. Schibilla, Brussels, EC
F. Stieve, Neuherberg, DE
D. Teunen, Luxembourg, EC
J. Pages, Brussels, BE
J. Zoetelief, Rijswijk, NL
A. Watt, Edinburgh, UK
F. Shannoun, Luxembourg, LU
C. Back, Luxembourg, LU
E. van der Kop, Nijmegen, NL

Executive summary

A prerequisite for a successful screening project is that the mammograms contain sufficient diagnostic information to be able to detect breast cancer, using as low a radiation dose as is reasonably achievable (ALARA). This quality demand holds for every single mammogram. *Quality control (QC)* therefore must ascertain that the equipment performs at a constant high quality level.

In the framework of 'Europe Against Cancer' (EAC), a European approach for mammography screening is chosen to achieve comparable high quality results for all centres participating in the mammography screening programme. Within this programme, *quality assurance (QA)* takes into account the medical, organisational and technical aspects. This chapter is specifically concerned with the quality control of physical and technical aspects and dosimetry.

The intention of this part of the guidelines is to indicate the basic test procedures, dose measurements and their frequencies. The use of these tests and procedures is essential for ensuring high quality mammography and comparison between centres. This document is intended as a minimum standard for implementation throughout the EC Member States and does not reduce more comprehensive and refined requirements for QC that are specified in local or national QA programmes. Therefore some screening programmes may implement additional procedures.

Quality control
Mammography screening should only be performed using modern dedicated X-ray equipment and appropriate image receptors.

QC of the physical and technical aspects in mammography screening starts with specification and purchase of the appropriate equipment, meeting accepted standards of performance. Before the system is put into clinical use, it must undergo acceptance testing to ensure that the performance meets these standards. This holds for the mammography X-ray equipment, image receptor, film processor and QC test equipment. After acceptance, the performance of all equipment must be maintained above the minimum level and at the highest level possible.

The QC of the physical and technical aspects must guarantee that the following objectives are met:
1. The radiologist is provided with images that have the best possible diagnostic information obtainable when the appropriate radiographic technique is employed. The images should at least contain the defined acceptable level of information, necessary to detect the smaller lesions (see CEC Document EUR 16260).
2. The image quality is stable with respect to information content and optical density and consistent with that obtained by other participating screening centres.
3. The breast dose is as low as reasonably achievable for the diagnostic information required.

QC measurements and frequencies
To attain these objectives, QC measurements should be carried out. Each measurement should follow a written QC protocol that is adapted to the specific requirements of local or national QA programmes. **The European protocol for the quality control of the physical**

and technical aspects of mammography screening gives guidance on individual physical, technical and dose measurements, and their frequencies, that should be performed as part of mammography screening programmes.

Several measurements can be performed by the local staff. The more elaborate measurements should be undertaken by medical physicists who are trained and experienced in diagnostic radiology and specifically trained in mammography QC. Comparability and consistency of the results from different centres is best achieved if data from all measurements, including those performed by local technicians or radiographers are collected and analysed centrally.

Image quality and breast dose depend on the equipment used and the radiographic technique employed. QC should be carried out by monitoring the physical and technical parameters of the mammographic system and its components. The following components and system parameters should be monitored:

- X-ray generator and control system
- Bucky and image receptor
- Film processing
- System properties (including dose)
- Viewing conditions

The probability of change and the impact of a change on image quality and on breast dose determine the frequencies with which the parameters should be measured. These frequencies are indicated for each test. The protocol also gives the acceptable and desirable limiting values for some QC parameters. The acceptable values indicate the minimal performance limits. The desirable values indicate the limits that are achievable. Limiting values are only indicated when consensus on the measurement method and parameter values has been obtained. The equipment required for conducting QC tests is listed together with the appropriate tolerances in table 2.

Diagnostic reference levels for mammography screening should be established according to the methods proposed in the '**European Protocol on Dosimetry in Mammography**' (EUR 16263, ISBN 92-827-7289-6). It provides accepted indicators for breast dose, from both measurements on a group of women and on test objects.

The first (1992) version of this document (EUR 14821) was produced by a Study Group, selected from the contractors of the CEC Radiation Protection Actions. The revised (1996) version is based on a critical review of recent QA and QC literature and includes the experience gained by users of the document and comments from manufacturers of equipment and film-screen systems (see literature and reference list, section 6, bibliography). This 2001 revision is based on further practical experience with the protocol, comments from manufacturers and the need to adapt to new developments in equipment and in the literature. Communication on this protocol can be directed to the

EUREF Office,
National Expert and Training Centre for Breast Cancer Screening,
PO Box 9101,
NL-6500 HB Nijmegen,
The Netherlands,
Tel: +31-(0)24-3616706
Fax: +31-(0)24-3540527
Web: www.euref.org

3.1 Introduction to the measurements

This protocol describes the basic techniques for the quality control of the physical and technical aspects of mammography screening. It has been developed from existing protocols (see 3.6, bibliography) and the experience of groups performing QC of mammography equipment. Since the technique of mammographic imaging and the equipment used are constantly improving, the protocol is subject to regular updates. In the near future digital mammography can be expected to replace film screen mammography. Some considerations on the implications for technical quality control are given in appendix 5.

Many measurements are performed using an exposure of a test object. All measurements are performed under normal working conditions; no special adjustments of the equipment are necessary.

Two standard types of exposures are specified:

- The **reference exposure** which is intended to provide information on the system under *defined* conditions, independent of the clinical settings.
- The **routine exposure** which is intended to provide information on the system under *clinical* settings.

For the production of the reference or routine exposure, an object is exposed using the machine settings as follows (unless otherwise mentioned):

	Reference exposure:	*Routine exposure:*
- test object thickness:	45 mm[1]	45 mm
- test object material:	PMMA	PMMA
- tube voltage:	28 kV	as used clinically
- target material:	molybdenum	as used clinically
- filter material:	molybdenum	as used clinically
- compression device:	in contact with test object	in contact with test object
- anti scatter grid:	present	present
- source-to-image distance:	matching with focused grid	matching with focused grid
- phototimer detector:	in position closest to chest wall	in position closest to chest wall
- automatic exposure control:	on	as used clinically
- optical density control:	as leading to the reference optical density	as leading to the target optical density

The optical density (OD) of the processed image is measured at the **reference point**, which lies 60 mm from the chest wall side and laterally centred. The **reference optical density** is preferably 1.4 OD, base and fog *excluded*.

All measurements should be performed with the same cassette to rule out differences between screens and cassettes except when testing individual cassettes as in section 3.2.2.

---

[1] This is the PMMA thickness most commonly used, but others may be specified in parts of this protocol.

Limits of acceptable performance are given, but often a better result would be desirable. Both the acceptable and desirable limits are summarised in 3.5, table 1. Occasionally no limiting value is given, but only a typical value as an indication of what may normally be expected. The measurement frequencies indicated in the protocol (summarised in table 1) are the minimum required. When the acceptable limiting value is exceeded the measurement should be repeated. If necessary, additional measurements should be performed to determine the origin of the observed problem and appropriate actions should be taken to solve the problem.

For guidance on the specific design and operating criteria of suitable test objects, see the Proceedings of the CEC Workshop on Test Phantoms (see 3.6, bibliography). Definition of terms, such as the 'reference point' and the 'reference density' are given in 3.4. The evaluation of the results of the QC measurements can be simplified by using the forms for QC reporting provided in appendix 6.

Staff and equipment

Several measurements can be performed by the local staff. The more elaborate measurements should be undertaken by medical physicists who are trained and experienced in diagnostic radiology and specifically trained in mammography QC. Comparability and consistency of the results from different centres is best achieved if data from all measurements, including those performed by local technicians or radiographers are collected and analysed centrally.

The staff conducting the daily/weekly QC-tests will need the following equipment[2] at the screening site:

- Sensitometer
- Densitometer
- Thermometer
- Standard test block[2] (45 mm PMMA)
- PMMA plates[3, 4]
- QC test object
- Reference cassette

The medical physics staff conducting the other QC-tests will need the following additional equipment and may need duplicates of many of the above[5]:

- Dosemeter
- kVp-meter
- Exposure time meter
- Light meter
- QC test objects
- Aluminium sheets
- Focal spot test device + stand
- Stopwatch
- Film-screen contact test device
- Tape measure
- Compression force test device
- Rubber foam
- Lead sheet
- Aluminium stepwedge

---

[2] The standard test block may be composed of several PMMA plates. See also 3.4.

[3] PMMA (polymethylmethacrylate) is commercially available under several brand names, e.g. Lucite, Plexiglas and perspex.

[4] ≥ 150 X 100 mm or semi-circular with a radius of ≥ 100 mm, and covering a total thickness range from 20 to 70 mm PMMA (normally PMMA of 180 X 240 mm is available).

[5] The specifications of the listed equipment are given, where appropriate, in 3.5, table 2.

3.2 Description of the measurements

Generally when absolute measurements of dose are performed, make sure that the proper corrections for temperature and air pressure are applied to the raw values. Use one and the same box of (fresh) film throughout the tests described in this protocol.

3.2.1 X-ray generation

3.2.1.1 X-ray source

The measurements to determine the focal spot size, source-to-image distance, alignment of X-ray field and image receptor, radiation leakage and tube output, are described in this section.

Focal spot size

The measurement of the focal spot size is intended to determine its physical dimensions at installation or when resolution has markedly decreased. The focal spot size must be determined for all available targets of the mammography unit. For routine quality control the evaluation of spatial resolution is considered adequate.

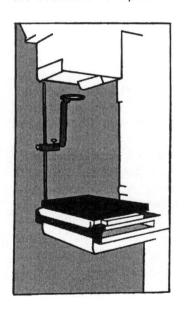

The focal spot dimensions can be obtained by using one of the following methods.
- star pattern method; a convenient method (routine testing)
- slit camera; a complex, but accurate method for exact dimensions (acceptance testing)
- pinhole camera; a complex, but accurate method to determine the shape (acceptance testing)
- multi-pinhole test tool; a simple method to determine the size across the field (routine/acceptance testing)

A magnified X-ray image of the test device is produced using a non-screen cassette. This can be achieved by placing a black film (OD ≥ 3) between screen and film. Select the focal spot size required, 28 kV tube voltage and a focal spot charge (mAs) to obtain an optical density between 0.8 and 1.4 OD base and fog excluded (measured in the central area of the image). The device should be imaged at the reference point of the image plane, which is located at 60 mm from the chest wall side and laterally centred. Remove the compression device and use the test stand to support the test device. Select about the same focal spot charge (mAs) that is used to produce the standard image of 45 mm PMMA, which will result in an optical density of the star pattern image in the range 0.8 to 1.4.

According the IEC/NEMA norm, a 0.3 nominal focal spot is limited to a width of 0.45 mm and a length of 0.65 mm. A 0.4 nominal focal spot is limited to 0.60 and 0.85 mm respectively. No specific limiting value is given here, since the measurement of imaging performance of the focal spot is incorporated in the limits for spatial resolution at high contrast (see 3.2.5.2).

Focal spot size: star pattern method

The focal spot dimensions can be estimated from the 'blurring diameter' on the image (magnification 2.5 to 3 times) of the star pattern. The distance between the outermost blurred regions is measured in two directions: perpendicular and parallel to the tube axis. Position the cassette on top of the bucky (no grid).

The focal spot is calculated by applying formula 1, which can also be found in the completion form.

$$f = \frac{\pi.\theta}{180} \frac{d_{blur}}{(m_{star}-1)}$$ (1)

where θ is the angle of the radiopaque spokes, and d_{blur} is the diameter of the blur.
The magnification factor (m_{star}) is determined by measuring the diameter of the star pattern on the acquired image (d_{image}) and the diameter of the device itself (d_{star}), directly on the star, and is calculated by:

$$m_{star}=d_{image}/d_{star}$$ (2)

Limiting value *None*
Frequency   *At acceptance and when resolution has changed*
Equipment   *Star resolution pattern (spoke angle 1° or 0.5°) and appropriate test stand*

Focal spot size: slit camera method

To determine the focal spot dimensions (f) with a slit camera, a 10 µm slit is used. Produce two magnified images (magnification 2.5 to 3 times) of the slit, perpendicular and parallel to the tube axis. Remove the compression device and use a test stand to support the slit.

The dimensions of the focal spot are derived by examining and measuring the pair of images through the magnifying glass. Make a correction for the magnification factor according to $f=F/m_{slit}$, where F is the width of the slit image. The magnification factor (m_{slit}) is determined by measuring the distance from the slit to the plane of the film ($d_{slit-to-film}$) and the distance from the focal spot to the plane of the slit ($d_{focal\ spot-to-slit}$). m_{slit} is calculated by:

$$m_{slit}=d_{slit-to-film}/d_{focal\ spot-to-slit}$$ (3)

Note: $m_{slit} = m_{image} - 1$, and the method requires a higher exposure than the star pattern method.
Limiting value *None*
Frequency   *At acceptance and when resolution has changed*
Equipment   *Slit camera (10 µm slit) with appropriate test stand and magnifying glass (5-10x), having a built-in graticule with 0.1 mm divisions*

Focal spot size: pinhole method

To determine the focal spot dimensions (f) with a pinhole, a 30 μm gold/platinum alloy pinhole is used. Produce a magnified image (magnification 2.5 to 3 times) of the pinhole. The dimensions of the focal spot are derived by examining the images through the magnifying glass and correcting for the magnification factor according to $f=F/m_{pinhole}$, where F is the size of the imaged focal spot. The magnification factor ($m_{pinhole}$) is determined by measuring the distance from the pinhole to the plane of the film ($d_{pinhole-to-film}$) and the distance from the focal spot to the plane of the pinhole ($d_{focal\ spot-to-pinhole}$). $m_{pinhole}$ is calculated by:

$$m_{pinhole}=d_{pinhole-to-film}/d_{focal\ spot-to-pinhole} \qquad (4)$$

Note: The method requires a higher exposure than the star pattern method.
Limiting value None
Frequency At acceptance and when resolution has changed
Equipment Pinhole (diameter 30 μm) with appropriate test stand and magnifying glass (5-10x), having a built-in graticule with 0.1 mm divisions

The *multi-pinhole* device is used similarly. It allows an estimate of the focal spot size at any position in the X-ray field. This method is not suitable for measuring the dimension of fine focus because of the relatively large size of the pinholes.

Source-to-image distance

Measure the distance between the focal spot indication mark on the tube housing and the top surface of the bucky. Add distance between bucky surface and the top of the image receptor.

Typical value The source-to-image distance should conform to the manufacturers' specification and typically is ≥ 600 mm
Frequency At acceptance only. When distance is adjustable: every six months
Equipment Tape measure

Alignment of X-ray field/image receptor

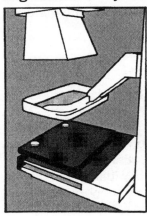

The alignment of the X-ray field and image receptor at the chest wall side can be determined with two loaded cassettes and two X-ray absorbers, e.g. coins.
Place one cassette in the bucky tray and the other on top of the breast support table. Make sure the second cassette has a film loaded with the emulsion side away from the screen. It must extend beyond the chest wall side about 30 mm. Mark the chest wall side of the bucky by placing the absorbers on top of the cassette. Automatic exposure will result in sufficient optical densities. Reposition the films on a light box using the imaged absorbers as a reference. The alignment between the film, X-ray field and chest wall edge of the bucky should be measured.

Note 1:   The lateral edges of the X-ray field should at least expose the image receptor. A slight extension beyond any edge of the image receptor is acceptable.

Note 2:   If more than one field size or target is used, the measurement should be repeated for each.

Limiting value   *For all focal spots: All sides: X-rays must cover the film by no more than 5 mm outside the film. On chest wall edge: distance between film edge and edge of the bucky must be ≤ 4 mm*

Frequency   *Yearly*

Equipment   *X-ray absorbers, e.g. coins, rulers, iron balls, tape measure*

Radiation leakage

The measurement of leakage radiation comprises two parts: firstly the location of leakage and secondly, the measurement of its intensity.

Position a beam stopper (e.g. lead sheet) over the end of the diaphragm assembly such that no primary radiation is emitted. Enclose the tube housing with loaded cassettes and expose to the maximum tube voltage and a high tube current (several exposures). Process the films and pinpoint any excessive leakage. Next, quantify the amount of radiation at the 'hot-spots' at a distance of 50 mm of the tube with a suitable detector. Correct the readings to air kerma rate in mGy/h (free in air) at the distance of 1 m from the focal spot at the maximum rating of the tube.

Limiting value   *Not more than 1 mGy in 1 hour at 1 m from the focus at the maximum rating of the tube averaged over an area not exceeding 100 cm^2, and according to local regulations*

Frequency   *At acceptance and after intervention on the tube housing*

Equipment   *Dosemeter and appropriate detector*

Tube output

The specific tube output (μGy/mAs) and the output rate (mGy/s) should both be measured at 28 kVp on a line passing through the focal spot and the reference point, in the absence of scatter material and attenuation (e.g. due to the compression plate). A tube load (mAs) similar to that required for the reference exposure should be used for the measurement. Correct for the distance from the focal spot to the detector and calculate the specific output at 1 meter and the output rate at a distance equal to the focus-to-film distance (FFD).

Typical values   *40-75 μGy/mAs at 1 meter*
    10-30 mGy/s at a distance equal to the FFD

Frequency   *Every six months and when problems occur*

Equipment   *Dosemeter, exposure timer*

Note: A high output is desirable for a number of reasons e.g. it results in shorter exposure times, minimising the effects of patient movement and ensures adequate penetration of large/dense breasts within the setting of the guard timer. In addition any marked changes in output require investigation.

3.2.1.2 Tube voltage

The radiation quality of the emitted X-ray beam is determined by tube voltage, anode material and filtration. Tube voltage and Half Value Layer (i.e. beam quality assessment) can be assessed by the measurements described below.

Reproducibility and accuracy

A tube voltage check over the range 25 - 31 kVp at 1 kV intervals should be performed. If other tube voltages are used clinically then these must be measured also. The reproducibility is measured by repeated exposures at one fixed tube voltage that is normally used clinically (e.g. 28 kVp).

Note: Consult the instruction manual of the kVp-meter for the correct positioning.

Limiting value *Accuracy for 25-31 kV: < ± 1 kV, reproducibility < ± 0.5 kV*
Frequency *Every six months*
Equipment *kVp-meter*

Half Value Layer

The Half Value Layer (HVL) can be assessed by adding thin aluminium (Al) filters to the X-ray beam and measuring the attenuation.

Position the exposure detector at the reference point (since the HVL is position dependent) on top of the bucky. Place the compression device halfway between focal spot and detector. Select 28 kV tube voltage and an adequate focal spot charge (mAs-setting), and expose the detector directly. The filters can be positioned on the compression device and must intercept the whole radiation field. Use the same tube load (mAs) setting and expose the detector through each filter. For higher accuracy (about 2%) a diaphragm, positioned on the compression paddle, limiting the exposure to the area of the detector may be used (see European Protocol on Dosimetry in Mammography). The HVL is calculated by applying formula 5.

$$HVL = \frac{X_1 \ln(\frac{2Y_2}{Y_0}) - X_2 \ln(\frac{2Y_1}{Y_0})}{\ln(\frac{Y_2}{Y_1})}$$

(5)

The direct exposure reading is denoted as Y_0; Y_1 and Y_2 are the exposure readings with added aluminium thickness of X_1 and X_2 respectively.

Note 1: The purity of the aluminium ≥ 99.9% is required. The thickness of the aluminium sheets should be measured with an accuracy of 1%.

Note 2: For this measurement the output of the X-ray machine needs to be stable.

Note 3: The HVL for other (clinical) tube voltages and other target materials and filters may also be measured for assessment of the mean glandular dose (see appendix 3 and the European Protocol on Dosimetry in Mammography).

Note 4: Alternatively a digital HVL-meter can be used, but correct these readings under extra filtration following the manufacturers' manual.

Limiting value   *For 28 kV Mo/Mo the HVL must be over 0.30 mm Al equivalent, and is typically < 0.40 mm Al. Typical values for other tube voltages, targets and filters, are shown in appendix 3*
Frequency   *Yearly*
Equipment   *Dosemeter, aluminium sheets 0.30 and 0.40 mm*

3.2.1.3 AEC-system

The performance of the Automatic Exposure Control (AEC) system can be described by the reproducibility and accuracy of the automatic optical density control under varying conditions, like different object thickness and tube voltages. Essential prerequisites for these measurements are a stable operating film-processor and the use of the reference cassette. If more than one breast support table, with a different AEC detector attached, is used then each system must be assessed separately.

Optical density control setting: central value and difference per step

To compensate for the long term variations in mean density due to system variations the central optical density setting and the difference per step of the selector are assessed. To verify the adjustment of the optical density control, produce exposures with a 45 mm PMMA test object with varying settings of the optical density control selector. Typical routine exposure factors should be used.

A target value for the mean optical density at the reference point should be established according to local preference, in the range: 1.3 – 1.8 OD, base and fog included.

Limiting value   *The optical density (base and fog included) at the reference point should remain within ± 0.15 OD of the target value. The change produced by each step in the optical density control should be about 0.10 OD; step-sizes within the range 0.05 to 0.20 OD are acceptable. The acceptable value for the range covered by full adjustment of the density control is > 1.0 OD*
Frequency   *Step-size and adjustable range: every six months*
                 Density and mAs-value for clinically used AEC setting: daily
Equipment   *Standard test block, densitometer*

Guard timer

The AEC system should also be equipped with a guard timer which will terminate the exposure in case of malfunctioning of the AEC system. Measure the tube load (mAs) at which the system terminates the exposure e.g. when using increasing thickness of PMMA plates.

Warning: an incorrect functioning of the guard timer could damage the tube. To avoid excessive tube load consult the manual for maximum permitted exposure time.

Limiting value   *None*
Frequency   *Yearly*
Equipment   *Sheet of lead*

Short term reproducibility

Position the dosemeter in the X-ray beam but without covering the AEC-detector. The short term reproducibility of the AEC system is calculated by the deviation of the exposure meter reading of ten routine exposures (45 mm PMMA).

Limiting value	*The deviations from the mean value of exposures must be < ± 5%. Desirable would be < ± 2%*
Frequency	*Every six months*
Equipment	*Standard test block, dosemeter*
Note:	For the assessment of the reproducibility, also compare these results from the short term reproducibility with the results from the thickness and tube voltage compensation and from the optical density control setting at 45 mm PMMA at identical settings. Any problem will be indicated by a mismatch between those figures.

Long term reproducibility

The long term reproducibility can be assessed from the measurement of optical density and tube load (mAs) resulting from the exposures of a PMMA block or the QC test object in the daily quality control. Causes of deviations can be found by comparison of the daily sensitometry data and tube load (mAs) recordings (see 3.2.3.2).

Limiting value	*The variation from the target value must be within < ± 0.20 OD; < ± 0.15 OD desirable*
Frequency	*Daily*
Equipment	*Standard test block or QC test object, densitometer*

Object thickness and tube voltage compensation

Compensation for object thickness should be measured by exposures of PMMA plates in the thickness range 20 to 70 mm, using a range of clinical settings (tube voltage, target, filter, modes) for the AEC corresponding to clinical practice. These settings include: full-automatic, semi-automatic as well as manual modes. In full-automatic mode all pre-programmed combinations of tube voltage, anode and filter should be chosen automatically when going through the range of PMMA thicknesses. When a combination is not chosen automatically then this combination must be selected manually, with the simulated breast thickness closest to the proper thickness (i.e. the PMMA thickness where this technique is appropriate). See appendix 5 for samples of such settings in the report forms.

Limiting value	*All optical density variations must be within ± 0.15 OD, with respect to the target optical density. Desirable: ± 0.10 OD*
Frequency	*Every six months: full test*
	Weekly: 20, 45, 65 mm PMMA exposed as for clinical settings
Equipment	*PMMA: plates 10x180x240 mm³, densitometer*

3.2.1.4 Compression

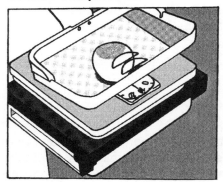

The compression of the breast tissue should be firm but tolerable. There is no optimal value known for the force, but attention should be given to the applied compression and the accuracy of the indication. All units must have motorised compression. See also the paragraph on compression in the radiography chapter.

Compression force

The compression force can be adequately measured with a compression force test device or a bathroom scale (use compressible material e.g. a tennis ball to protect the bucky and compression device).

When compression force is indicated on the console, it should be verified whether the figure corresponds with the measured value. It should also be verified whether the applied compression force is maintained over a period of 1 minute. A loss of force over this time may be explained, for example, by a leakage in the pneumatic system.

Limiting value   *Maximum automatically applied force: 130 - 200 N. (~ 13-20 kg), and must be maintained unchanged for at least 1 minute*
Frequency   *Yearly*
Equipment   *Compression force test device*

Compression plate alignment

The alignment of the compression device at maximum force can be visualised and measured when a piece of foam-rubber is compressed. Measure the distance between bucky surface and compression device on each corner. Normally, those four distances are equal. Misalignment normal to the chest wall side is less disturbing than in the parallel direction, as it compensates for the heel effect. The upright edge of the device must be projected outside the receptor area and optimally within the chest wall side of the bucky.

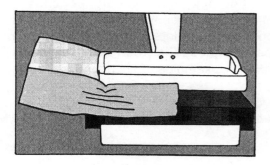

Limiting value   *Minimal misalignment is allowed, $\leq$ 15 mm is acceptable for asymmetrical load and in the direction towards the nipple, $\leq$ 5 mm for symmetrical load*
Frequency   *Yearly*
Equipment   *Foam rubber (specific mass: about 30 mg/cm^3), tape measure*

3.2.2 Bucky and image receptor

If more than one bucky and image receptor system is attached to the imaging chain than each system must be assessed separately.

3.2.2.1 Anti scatter grid

The anti scatter grid is composed of strips of lead and low density interspace material and is designed to absorb scattered photons. The grid system is composed of the grid, a cassette holder, a breast support table and a mechanism for moving the grid.

Grid system factor

The grid system factor can be determined by dose measurements. Produce two images, one with and one without the grid system. Use manual exposure control to obtain images of about reference optical density. The first image is made with the cassette in the bucky tray (imaged using the grid system) and PMMA on top of the bucky. The second with the cassette on top of the bucky (imaging not using the grid system) and PMMA on top of the cassette. The grid system factor is calculated by dividing the dosemeter readings, corrected for the inverse square law and optical density differences.

Note: *Not correcting the doses for the inverse square law will result in an over estimation of 5%.*
Typical value   *< 3*
Frequency   *At acceptance and when dose or exposure time increases suddenly*
Equipment   *Dosemeter, standard test block and densitometer*

Grid imaging

To assess the homogeneity of the grid in case of suspected damage or looking for the origin of artefacts, the grid may be imaged by automatic exposure of the bucky at the lowest position of the AEC-selector, without any added PMMA. This in general gives a good image of the gridlines.

Limiting value   *No significant non uniformity*
Frequency   *Yearly*
Equipment   *None*

3.2.2.2 Screen-film

The current image receptor in screen-film mammography consists of a cassette with one intensifying screen in close contact with a single emulsion film. The performance of the stock of cassettes is described by the inter cassette sensitivity variation and screen-film contact.

Inter cassette sensitivity and attenuation variation and optical density range

The differences between cassettes can be assessed with the reference exposure (section 1). Select an AEC setting (should be the normal position and using a fixed tube voltage, target and filter) to produce an image having about the clinically used mean optical density on the processed film. Repeat for each cassette using films from the same box or batch. Make sure the cassettes are identified properly. Measure the exposure (in terms of mGy or mAs) and the corresponding optical densities on each film at the reference point. To ensure that the cassette tests are valid the AEC system in the mammography unit needs to be sufficiently stable. It will be sufficient if the variation in repeated exposures selected by the AEC for a single cassette is (in terms of mGy and mAs) $<\pm$ 2%.

Limiting value	*The exposure, in terms of mGy (or mAs), must be within ± 5% of the mean for all cassettes*
	The maximum difference in optical density between all cassettes: ± 0.10 OD is acceptable, ± 0.08 OD is desirable
Frequency	*Yearly, and after introducing new screens*
Equipment	*Standard test object, dosemeter, densitometer*

Screen-film contact

Clean the inside of the cassette and the screen. Wait for at least 5 minutes to allow air between the screen and film to escape. Place the mammography contact test device (about 40 metal wires/inch, 1.5 wires/mm) on top of the cassette and make a non grid exposure to produce a film with an average optical density of about 2 OD at the reference point. Regions of poor contact will be blurred and appear as dark spots in the image. Reject cassettes only when they show the same spots when the test is repeated after cleaning. View at a distance of 1 meter. Additionally the screen resolution may be measured by imaging a resolution pattern placed directly on top of a cassette.

Limiting value	*No significant areas (i.e. > 1 cm²) of poor contact are allowed in the diagnostically relevant part of the film*
Frequency	*Every six months and after introducing new screens*
Equipment	*Mammography screen-film contact test device, densitometer and viewbox*

3.2.3 Film processing

The performance of the film processing greatly affects image quality. The best way to measure the performance is by sensitometry. Measurements of temperature and processing time are performed to establish the baseline performance.

3.2.3.1 Baseline performance of the processor

Temperature verification and baseline

To establish a baseline performance of the automatic processor, the temperature of developer and fixer are measured. Take care that the temperature is measured at a fixed point, as recommended by the manufacturers. The measured values can be used as background information when malfunction is suspected. Do not use a glass thermometer because of the contamination risk in the event of breakage.

Limiting value   *Compliance with the manufacturer's recommendations*
Frequency   *Every six months*
Equipment   *Electronic thermometer*

Processing time

The total processing time can be measured with a stopwatch. Insert the film into the processor and start the timer when the signal is given by the processor. When the processed film is available, stop the timer. When malfunction of the processor is suspected, measure this processing time exactly the same way again and check to see if there is any difference.

Limiting value   *Compliance with the manufacturer's recommendations*
Frequency   *At acceptance and when problems occur*
Equipment   *Stopwatch*

3.2.3.2 Film and processor

The films used in mammography should be specially designed for that purpose. Light sensitometry is a suitable method to measure the performance of the processor. Disturbing processor artefacts should not be present on the processed image.

Sensitometry

Use a sensitometer to expose a film with light and insert the exposed side into the processor first. Before measuring the optical densities of the stepwedge, a visual comparison can be made with a reference strip to rule out a procedure fault, like exposure with a different colour of light or exposure of the base instead of the emulsion side.
From the characteristic curve (the graph of measured optical density against the logarithm of exposure by light) the values of base and fog, maximum density, speed and film gradients can be derived. These parameters characterise the processing performance. A detailed description of these ANSI-parameters and their clinical relevance can be found in appendix 1, film parameters.

Typical values: base and fog: 0.15 – 0.25 OD
           contrast: Mgrad: 3.0 – 4.0
                 Grad $_{1-2}$: 3.5 – 5.0
Frequency   *Daily*
Equipment   *Sensitometer, densitometer*
Note: There is no clear evidence for the optimal value of film gradient; the ranges quoted are based on what is typical of current practice. At the top end of these ranges the high film gradient may lead to under and over exposure of parts of the image for some types of breast, thereby reducing the information content.
           A further complication of using a very high film contrast is that stable conditions with very low variability of the parameters are required to achieve any benefit in terms of overall image quality (see appendix 1).

Daily performance

The daily performance of the processor is assessed by sensitometry. After the processor has been used for about one hour each morning, perform the sensitometry as described above. The variability of the parameters can be calculated over a period of time e.g. one month (see calculation of film parameters in appendix 1).

Limiting value   See table below
Frequency   Daily and more often when problems occur
Equipment   Sensitometer, densitometer

The assessment of variations can be found in the use of the following table, where the values are expressed as a **range** (Max value - Min value). Acceptable and desirable ranges are quoted in the table below for speed and contrast indices for centres where computer facilities for calculating speed and film gradient (Mgrad and Grad$_{1,2}$) are not available. However this approach is less satisfactory as these indices are not pure measures of speed and contrast.

Assessment of variations

	acceptable	desirable	
base and fog	< 0.03	< 0.02	OD
max. density	< 0.30	< 0.20	OD
speed	< 0.05	< 0.03	
mean gradient (Mgrad)	< 0.30	< 0.15	
mid gradient (Grad$_{1,2}$)	< 0.40	< 0.20	
speed index	< 0.30	< 0.20	OD
contrast index	< 0.30	< 0.20	OD
temperature displayed	< 2	< 1	°C

Artefacts

An image of the standard test block obtained daily, using a routine exposure should be inspected. This should show a homogeneous density, without significant scratches, shades or other marks indicating artefacts.

Limiting value   No artefacts
Frequency   Daily
Equipment   Standard test block or PMMA plates 40-60 mm and area 18X24 cm, viewing box

3.2.3.3 Darkroom

Light tightness of the darkroom should be verified. It is reported, that about half of darkrooms are found to be unacceptable. Cassettes and film hopper should also be light tight. Extra fogging by the safelights must be within given limits.

Light leakage

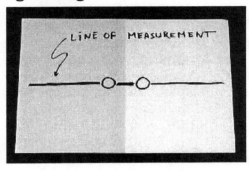

Remain in the darkroom for a minimum of five minutes with all the lights, including the safelights, turned off. Ensure that adjacent rooms are fully illuminated. Inspect all those areas likely to be a source of light leakage. To measure the extra fog as a result of any light leakage or other light sources, a pre-exposed film of about 1.2 OD is needed. This film can be obtained by a reference exposure of a uniform PMMA block. Always measure the optical density differences in a line perpendicular to the tube axis to avoid influence of the heel effect.

Open the cassette with pre-exposed film and position the film (emulsion up) on the (appropriate part of the) workbench. Cover half the film and expose for two minutes. Position the cover parallel to the tube axis to avoid the influence of the heel effect in the measurements. Measure the optical density difference of the background (D_{bg}) and the fogged area (D_{fogged}). The extra fog (ΔD) equals:

$$\Delta D = D_{fogged} - D_{bg}$$

(6)

Limiting value   *Extra fog: $\Delta D \leq 0.02$ OD in 2 minutes*
Frequency   *Every six months and when light leakage is suspected*
Equipment   *Film cover, densitometer*

Safelights

Perform a visual check that all safelights are in good working order (filters not cracked). To measure the extra fog as a result of the safelights, repeat the procedure for light leakage but with the safelights on. Make sure that the safelights were on for more than 5 minutes to avoid start-up effects.

Limiting value   *Extra fog: $\Delta D \leq 0.05$ OD in 2 minutes*
Frequency   *At acceptance, every six months and every time the darkroom environment*
               has changed
Equipment   *Film cover, densitometer*

Film hopper

Fogged edges on unexposed (clear) films may indicate that the film hopper is no longer light tight. Place one fresh sheet of film in the hopper. Leave it there for several hours with

---

full white light illumination in the darkroom. Inspect the processed film for light leakage of the hopper.

Limiting value Extra fog: < 0.02
Frequency   When light leakage is suspected
Equipment   None

Cassettes
Dark edges on radiographs indicate a need to perform light leakage tests on individual cassettes. Reload the suspect cassette with a fresh sheet of film and place it in front of a viewing box for several hours, making sure that each side of the cassette is exposed to bright light by turning it over. Inspect the processed film for dark edges due to light leakage of the cassette.

Limiting value No extra fogging
Frequency   This test should be performed at acceptance and when light leakage is
                suspected
Equipment   None

3.2.4 Viewing conditions

Since good viewing conditions are important for the correct interpretation of the diagnostic images, they must be optimised. Although the need for relatively bright light boxes is generally appreciated, the level of ambient lighting is also very important and should be kept low. In addition it is imperative that glare is minimised by masking the film.

As regards light levels the procedures for photometric measurements and the values required for optimum mammographic viewing are not well established. However there is general agreement on the parameters that are important. The two main measurements in photometry are luminance and illuminance. The luminance of viewing boxes is the amount of light emitted from a surface measured in candela/m^2. Illuminance is the amount of light falling on a surface and is measured in lux (lumen/m^2). The illuminance that is of concern here is the light falling on the viewing box, i.e. the ambient light level. (An alternative approach is to measure the light falling on the film reader's eye by pointing the light detector at the viewing box from a suitable distance with the viewing box off.) Whether one is measuring luminance or illuminance one requires a detector and a photometric filter. This combination is designed to provide a spectral sensitivity similar to the human eye. The collection geometry and calibration of the instrument is different for luminance and illuminance. To measure luminance a lens or fibre-optic probe is used, whereas a cosine diffuser is fitted when measuring illuminance. Where the only instrument available is an illuminance meter calibrated in lux it is common practice to measure luminance by placing the light detector in contact facing the surface of the viewing box and converting from lux to cd/m^2 by dividing by π. Since this approach makes assumptions about the collection geometry, a correctly calibrated luminance detector is preferred.

There is no clear consensus on what luminance is required for viewing boxes. It is generally thought that viewing boxes for mammography need to be higher than for general radiography. In a review of 20 viewing boxes used in mammographic screening in the UK, luminance averaged 4500 cd/m^2 and ranged from 2300 to 6700 cd/m^2. In the USA the ACR recommends a minimum of 3500 cd/m^2 for mammography. However some experts have suggested that the viewing box luminance need not be very high provided the ambient light is sufficiently low and that the level of ambient light is the most critical factor. The limiting values suggested here represent a compromise position until clearer evidence is available.

3.2.4.1 Viewing box

Luminance
The tendency to use a high optical density for mammography means that one must ensure that the luminance of the viewbox is adequate. Measure the luminance close to the centre of the illuminated area of each panel using a luminance meter calibrated in cd/m^2. An upper limit is included to minimise glare where films are imperfectly masked.

Limiting value *Luminance should be in the range 3000-6000 cd/m^2*
Frequency   *Yearly*
Equipment   *Luminance meter*

Homogeneity
The homogeneity of a single viewing box is measured by multiple readings of luminance over the surface of the illuminator, compared with the mean value of readings in the middle of the viewing area. Readings very near the edges (e.g. within 5 cm) of the viewing box should be avoided. Gross mismatch between viewing boxes or between viewing conditions used by the radiologist and those used by the radiographer should be avoided. If a colour mismatch exists, check to see that all lamps are of the same brand, type and age. Change all tubes at the same time. To avoid inhomogeneities as a result of dust, clean the light boxes regularly inside and out.

Limiting value *The uniformity of luminance across a single light box should be within ± 30% in the area 5 cm in from the edge of the pane. The intensity of different light boxes at one department should be within 15% of the average (measured in the middle of the viewing area)*
Frequency   *Yearly*
Equipment   *Luminance meter*

3.2.4.2 Ambient light

Level
When measuring the ambient light level (illuminance), the viewing box should be switched off. Place the detector against the viewing area and rotate away from the surface to obtain a maximal reading. This value is denoted as the ambient light level.

Limiting value   Ambient light level < 50 lux
Frequency   Yearly
Equipment   Illuminance meter

3.2.5 System properties

The success of a screening programme is dependent on the proper information transfer and therefore on the image quality of the mammogram. Decreasing the dose per image for reasons of radiation protection is only justified when the information content of the image remains sufficient to achieve the aim.

3.2.5.1 Dosimetry

The measurement of exposure and the calculation of the mean glandular dose in mammography are described in detail in the European Protocol on Dosimetry in Mammography (see 3.6, bibliography). Only the measurement of entrance surface air kerma is described here for convenience.

Entrance surface air kerma

This measurement is performed under reference conditions (28 kV, Mo target material, 30 µm Mo filter) either with AEC or manual exposure. Produce two exposures of the standard test block with an optical density under and over 1.4 OD (excluding base and fog). The corresponding entrance surface dose should be measured as close to the reference point as possible. The value for the entrance surface air kerma at the reference density should be interpolated linearly from these data. From this value the average glandular dose can be calculated (see page 29, European Protocol on Dosimetry). The average glandular dose for a 4.5 cm thick breast is typically less than 2.0 mGy.

Limiting value ≤ 15 mGy (for other OD's and thicknesses: see appendix 3)
Frequency   Yearly
Equipment   Dosemeter, standard test block, densitometer

3.2.5.2 Image quality

The information content of an image may best be defined in terms of just visible contrasts and details, characterised by its contrast-detail curve. The basic conditions for good performance and the constancy of a system can be assessed by measurement of the following: resolution, contrast visibility, threshold contrast and exposure time.

Spatial resolution

One of the parameters which determine image quality is the system spatial resolution. It can be adequately measured by imaging two resolution lead bar patterns, up to 20 line pairs per mm (lp/mm) each. They should be placed on top of PMMA plates with a total thickness of 45 mm. Image the patterns at the reference point both parallel and perpendicular to the tube axis, and determine these resolutions.

Note:	If the resolution is measured at different heights between 25 and 50 mm from the tabletop it can differ by as much as 4 lp/mm. The distance from the chest wall edge is critical, but the position parallel to the thorax side is not critical within ± 5 cm from the reference point. Resolution is generally worse parallel to the tube axis due to the asymmetrical shape of the focal spot.
Limiting value	*> 10 lp/mm acceptable, > 13 lp/mm desirable at the reference point in both directions*
Frequency	*Weekly*
Equipment	*PMMA plates 180x240 mm, resolution pattern(s) up to 20 lp/mm, densitometer*

Image contrast

Since image contrast is affected by various parameters (like tube voltage, film contrast etc.) this measurement is an effective method to detect a range of system faults. Make a reference exposure of an aluminium or PMMA stepwedge and measure the optical density of each step in the stepwedge. Draw a graph of the readings at each step against the stepnumber. The graph gives an impression of the image contrast. Since this graph includes the processing conditions, the film curve has to be excluded to find the radiation contrast, see appendix 2.

Note:	The value for image contrast is dependent on the whole imaging chain, therefore no absolute limits are given. Ideally the object is part of, or placed on top of, the daily quality control test object.
Limiting value	*± 10% acceptable, ± 5% desirable*
Frequency	*Weekly, and when problems occur*
Equipment	*PMMA or aluminium stepwedge, densitometer*

Threshold contrast visibility

This measurement should give an indication of the lowest detectable contrast of 'large' objects (diameter > 5 mm). Therefore a selection of low contrast objects has to be embedded in a PMMA test object to mimic clinical exposures. There should be at least two visible and two non-visible objects. Note, that the result is dependent on the mean OD of the image and on noise.

Produce a routine exposure and let two or three observers examine the low contrast objects. The number of visible objects is recorded. Ideally the object is part of, or placed on top of, the daily quality control test object.

Limiting value	*Minimum detectable contrast for a < 6 mm detail < 1.5% (see appendix 4)*
Frequency	*Weekly*
Equipment	*Test object with low contrast details plus PMMA plates, to a thickness of 45 mm, densitometer*

Exposure time

Long exposure times can give rise to motion unsharpness. Exposure time may be measured by some designs of kVp and output meters. Otherwise a dedicated exposure timer has to be used. The time for a routine exposure is measured.

Limiting value Acceptable: < 2 sec.; desirable: < 1.5 sec.
Frequency   Yearly and when problems occur
Equipment   Exposure time meter, standard test block

3.3 Daily and weekly QC tests

To ascertain that the performance of the equipment is likely to be unchanged with respect to former measurements a number of tests should be conducted daily. For this purpose, a dedicated QC test object or set of test objects are convenient. The actual frequencies recommended for each measurement are specified in 3.5 and summarised in table 1. The procedure must facilitate the measurement of some essential physical quantities, and it should be designed to evaluate:

- AEC reproducibility
- tube output
- reference optical density
- spatial resolution
- image contrast
- threshold contrast visibility
- homogeneity, artefacts
- sensitometry (speed, contrast, gross fog)

Practical considerations:
- Ideally the sensitometric stepwedge should be on the same film as the image of the test object, to be able to correct optimally for the processing conditions.
- To improve the accuracy of the daily measurement, the test object should be designed in such a way that it can be positioned reproducibly on the bucky.
- The shape of the test object does not have to be breast-like. To be able to perform a good homogeneity check, the test object should cover the normally imaged area on the image receptor (180x240 mm).
- For testing the AEC reproducibility, the PMMA test object may comprise several layers of PMMA, 10 or 20 mm thick. It is important to use the same PMMA blocks since variations in thickness of the PMMA plates will influence the tube load (mAs) read-out. Sufficient blocks are required to make up a thickness in the range 20-70 mm to adequately simulate the range of breast thickness found clinically.

3.4 Definition of terms

The definitions given here specify the meaning of the terms used in this document.

Accuracy: This is the closeness of an observed value of a quantity to the true value. It is calculated here as the difference between measured value (m) and true value (t) according to (m/t -1). When expressed as a percentage use (m/t -1) X 100%.

Air kerma: The quotient of dE_{tr} by dm, measured in Gray, where dE_{tr} is the sum of initial kinetic energies of all the charged ionising particles liberated by uncharged ionising particles in a mass of air dm (adapted from ICRU 1980).

Automatic exposure control (AEC): A mode of operation of an X-ray machine by which the tube loading is automatically controlled and terminated when a pre-set radiation exposure to the image receptor is reached. The tube potential (kV), target and filter material may also be automatically selected.

Average glandular dose: Reference term (ICRP 1987) for radiation dose estimation from X-ray mammography i.e. the average absorbed dose in the glandular tissue (excluding skin) in a uniformly compressed breast of, e.g., 50% adipose, 50% glandular tissue composition. The reference breast thickness and composition should be specified.

Baseline value: The observed value of a parameter that is typical for a system.

Breast compression: The application of pressure to the breast during mammography so as to immobilise the breast and to present a lower and more uniform breast thickness to the X-ray beam.

Compression paddle: An approximately rectangular plate, positioned parallel to and above the breast table of a mammography X-ray machine, which is used to compress the breast.

Deviation (± %): The percentage of difference between measured value (m) and prescribed value (p) according to (m/p -1) x 100% .

Dmin: Minimum density achievable with an exposed film; usually the density of the first step of a sensitometric strip.

Dmax: Maximum density achievable with an exposed film; usually the density of the highest step of a sensitometric strip.

Entrance surface air kerma (ESAK): The air kerma measured free-in-air (without backscatter) at a point in a plane corresponding to the entrance surface of a specified object e.g., a patient's breast or a standard test object.

Film gradient: The film gradient provides a measure of the film contrast.

Mgrad Mean Gradient; the property which expresses the film contrast in the diagnostic range. Mgrad is calculated as the slope of the line through the points D_1=Dmin+0.25 OD and D_2=Dmin+2.00 OD. Since the film curve is constructed from a limited number of points, D_1 and D_2 must be interpolated. Linear interpolation of the construction points of the film curve will result in sufficient accuracy.

Grad$_{1,2}$ Middle Gradient; the property which expresses the film contrast in the middle of the diagnostic range. Grad$_{1,2}$ is calculated as the slope of the line through the points D_1=Dmin+1.00 OD and D_2=Dmin+2.00 OD. Since the film curve is constructed from a limited number of points, D_1 and D_2 must be interpolated. Linear interpolation of the construction points of the film curve will result in sufficient accuracy.

Grad: See: film gradient.

Grid: A device which is positioned close to the entrance surface of an image receptor to reduce the quantity of scattered radiation reaching the receptor.

Half value layer (HVL): The thickness of absorber which attenuates the air kerma of a collimated X-ray beam by half. The absorber used normally is high purity aluminium.

Heel effect: The non-uniform distribution of air kerma rate in an X-ray beam in a direction parallel to the cathode-anode axis.

Inverse square law: The physical law which states that the X-ray beam intensity reduces in inverse proportion to the square of the distance from the point of measurement to the X-ray tube focus.

Image quality: Information content of the image in terms of just visible contrasts and details.

Laterally centred: Centred on a line perpendicular to the cathode-anode axis, not necessarily in the middle of the image.

Limiting value: A value of a parameter which, if exceeded, indicates that corrective action is required, although the equipment may continue to be used clinically. Limiting values for dose or air kerma are derived differently from reference values, i.e., reference ESD is based on third quartile values derived during surveys whereas limiting values of other parameters are derived from standard good practice.

Mammography: The X-ray examination of the breast. This may be undertaken for health screening of a population (mammography screening) or to investigate symptoms of breast disease (symptomatic diagnosis).

Net optical density: Optical density excluding base and fog.

Optical density (OD): The logarithm of the ratio of the intensity of perpendicularly incident light (I_o) on a film to the light intensity (I) transmitted by the film: $OD = \log_{10}(I_o/I)$. Optical density differences should be measured in a line perpendicular to the tube axis to avoid influences by the heel effect.

Patient: Any woman attending a facility for mammography whether for screening or for symptomatic diagnosis.

Patient dose: A generic term for a variety of radiation dose quantities applied to a (group of) patient(s).

PMMA: The synthetic material polymethylmethacrylate. Trade names include Lucite, Perspex and Plexiglas.

Precision: The variation (usually relative standard deviation) in observed values. A synonym is repeatability.

QC test object: Object made of tissue simulating material (usually PMMA) with embedded measuring devices (e.g. resolution pattern, stepwedge).

Quality assurance   as defined by the WHO (1982): 'All those planned and systematic actions necessary to provide adequate confidence that a structure, system or component will perform satisfactorily in service (ISO 6215-1980). Satisfactory performance in service implies the optimum quality of the entire diagnostic process-i.e., the consistent production of adequate diagnostic information with minimum exposure of both patients and personnel.'

Quality control   as defined by the WHO (1982): 'The set of operations (programming, co-ordinating, carrying out) intended to maintain or to improve [. . .] (ISO 3534-1977). As applied to a diagnostic procedure, it covers monitoring, evaluation, and maintenance at optimum levels of all characteristics of performance that can be defined, measured, and controlled.'

Radiation detector: An instrument indicating the presence and amount of radiation.

Radiation dose: A generic term for a variety of radiation quantities.

Radiation dosemeter: A radiation detector, connected to a measuring and display unit, which has a geometry, size, energy response and sensitivity suitable for measurements of the radiation generated by an X-ray machine.

Radiation output: The air kerma measured free-in-air (without backscatter) per unit of tube loading at a specified distance from the X-ray tube focus and at stated radiographic exposure factors.

Radiation quality: A measure of the penetrating power of an X-ray beam, usually characterised by a statement of the tube potential and the half value layer (HVL).

Range: The absolute difference of minimum and maximum values of measured quantities.

Reference cassette:	The identified cassette that is used for the QC tests.
Reference exposure:	The exposure of the test object to provide an image at the reference optical density.
Reference optical density:	The optical density of 1.4 OD, base and fog excluded, measured in the reference point.
Reference point:	A measurement position in the plane occupied by the entrance surface of a 45 mm thick test object, 60 mm perpendicular to the chest wall edge of the table and centred laterally.
Reference value (for dose):	The value of a quantity obtained for patients which may be used as a guide to the acceptability of a result. In the 1996 version of the 'European Guidelines on Quality Criteria for Diagnostic Radiographic Images' it is stated that the reference value can be taken as a ceiling from which progress should be pursued to lower dose values in line with the ALARA principle. This objective is also in line with the recommendations of ICRP Publication 60 (1991) that consideration be given to the use of 'dose constraints and reference or investigation levels' for application in some common diagnostic procedures.
Reproducibility	indicates the reliability of a measuring method or tested equipment. The results under identical conditions should be constant.
Resolution (at high or low contrast)	describes the smallest detectable detail at a defined high or low contrast to a given background.
Routine exposure:	The exposure of the standard test object under the conditions that would normally be used to produce a mammogram. It is used to determine image quality and dose under clinical conditions.
Speed:	See appendix 1: 'Film-parameters'.
Standard breast:	A model used for calculations of glandular dose consisting of a 40 mm thick central region comprising a 50%: 50% mixture by weight of adipose tissue and glandular tissue surrounded by a 5 mm thick superficial layer of adipose tissue. The standard breast is semicircular with a radius ≥ 80 mm and has a total thickness of 50 mm. (Note that other definitions of a standard breast have

been used in other protocols e.g. in the U.K. the standard breast has a total thickness of 45 mm with a 35 mm thick central region.)

Standard test block: A PMMA test object to represent approximately the average breast (although not an exact tissue-substitute) so that the X-ray machine operates correctly under automatic exposure control and the dosemeter readings may be converted into dose to glandular tissue. The thickness is 45 ± 0.5 mm and the remaining dimensions are either rectangular ≥ 150 mm x 100 mm or semi-circular with a radius of ≥ 100 mm.

Target OD: The optical density (OD) at the reference point of a routine exposure, chosen by the local staff as the optimal value for their imaging system. The target OD chosen should be in the range 1.3 - 1.8 OD, base and fog included.

Test object: See QC test object.

Threshold contrast: The contrast that produces a just visible difference between an object and the background.

Tube-current exposure-time product (mAs): The product of the X-ray tube current (milliampere, mA) and the radiographic exposure time (second, s).

Tube loading: The tube-current exposure-time product (mAs) that applies during a particular exposure.

Tube potential: The potential difference (kilovolt, kV) applied across the anode and cathode of the X-ray tube during a radiographic exposure.

Typical value: The value of a parameter that is found in most facilities in comparable measurements. The statement of such a value is an indication of what to expect, without any limits attached to that.

X-ray spectrum: The distribution of photon energies in an X-ray beam.

3.5 Tables

Table 1: Radiographic technique parameters, frequency of quality control, measured and limiting values.

	frequency	typical value	limiting value acceptable	desirable	unit
3.2.1 X-ray generation and control					
X-ray source					
- focal spot size	i	0.3	IEC/NEMA	-	-
- source-to-image distance	i	≥ 600	-	-	mm
- alignment of X-ray field/ image receptor	12	-	< 5	< 5	mm
- film/bucky edge	12	-	< 4	< 4	mm
- radiation leakage	i	-	< 1	< 1	mGy/hr
* output	6	40 - 75	> 30	> 40	µGy/mAs
* output rate	6	10 - 30	> 7.5	> 10	mGy/s
tube voltage					
- reproducibility	6	-	< ± 0.5	< ± 0.5	kV
- accuracy (25 – 31 kV)	6	-	< ± 1.0	< ± 1.0	kV
- HVL (Mo/Mo)	12	0.3 - 0.4	> 0.3	> 0.3	mm Al
AEC					
* central opt. density control setting [1]	6	-	< ± 0.15	< ± 0.15	OD
- opt. dens. control step	6	-	< 0.20, > 0.05	< 0.10, > 0.05	OD
- adjustable range	6	-	> 1.0	> 1.0	OD
* short term reproducibility	6	-	< ± 5%	< ± 2%	OD
* long term reproducibility	d	-	< ± 0.20	< ± 0.15	OD
- object thickness compensation	w	-	< ± 0.15	< ± 0.10	OD
and tube voltage compensation	6	-	< ± 0.15	< ± 0.10	OD
compression					
- compression force	12	130 - 200	-	-	N
- maintain force for	12	-	1	1	min
- compression plate alignment, asymmetric to nipple	12	-	< 15	< 15	mm
- compression plate alignment, laterally symmetric	12	-	< 5	< 5	mm

This table is continued on next page.

i = at acceptance; d = daily; w = weekly; 6 = every 6 months; 12 = every 12 months

* standard measurement conditions

[1] for standard blue based films only

Table 1, continued: Radiographic technique parameters, frequency and limiting values.

	frequency	typical value	limiting value		unit
			acceptable	desirable	
3.2.2 Bucky and image receptor					
anti scatter grid					
* grid system factor	i	< 3	-	-	-
screen-film					
* inter cassette sensitivity variation (mAs)	12	-	< ± 5%	< ± 5%	mGy
* inter cassette sensitivity variation (OD range)	12	-	< ± 0.10	< ± 0.08	OD
- screen-film contact	12	-	-	-	-
3.2.3 Film processing					
processor					
- temperature	i	34 - 36	-	-	°C
- processing time	i	90	-	-	s
film					
- sensitometry: base and fog	d	0.15 - 0.25[1]	-	-	OD
speed	d	-	-	-	-
contrast Mgrad:	d	3.0 - 4.0	-	-	-
$Grad_{1,2}$	d	3.5 - 5.0	-	-	-
- daily performance (see 3.2.3.2)	d	-	< 10%	< 5%	-
- artefacts	d	-	-	-	-
darkroom					
- light leakage (extra fog in 2 minutes)	12	-	< + 0.02[2]	< + 0.02[2]	OD
- safelights (extra fog in 2 minutes)	12	-	< + 0.10[2]	< + 0.10[2]	OD
- film hopper	i	-	< + 0.02[2]	< + 0.02[2]	OD
- cassettes	i	-	-	-	-

This table is continued on next page.

i = at acceptance; d = daily; w = weekly; 6 = every 6 months; 12 = every 12 months
* standard measurement conditions
[1] for standard blue based films only
[2] at net optical density 1.00 OD

Table 1, continued: Radiographic technique parameters, frequency and limiting values.

	frequency	typical value	limiting value		unit
			acceptable	desirable	
3.2.4 Viewing conditions					
viewing box					
- brightness	12	-	3000 - 6000	3000 - 6000	cd/m^2
- homogeneity	12	-	< ± 30%	< ± 30%	cd/m^2
- difference throughout department	12	-	-	< ± 15%	cd/m^2
environment					
- ambient light level	12	-	< 50	< 50	lux
3.2.5 System properties					
reference dose image quality					
* entrance surface dose; 45 mm test object	12	-	< 15	< 14	mGy
* spatial resolution, reference point	w	-	> 10	> 13	lp/mm
* image contrast variation	w	-	< ± 10%	< ± 5%	-
* threshold contrast visibility	w	-	1.5%	1.5%	-
* exposure time	12	-	< 2	< 1.5	s

i = at acceptance; d = daily; w = weekly; 6 = every 6 months; 12 = every 12 months

* standard measurement conditions

Table 2: QC equipment and calibration requirements

QC equipment	accuracy	reproducibility	unit
sensitometer	-	± 2%	OD
densitometer	±0.02 at 1.00 OD	± 1%	OD
dosemeter	± 5%	± 1%	mGy
thermometer	± 0.3	± 0.1	°C
kVp-meter for mammographic use	± 2%	± 1%	kV
exposure time meter	± 5%	± 1%	s
luminance meter	± 10%	± 5%	$Cd.m^{-2}$
illuminance meter	± 10%	± 5%	klux
test objects, PMMA	± 2%	-	mm
compression force test device	± 10%	± 5%	N

aluminium filters (purity ≥ 99.9%)			
aluminium stepwedge			
resolution pattern (> 15 lp/mm)			
focal spot test device			
stopwatch			
film-screen contact test tool			
tape measure			
rubber foam for compression plate alignment			
lead sheet			

3.6 Bibliography

CEC-Reports

1   *Technical and Physical Parameters for Quality Assurance in Medical Diagnostic Radiology; Tolerances, Limiting Values and Appropriate Measuring Methods*
    1989: British Institute of Radiology; BIR-Report 18, CEC-Report EUR 11620.

2   *Optimisation of Image Quality and Patient Exposure in Diagnostic Radiology*
    1989: British Institute of Radiology; BIR-Report 20, CEC-Report EUR 11842.

3   *Dosimetry in Diagnostic Radiology*
    Proceedings of a Seminar held in Luxembourg, March 19-21, 1991.
    1992: Rad. Prot. Dosimetry vol 43, nr 1-4; CEC-Report EUR 14180.

4   *Test Objects and Optimisation in Diagnostic Radiology and Nuclear Medicine*
    Proceedings of a Discussion Workshop held in Würtzburg (FRG), June 15-17, 1992
    1993: Rad. Prot. Dosimetry vol 49, nr 1-3; CEC-Report EUR 14767.

5   *Quality Control and Radiation Protection of the Patient in Diagnostic Radiology and Nuclear Medicine*
    1995: Rad. Prot. Dosimetry vol 57, nr 1-4; CEC-Report EUR 15257.

6   *European Guidelines on Quality Criteria for Diagnostic Radiographic Images*
    1996: CEC-Report EUR 16260.

Protocols

1   *The European Protocol for the Quality Control of the Technical Aspects of Mammography Screening.*
    1993: CEC-Report EUR 14821.

2   *European Protocol on Dosimetry in Mammography.*
    1996: CEC-Report EUR 16263.

3   *Protocol acceptance inspection of screening units for breast cancer screening, version 1993.*
    National Expert and Training Centre for Breast Cancer Screening, University Hospital Nijmegen (NL)
    1996 (translated in English).

4   *Protocol of quality control in mammography.*
    LNETI/DPSR, 1991.

5   ISS: *Controllo di Qualità in Mammografia: aspetti technici e clinici.*
    Instituto superiore de sanità (in Italian),
    1995: ISTASAN 95/12.

6   IPSM: *Commissioning and Routine Testing of Mammographic X-Ray Systems - second edition*
    The Institute of Physical Sciences in Medicine, York
    1994: Report no. 59/2.

7   American College of Radiology (ACR), Committee on Quality Assurance in Mammography: *Mammography quality control.*
    1994, revised edition

8   American Association of Physicists in Medicine (AAPM): *Equipment requirements and quality control for mammography*
    1990: report No. 29

9   *Quality Control in Mammography,*
    1995: Physics consulting group Ontario Breast Screening Programme

10 *Belgisch Protocol voor de kwaliteitszorg van de fysische en technische aspecten bij mammografische screening.*
    QARAD/LUCK (in Dutch), 1999

Publications

1   Chakraborty D.P.: *Quantitative versus subjective evaluation of mammography accreditation test object images.*
    1995: Med. Phys. 22(2):133-143

2   Wagner A.J.: *Quantitative mammography contrast threshold test tool.*
    1995: Med. Phys. 22(2):127-132

3   Widmer J.H.: *Identifying and correcting processing artefacts.*
    Technical and scientific monograph
    Health Sciences Division
    Eastman Kodak Company, Rochester, New York, 1994

4   Caldwell C.B.: *Evaluation of mammographic image quality: pilot study comparing five methods.*
    1992: AJR 159:295-301

5   Wu X.: *Spectral dependence of glandular tissue dose in screen-film mammography.*
    1991: Radiology 179:143-148

6   Hendrick R.E.: *Standardization of image quality and radiation dose in mammography.*
    1990: Radiology 174(3):648-654

7   Baines C.J.: *Canadian national breast screening study: assessment of technical quality by external review.*
    1990: AJR 155:743-747

8   Jacobson D.R.: *Simple devices for the determination of mammography dose or radiographic exposure.*
1994: Z. Med. Phys. 4:91-93

9   Conway B.J.: *National survey of mammographic facilities in 1985, 1988 and 1992.*
1994: Radiology 191:323-330

10 Farria D.M.: *Mammography quality assurance from A to Z.*
1994: Radiographics 14: 371-385

11 Sickles E.A.: *Latent image fading in screen-film mammography: lack of clinical relevance for batch-processed films.*
1995: Radiology 194:389-392

12 Sullivan D.C.: *Measurement of force applied during mammography.*
1991: Radiology 181:355-357

13 Russell D.G.: *Pressures in a simulated breast subjected to compression forces comparable to those of mammography.*
1995: Radiology 194:383-387

14 Faulkner K.: *Technical note: perspex blocks for estimation of dose to a standard breast - effect of variation in block thickness.*
1995: Br. J. Radiol. 68:194-196

15 Faulkner K.: *An investigation into variations in the estimation of mean glandular dose in mammography.*
1995: Radiat. Prot. Dosimet. 57:405-407

16 K.C. Young, M.G. Wallis, M. L. Ramsdale*: Mammographic Film Density and Detection of Small Breast cancers*, 1994 Clin. Radiol (49) 461-465

17 Tang S.: *Slit camera focal spot measurement errors in mammography.*
1995: Med. Phys. 22:1803-1814

18 Hartmann E.: *Quality control of radiographic illuminators and associated viewing equipment. Retrieval and viewing conditions.*
1989: BIR report 18:135-137

19 Haus A.G.: *Technologic improvements in screen-film mammography.*
1990: Radiology 174(3):628-637

20 L.K. Wagner, B.R. Archer, F. Cerra; *On the measurement of half-value layer in film-screen mammography.*
1990: Med. Phys. (17):989-997.

21 J.D. Everson, J.E. Gray: *Focal-Spot Measurement: Comparison of Slit, Pinhole, and Star Resolution Pattern Techniques.*
1987: Radiology (165):261-264.

22 J. Law: *The measurement and routine checking of mammography X-ray tube kV.*
1991: Phys.Med.Biol. (36):1133-1139.

23 J. Law: *Measurements of focal spot size in mammography X-ray tubes.*
1993: Brit. J. Of Radiology (66):44-50

24 M. Thijssen et al: *A definition of image quality: the image quality figure.*
1989: Brit. Inst. Radiology, BIR-report 20: 29-34

25 R.L. Tanner: *Simple test pattern for mammographic screen-film contact measurement.*
1991: Radiology (178):883-884.

26 K.C. Young, M.L. Ramsdale, A. Rust: *Mammographic dose and image quality in the UK breast screening programme.* 1998, NHSBSP report 35

27 J. Zaers, S. van Woudenberg, G. Brix: *Qualitätssicherung in der Röntgen-mammographie*
1997: Der Radiologe (37):617-620

28 J. Law: *Checking the consistency of sensitometers and film processors in a mammographic screening programme.* 1996 Brit. J. Of Radiology (69) 143-147

29 K. J. Robson, C.J. Kotre, K. Faulkner: *The use of a contrast-detail test object in the optimization of optical density in mammography,*
1995 Brit. J. Of Radiology (68) 277-282

30 J.A. Terry, R.G. Waggener, M.A. Miller Blough: *Half-value layer and intensity variations as a function of position in the radiation field for film screen mammography,* 1999 Med. Phys. 26 259-266

31 S. Tang, G.T. Barnes, R.L. Tanner: *Slit camera focal spot measurement errors in mammography,*
1995 Med. Phys. (22) 1803-1814

32 J. Coletti et al.: *Comparison of exposure standards in the mammography x-ray region,*
1997 Med. Phys (8) 1263-1267

33 C. Kimme Smith et al. *Mammography film processor replenishment rate: Bromide level monitoring,*
1997 Med. Phys. (3) 369-372

35 M. Goodsitt, H. Chan, B. Liu: *Investigation of the line-pair method for evaluating mammographic focal spot performance,* 1997 Med. Phys. (1) 11-15

34 A. Krol et al. *Scatter reduction in mammography with air gap,*
1996 Med. Phys. (7) 1263-1270

35 D. McLean, J. Gray: *K-characteristic photon absorption from intensifying screens and other materials: Theoretical calculations and measurements,*
1996 Med. Phys. (7) 1253-1261

36 P. Rezentes, A. de Almeida, G. Barnes: *Mammographic Grid Performance,*
1999 Radiology 210:227-232

37 J. Hogge et al. *Quality assurance in Mammography: Artifact Analysis,*
1999 Radiographics 19:503-522

38 J. Byng et al.: *Analysis of Mammographic Density and Breast Cancer Risk from Digitized Mammograms,*
1998 Radiographics 18:1587-1598

Other reports

1 International Electrotechnical Commission (IEC), Geneva, Switzerland: *Characteristics of focal spots in diagnostic X-ray tube assemblies for medical use,*
1982: IEC-Publication 336.

2 *Quality assurance in mammography - quality control of performance and constancy,*
1990: Series of Nordic Reports on radiation Safety No. 1, Denmark, Finland, Iceland, Norway and Sweden.

3 Société française des physiciens d'hôpital, Nancy: *Contrôle de qualité et mesure de dose en mammographie - aspects théoriques et pratiques* (in French),
1991.

4 Department Health & Social Security, Supplies Technology Division (DHSS): *Guidance notes for health authorities on mammographic equipment requirements for breast cancer screening,*
1987: STD

5 Department of Radiodiagnostic Radiology, University of Lund, Sweden: *Quality Assurance in Mammography,*
1989.

6 *Sicherung der Bildqualität in röntgendiagnostischen Betrieben - Filmverarbeitung* (in German),
1985: DIN 6868 teil 2: Beuth Verlag GmbH, Berlin.

7 American Association of Physicists in Medicine (AAPM): *Basic quality control in diagnostic radiology,*
1978: report No. 4

8 ECRI: *Special issue: Mammography Units,*
1989: Health Devices:Vol.18:No.1:Plymouth Meeting (PA)

9   ECRI: *Double issue: Mammography Units*,
     1990: Health Devices:Vol.19:No.5-6:Plymouth Meeting (PA)

10   Siemens Medical Systems Inc., New Jersey: *Mammography QA - Doc.# 54780/up*,
     1990

11   *ANSI: Determination of ISO speed and average gradient*,
     American National Standards Institute (ANSI).
     1983: Nr. PH2.50.

12   *Sicherung der Bildqualität in röntgendiagnostischen Betrieben - Konstantzprüfung für
     die Mammographie* (in German),
     1989: DIN-1:6868 teil 7:Beuth Verlag GmbH, Berlin.

13   *Sicherung der Bildqualität in röntgendiagnostischen Betrieben - Abnahmeprüfung an
     Mammographie-Einrichtungen* (in German),
     1989: DIN-2:6868 teil 52: Beuth Verlag GmbH, Berlin.

14   *ICRP Publication 52, including the Statement from the Como Meeting of the ICRP*,
     1987: Annals of the ICRP 17 (4), i-v, Pergamon Press, Oxford, UK.

15   *ICRP Publication 60, 1990 Recommendations of the ICRP*,
     (Adopted by the Commission in November 1990);
     1991: Annals of the ICRP 21 (1-3), Pergamon Press, Oxford, UK.

Colaborating institutes

Quality in Radiology, Belgium (QUARAD)
Leuvens Universitair Centrum voor Kankerpreventie, Belgium (LUCK)
Association pour la Recherche et le Dépistage des Cancers du Sein, France (ARCADES)
Landelijk Referentiecentrum voor bevolkingsonderzoek op Borstkanker, the Netherlands
(LRCB)
European Medical Imaging Film Manufacturers Association, Belgium (EMIFMA)
National Coordinating Centre fot the Physics of Mammography, UK (NCCPM)
Programme Mammographie, Luxembourg (PM)

Appendix 1
Film-parameters

The film curve can be characterised by a few parameters. Most important items are contrast, sensitivity and base and fog. There are different methods to calculate the film-parameters. Existing normalisations differ so much that the following method is suggested, derived from the Dutch protocol (1991), which is based on the ANSI (1983) norm.

Very high contrast can be a problem because of an associated reduction in dynamic range which may result in dense breast tissue being imaged in relatively low film densities where the film performance is relatively poor. To some extent this can be compensated for by setting relatively high average film densities, but even then a lower film contrast may better image local areas of dense tissue. Conversely a very low overall film contrast may indicate an inadequately processed film and subtle details may be missed by the radiologist.

Research has shown that film gradient measured by light sensitometry correlates well with film gradient measured by X-ray sensitometry using a fixed kV and target filter combination. One must bear in mind that film emulsions may respond slightly differently to the light from a sensitometer as opposed to the light from the screen used for imaging.

Dmin   Base and fog; the optical density of a non exposed film after developing. The minimum optical density can be visualised by fixation only of an unexposed film. The extra fog is a result of developing the (unexposed) emulsion.

Dmax   The maximum density achievable with an exposed film; i.e. the highest density step.

Mgrad   Mean gradient; the property which expresses the filmcontrast in the diagnostic range. MGrad is calculated as the slope of the line through the points D_1=Dmin+0.25 OD and D_2=Dmin+2.00 OD. Since the film curve is constructed from a limited number of points, D_1 and D_2 must be interpolated. Linear interpolation of the construction points of the film curve will result in sufficient accuracy.

Grad$_{1,2}$ Middle gradient; the property which expresses the filmcontrast in the diagnostic range. Grad$_{1,2}$ is calculated as the slope of the line through the points D_1=Dmin+1.00 OD and D_2=Dmin+2.00 OD. Since the film curve is constructed from a limited number of points, D_1 and D_2 must be interpolated. Linear interpolation of the construction points of the film curve will result in sufficient accuracy.

Grad$_{gland}$ The glandular tissue gradient can be defined as an alternative. This is the gradient at glandular densities 0.8 – 1.5 OD. This gradient is used in combination with the Grad$_{fat}$.

Grad$_{fat}$ The alternative fat tissue gradient is defined between densities of 1.8 and 2.5 OD. This gradient is used in combination with the Grad$_{gland}$.

Speed Sensitivity; the property of the film emulsion directly related to the dose. The Speed is calculated as the x-axis cut-off at optical density 1.00+Dmin, also called 'Speedpoint'. The higher the figure for Speed, the more dose is needed to obtain the right optical density. Since the film curve is constructed from a limited number of points, the Speed must be interpolated. Linear interpolation will result in sufficient accuracy.

Since these parameters are derived from the characteristic curve by interpolation they are not very practical if a computer is not available. A simpler procedure is to use the parameters below which are based on density measurements of particular sensitometric steps.

Speed Index The density of the step near to the speedpoint density 1.0 OD, base and fog excluded. Usually this is the density of step 11 of the sensitometric stepwedge.

Contrast Index 1 The difference in density found between the step nearest to the speedpoint density (1.0 OD, base and fog excluded) and the one with a 0.6 log E (factor 4) higher light exposure (normally 4 density steps) (ACR).

Contrast Index 2 The difference in density steps found between the step nearest to the speedpoint and the step nearest to a density at 2.0 OD, base and fog excluded (IPSM, see bibliography).

Appendix 2
A method to discriminate between processing and exposure variations by correction for the film curve

The optical density of a film is the result of X-ray exposure and processing. The film is mainly exposed by light emitted by the intensifying screen. The light emission of the screen is proportional with the incident X-ray exposure. Primary X-rays only contribute up to 5% of the total exposure. The developing process determines the optical density of the exposed area.

When an optical density in any given film is measured, the corresponding exposure is unknown. However, the film curve (measured with light sensitometry) describes the relation between light exposure and optical density. Any measured optical density can be converted into a relative log(light exposure) or log(I') by interpolation of the film curve. This figure log(I') is a relative value and strongly depends on the sensitometer used. But still it is a useful value, closely related with the radiation dose applied and is therefore suitable to calculate the mass attenuation coefficient of an arbitrary X-ray stepwedge. Note that recently available films, using a different type of sensitising and grains, in some cases show a discrepancy between the gradient as a result of light and by X-rays.

When the optical density of several images, taken under identical conditions, is measured, there will be a range of optical densities. This can either be the result of a change in exposure or a change in developing conditions. By calculating the relative figure log(I') we are able to distinguish between processor faults and tube malfunctions.

Approximation of X-ray contrast
To assess the X-ray contrast, correct the OD-readings of an Al-stepwedge for the processing to conditions by converting the optical densities into a fictional 'exposure', log(I'), according to the film curve. Now, a graph of the stepwedge number against 'exposure' will result in an almost straight line. The slope of this line is a measure for the X-ray contrast.

Appendix 3
Typical values for other spectra and densities

Other spectra
The techniques used to produce a mammographic image are constantly optimised. New anode materials, in combination with filters of different composition and thickness, may be explored to improve image quality or to reduce patient dose. Some of these new techniques are used in mammography screening. The typical values of the HVL of some of these combinations are listed below (appendix 3, European Protocol on Dosimetry in Mammography).

Table 1: HVL values for common anode-filter combinations in mammography. Numbers in brackets refer to a HVL with a 3 mm compression plate in the beam.

Anode and filter materials	HVL at 25 kVp mm Al	HVL at 28 kVp mm Al
Mo + 30 µm Mo	0.28 (0.34)	0.32 (0.37)
Mo + 25 µm Rh	0.36 (0.40)	0.40 (0.44)
W + 60 µm Mo	0.35 (0.39)	0.37 (0.41)
W + 50 µm Rh	0.48 (0.51)	0.51 (0.54)
W + 40 µm Pd	0.44 (0.48)	0.48 (0.53)
Rah + 25 µm Rh	0.34 (0.40)	0.39 (0.45)

Other densities
The mean optical density of a mammogram affects the dose imparted in the tissue. Applying a different mean OD in the mammogram changes the exposure and the glandular dose. An indication of the changes expected in respect to the reference exposure (28 kV) are listed below as adaptation of the limiting value for the Entrance Surface Air Kerma (ESAK) and standard Average Glandular Dose (sAGD). The film is expected to fulfil the limiting value by having an Mgrad of 3.0 (see table 2.3 and table 3.2 in the European Protocol on Dosimetry in Mammography).

Table 2: Values for ESAK, AGD, at a given density

Net film density (OD)	0.8	1.0	1.2	1.4	1.6	1.8
ESAK (mGy)	9	11	13	15	17	19
Standard AGD (mGy)	1.8	2.3	2.8	3.2	3.6	4.0

Note: The values refer to the 5 cm thick 'standard breast' as defined in the European Protocol on Dosimetry in Mammography.

Appendix 4
Low contrast visibility

The visibility of an object in respect to its background is dependent on three main properties of the object in the image:

- the size of the object (detail size, D)
- the noise in both object and background
- the difference in mean optical density between object and background (contrast, C)

Theory predicts that the threshold of visibility, i.e. the relation between the size (D) and the contrast (C) of the just visible object, will follow a simple rule:

$$C*D = constant$$

In practice this only holds true for a certain range of diameters and performance diverges from theory at large and small diameters. In general it is observed that whereas a large object may be visible at a low contrast, a small object of the same contrast may not be seen at all. Conversely, the contrast that is necessary to just visualise that small object, would make a large object show up as a bright white spot. When noise is involved, as in an X-ray image, the value of the constant is increased, leading to the need for greater contrast in order to visualise an object. Thus it is the contrast-to-noise ratio that determines whether an object can be seen. Increasing film contrast will not improve visibility unless steps are taken to prevent the overall noise from increasing by the same amount (e.g. by reducing film granularity). Using lower energy X-rays (e.g. by lowering the kVp) or increasing the dose may improve the contrast-to-noise ratio. But lowering the X-ray energy or increasing the dose may lead to a higher risk for the women. To obtain an optimal diagnostic quality at an acceptable risk, limits are set to the noise by defining the minimum detectable contrast for a certain detail size within acceptable dose limits. An object ≤ 6 mm must to be visible when it has a 1.5% contrast in the image.
The 1.5% contrast can be obtained, when a disk of 0.3 mm PMMA or 0.1 μm gold is put on top of or inside the 45 mm PMMA test object. To facilitate comparison with other object contrasts, disks of the same diameter with 15%-20% higher and lower contrast should be positioned next to that disk.

Appendix 5
Digital mammography

The introduction of mammography systems that do not use a screen-film combination as the detector and storage medium but that produce a digital image, allows the visualisation of contrasts beyond the limitations of film. That gives rise to a different approach to the quality demands that are stated in this document. A separate part will have to deal with these aspects in future editions.

Some considerations on the subject are given here:

Spatial resolution
In film-screen systems it is sufficient to characterise the information transfer at lower frequencies by its spatial resolution at higher frequencies: a maximal resolution of 12 lp/mm ensures sufficient contrast at frequencies about 2-5 lp/mm, where the human eye is most sensitive.

In digital systems the resolution is limited by the properties of the detecting medium, the pixel size used in the detector and by the imaging system. As a result, the resolution that is given by the pixel size of the imaging system is not the right measure to characterise the imaging capabilities of the digital system.

Since the detection of an object is dependent on its contrast to the background, the contrast-detail (CD) curve or other contrast based transfer functions of the system might be a more appropriate measure than the currently used Modulation Transfer Function (MTF). Adequate test devices are readily available but need a more complicated evaluation than resolution patterns.

The use of digital systems allows the adjustment of very low contrasts to the sensitivity of the human eye. This will make the demand of a resolution better than 10 lp/mm obsolete for digital systems (3.2.5.2).

X-ray generation
The information needed to produce images of sufficient diagnostic quality is produced by the X-ray part of the system. This can lead to the conclusion that no reduction in the demands on geometry and focal spot size are allowed. The influence of the stability in X-ray production, the reproducibility of the automatic exposure system and kVp-thickness compensations however may become less important.

Threshold contrast visibility
Since most of the digital systems make use of detectors with a higher detective quantum efficiency (DQE) than the film-screen systems, this will set new standards for the threshold contrast visibility of 'large' objects (3.2.5.2). Also the computing power of these systems might give detecting results beyond the capabilities of the human eye, by using image improvement algorithms and computer aided diagnosis (CAD).

Grid

The contrast in film-screen systems is strongly affected by scatter, since this adds to an offset optical density of both the object and its background. This leads to the strong benefit of the use of an anti-scatter grid. In digital systems these relations change due to the properties of the detector and the ability to adjust for this offset. This might allow the use of a grid with reduced selectivity for primary radiation or no grid at all, which has a great benefit to the dose per image.

Dose

Since the threshold contrast visibility improves by allowing a higher dose per image to the detector due to the better signal-to-noise ratio, and since the digital systems are able to process a wide range of intensities, there will be a tendency to increase the exposure per image. This leads to a higher absorbed dose in the glandular tissue, which increases the risk for the woman. Great care should be taken in the techniques chosen to make the exposures, since they can be chosen freely, where in screen-film systems the mean optical density and the risk of under or overexposure of the film limit the dose to the women. The dose constraint (3.2.5.1) also holds for digital systems. Exposure parameters or system sensitivity therefore should be included in the image and in the file information.

Summary

The introduction of digital mammography will lead to different measures and limitations in the quality control for these systems in respect to screen-film systems. Since many aspects are still developing or not yet fully understood, research has to be done on the aspects of quality control of digital mammography systems. The dose per image must be monitored carefully.

Appendix 6
Completion forms for QC reporting

QC report

based on

The European protocol for the quality control of the physical and technical aspects of mammography screening

Third edition

Date: _____

Contact: _____

Institute: _____

Address: _____

Telephone: _____

Conducted by: _____

3.2.1 X-ray generation

3.2.1.1 X-ray source

Focal spot size

Class (large) focal spot: _____ (IEC)

* *star pattern method*

diameter star pattern	D_{star}	____ mm
spoke angle θ	θ	____ °
diameter magnified star image	D_{mag}	____ mm
diameter first MTF zero $\perp$ AC axis	$D_{blur, \perp}$	____ mm
diameter first MTF zero // AC axis	$D_{blur, //}$	____ mm

$$m_{star} = \frac{d_{mag}}{d_{star}} \; ; \; f = \frac{\pi \times \theta}{180} \times \frac{d_{blur}}{(m-1)}$$

* *slit camera method*

width slit		____ mm
distance slit-to-film	$d_{slit\text{-}film}$	____ mm
distance focus-to-slit	$d_{focus\text{-}slit}$	____ mm
width slit image $\perp$ AC axis	$F\perp$	____ mm
width slit image // AC axis	F //	____ mm

$$m_{slit} = \frac{d_{slit\text{-}film}}{d_{focus\text{-}slit}} \; ; \; f = \frac{F}{m_{slit}}$$

* *pinhole method*

diameter pinhole		____ μm
distance pinhole-to-film	$d_{pinhole\text{-}film}$	____ mm
distance focus-to-pinhole	$d_{focus\text{-}pinhole}$	____ mm
diameter pinhole $\perp$ AC axis	$f\perp$	____ mm
diameter pinhole // AC axis	f //	____ mm

$$m_{pinhole} = \frac{d_{pinhole\text{-}film}}{d_{focus\text{-}pinhole}} \; ; \; f = \frac{F}{m_{pinhole}}$$

Focal spot size **$f\perp$ = _____ mm**

f// = _____ mm   **Accepted: yes / no**

Source-to-image distance

Nominal value:	____ mm
Measured value :	
- Focus indication to bucky:	____ mm
- Bucky to cassette:	____ mm
Source-to-image distance:	____ mm

Alignment of X-ray field / image receptor

Distance at chest wall side film: inside/outside image receptor:
position

left:	____ mm, in / out
nipple:	____ mm, in / out
right :	____ mm, in / out
chest :	____ mm, in / out
Distance between film edge and bucky edge	____ mm

Accepted: yes / no

Radiation leakage

Description of position of 'hot spots'

1 _____
2 _____
3 _____

detector surface area: ____ mm^2

	measured:	calculated for
distance from tube:	50 mm	1000 mm,
surface area:	____ mm^2	100 cm^2:
nr:		
1. _____	____	____ mGy/hr
2. _____	____	____ mGy/hr
3. _____	____	____ mGy/hr

Accepted: yes / no

Tube output

focus to detector distance:	____ mm
surface air kerma:	____ mGy
focal spot charge:	____ mAs
specific tube output at 1 m	____ µGy/mAs
output rate at FFD	____ mGy/s

Accepted: yes / no

3.2.1.2 Tube voltage

Reproducibility and accuracy

Pre-set tube load: _____ mAs
Clinically most relevant kV: _____ kV

Accuracy

Setting	25	26	27	28	29	30	31	kV
Measured	____	____	____	____	____	____	____	kV
Deviation	____	____	____	____	____	____	____	kV

Accepted: yes / no

Accuracy at other clinical values

Setting	22	23	24	32	33	34	35	kV
Measured	____	____	____	____	____	____	____	kV
Deviation	____	____	____	____	____	____	____	kV

Reproducibility at the clinically most relevant value
Measured value: 1.____ 2.____ 3.____ 4.____ 5.____ kV
Reproducibility (max difference from the mean):   ____ kV

Accepted: yes / no

Half Value Layer

Anode/filter:	<u>Mo/Mo</u>			
Measured tube voltage:	____ kV			
Pre-set tube load:	____ mAs			
Filtration:	0.0	0.30	0.40	mm Al
Exposure:	Y_0	Y_1	Y_2	

		Y_0	Y_1	Y_2	
	1.	____	____	____	mGy
	2.	____	____	____	mGy
	3.	____	____	____	mGy

Average exposure: ____   ____   ____   mGy

$$HVL = \frac{X_1 \ln(\frac{2Y_2}{Y_0}) - X_2 \ln(\frac{2Y_1}{Y_0})}{\ln(\frac{Y_2}{Y_1})} = \_\_\_\_ \; mm \; Al$$

Deviation exposure at 0 mm Al :   ____ %

Accepted: yes / no

Half Value Layer for alternative filtration

Anode/filter: Mo/Rh

Measured tube voltage: ____ kV

Pre-set tube load: ____mAs

Filtration:	0.0	0.30	0.40	mm Al
Exposure:	Y_0	Y_1	Y_2	
1.	____	____	____	mGy
2.	____	____	____	mGy
3.	____	____	____	mGy

Average exposure: ____ ____ ____ mGy

HVL: ____ mm Al
Deviation exposure at 0 mm Al :   ____ %

Accepted: yes / no

3.2.1.3 AEC-system

Optical density control setting: central value and difference per step

Target density value: ____ OD

Setting	Exposure mGy	Tube load mAs	Density OD	Density incr. OD
-3	____	____	____	
-2	____	____	____	____
-1	____	____	____	____
0	____	____	____	____
1	____	____	____	____
2	____	____	____	____
3	____	____	____	____

Accepted: yes / no

Adjustable range: ____ OD

Accepted: yes / no

Optical density control setting for reference density: ____
Optical density control setting for target density: ____

Guard timer
Exposure terminates by exposure limit :   yes/no
Alarm or error code: yes/no
Exposure: ____ mGy
Tube load: ____ mAs

Short term reproducibility

Optical density control setting: ____

Exp. #	Exposure (mGy)	Tube load (mAs)
1	____	____
2	____	____
3	____	____
4	____	____
5	____	____
6	____	____
7	____	____
8	____	____
9	____	____
10	____	____

Deviation in tube load: ____ % (= 100 x (max-min)/mean)

Accepted: yes / no

Long term reproducibility: forms should be made to suit the local preferences

Object thickness and tube voltage compensation

Optical density control setting: ____

If there is an automatic kV/anode/filter mode find out for each mode
where the switchpoints are:

Switchpoint	from thickness [cm]	to thickness [cm]	kV	anode	filter
A:	____	____	____	____	____
B:	____	____	____	____	____
C:	____	____	____	____	____
D:	____	____	____	____	____
E:	____	____	____	____	____

At these switchpoints take two additional images with 1 cm extra and one with 1 cm
perspex less, while fixing the kV/filter/anode.

Optical density control setting: ____
Mode name: ____

OD thickness	anode/filter	kV 24	25	26	27	28	29	30	31
10 mm	_____	____	____	____	____	____			
20 mm	_____	____	____	____	____	____	____		
30 mm	_____	____	____	____	____	____	____	____	
40 mm	_____		____	____	____	____	____	____	____
50 mm	_____			____	____	____	____	____	____
60 mm	_____				____	____	____	____	____
70 mm	_____					____	____	____	____

Variation in optical density: ____ OD

3.2.1.4 Compression

Compression force

Force indication: ____ N
Measured compression force: ____ N
Compression force after 5 min: ____ N

Compression plate alignment

Attachment compression plate: in order / out of order

Symmetric load
Thickness indication: ____ cm

Height of compression plate above the bucky at full compression:

	left	right	difference(l/r)	
Rear :	____	____	____	cm
Front :	____	____	____	cm
Difference(r/f)	____	____		cm

Accepted: yes / no

Asymmetric load left-right
Height of compression plate above the bucky at full compression:

	left	right	difference(l/r)	
Rear :	____	____	____	cm
Front :	____	____	____	cm
Difference(r/f)	____	____		cm

Accepted: yes / no

Asymmetric load front-rear
Height of compression plate above the bucky at full compression:

	left	right	difference(l/r)	
Rear :	____	____	____	cm
Front :	____	____	____	cm
Difference(r/f)	____	____		cm

Accepted: yes / no

3.2.2 Bucky and image receptor

3.2.2.1 Anti scatter grid

Grid system factor

	exposure [mGy]	tube load [mAs]	density [OD]
Present:	____	____	____
Absent:	____	____	____
Grid system factor:	____		

Accepted: yes / no

Grid imaging
Additional grid images made:

#	added PMMA	description of artefacts
1.	yes/no	_____
2.	yes/no	_____
3.	yes/no	_____

Accepted: yes / no

3.2.2.2 Screen-film

Inter cassette sensitivity and attenuation variation and optical density range

AEC setting: ____

Cassette id	exposure [mGy]	tube load [mAs]	density [OD]
1	____	____	____
2	____	____	____
3	____	____	____
4	____	____	____
5	____	____	____
6	____	____	____
7	____	____	____
8	____	____	____
9	____	____	____
10	____	____	____
11	____	____	____
12	____	____	____

Average values: ____ mAs   ____ OD

Max. deviation: ____ %   ____ mAs   ____ OD

Reference cassette: ____

Accepted: yes / no

Screen-film contact

Cassette id: Description of artefacts:

____   _____

____   _____

____   _____

____   _____

____   _____

____   _____

____   _____

____   _____

____   _____

____   _____

____   _____

Accepted: yes / no

3.2.3 Film processing

3.2.3.1 Baseline performance of the processor

Temperature

Point of measurement in bath: _____

	Developer	Fixer
reference/nominal:	____	____
thermometer		
reference:	____	____
local:	____	____
console:	____	____

Process time

Time from processor signal to film available: ____ s

3.2.3.2 Film and processor

Sensitometry, daily performance, artefacts:
forms should be made to suit the local preferences

3.2.3.3 Darkroom

Light leakage

Fog (after 2 min.) of a pre-exposed film on the workbench:

point:	1	2	3	4	5	
D(point):	____	____	____	____	____	OD
D(background):	____	____	____	____	____	OD
Difference:	____	____	____	____	____	OD
Average difference:	____ OD					

Accepted: yes / no

Positions of light sources and leaks in the darkroom:

- _____

- _____

Safelights

Type of lighting:	direct/indirect
Height :	± ____ meter above workbench
Setting:	____

Filter condition :   good/ insufficient / absent / not checked

Fog (after 2 min.) of a pre-exposed film on the workbench:

point:	1	2	3	4	5	
D(point)	___	___	___	___	___	OD
D(background):	___	___	___	___	___	OD
Difference:	___	___	___	___	___	OD

Average difference: ___ OD

Accepted: yes / no

Film hopper
Fogging due to light leakage in film hopper is absent: yes/no

Accepted: yes / no

Cassettes
The following cassettes show light leakage:
Cassette id: leaking position

___	_____
___	_____
___	_____

Accepted: yes / no

3.2.4 Viewing conditions

3.2.4.1 Viewing box

Viewing box luminance
Reading from the luminance meter
(detector at the centre of the image plane): ___ Cd/m^2

Homogeneity
Cover the view box pane with mammography films, measure the luminance (remove films first) at all centre positions of these films.

Position	1	2	3	4	5
Top	___	___	___	___	___
Bottom	___	___	___	___	___

Homogeneity: ___ % (= 100% .$(L_{max} - L_{min}) / L_{centre}$)

Accepted: yes / no

3.2.4.2 Ambient light level

Reading from the illuminance meter (detector at the image plane, box is off): ____ lux

Accepted: yes / no

3.2.5 System properties

3.2.5.1 Dosimetry

Entrance surface air kerma for D = 1.4 OD (excl. base + fog)

exposure [mGy]	tube load [mAs]	density [OD]
____	____	____
____	____	____

Exposure for D = 1.4 OD (excl. b+s):　　　____ mGy

Accepted: yes / no

3.2.5.2 Image quality

Spatial resolution

Position of the centre of the pattern:
Height above the bucky surface:　　　____ mm
Distance from thorax side of the bucky:　　____ mm
Distance from AC axis:　　　____ mm

Resolution	R⊥ AC-axis	R// AC-axis
image 1	____	____
image 2	____	____
image 3	____	____
image 4	____	____

Accepted: yes / no

Image contrast

image	mAs	#1	#2	#3	#4	#5	#6	#7	#8	#9	#10
1	___	___	___	___	___	___	___	___	___	___	___
2	___	___	___	___	___	___	___	___	___	___	___
3	___	___	___	___	___	___	___	___	___	___	___
4	___	___	___	___	___	___	___	___	___	___	___
5	___	___	___	___	___	___	___	___	___	___	___

Present data in graph

Threshold contrast visibility

Observer	# objects identified
1	___
2	___
3	___

Accepted: yes / no

Exposure time

AEC setting for a routine image: ___
Tube load obtained: ___ mAs
Exposure time: ___ s

Accepted: yes / no

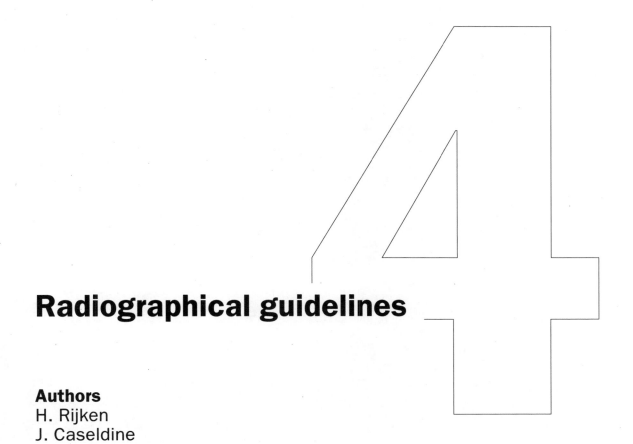

Radiographical guidelines

Authors
H. Rijken
J. Caseldine

4.1 Introduction

Screening for breast cancer by means of mammography has been proven to reduce mortality from breast cancer. Mammography as a screening test has to meet stringent quality requirements. These requirements can only be met when a comprehensive quality assurance programme is in place.

High quality screening demands high quality mammography carried out in a manner which is acceptable to the women. The role of the radiographer is central to the success of the breast screening programme in producing high quality mammograms which are crucial for the early diagnosis of breast cancer.

The image quality can be affected by the following factors, which are of equal importance:
• the ambience
• the X-ray equipment
• the image production chain
• how the radiographer relates to the woman
• the training, experience and motivation of the radiographer

4.2 Technical quality control

Quality control as defined by the World Health Organisation (WHO) is the 'set of operations (programming, coordinating, carrying out) intended to maintain or to improve [...] (ISO 3534-1977). As applied to a diagnostic procedure, it covers monitoring, evaluation, and maintenance at optimum levels of all characteristics of performance that can be defined, measured and controlled.'

In mammography this is the technical part of the quality assurance programme and comprises the operational techniques and activities required to maintain the quality of the performance. Quality control is required in order to produce a technically optimum mammogram and is dependent on a number of factors within the image production chain. Image quality standards must be established in order to guarantee a high level of technical quality. It is the radiographers' duty to carry out quality control procedures, monitor, evaluate and take corrective action to maintain these standards. These are laid down in the European Protocol for the Quality Control of the Physical and Technical Aspects of Mammography Screening (see chapter 3).

In quality control the radiographers must be involved in:
• equipment specification and selection
• commissioning and acceptance tests
• in-service consistency testing
• image quality assessment - using a recognised phantom

Several measurements can be performed by the local staff. The more elaborate measurements should be undertaken by medical physicists who are trained and experienced in diagnostic radiology and specifically trained in mammography quality control. Comparability and consistency of the results from different centres is best achieved if data from all measurements, including those performed by local radiographers are collected and analysed centrally.

In a screening facility there will be more than one radiographer carrying out mammography and quality control. One nominated radiographer in each unit should be assigned the overall responsibility for quality control. One radiographer should also have responsibility for ensuring that essential servicing, maintenance and repairs are carried out satisfactorily by relevant equipment engineers. This may or may not be the same person. A further important duty is to provide notification of significant equipment problems, breakdown and unacceptable variances in performance to the appropriate persons.

In each unit a quality control reference document must contain acceptable tolerance limits and guidelines to be followed should these tolerances be exceeded.

Time must be set aside to allow all radiographic quality control procedures to be carried out and for data arising from these procedures to be analysed, evaluated and acted upon.

A suggested list of tests and frequencies

			paragraph no. European Protocol
Daily	X-ray machine	automatic exposure control reproducibility	3.2.1.3
	film processor	sensitometry	3.2.3.2
	cassettes	screen inspection and cleaning	
Daily or weekly	film-processor	cleaning	
	X-ray machine	automatic exposure control repeatability	3.2.1.3
		AEC changing thickness	3.2.1.3
		image quality	3.2.5.2
Yearly	cassettes	film-screen contact	3.2.2.2
		sensitivity and radiation absorption	3.2.2.2

			paragraph no. European Protocol
	illuminators	output	3.2.4
Ongoing operator observations	all equipment	sharp edges	
		freedom of movement	
		brakes/locks	
		cassette robustness	
		foot switches	
		cables wear and tear	
		emergency compression release	
		warning lights	

Individual centres should draw up their own specific list of tests and frequencies. Attention should also be paid to the appropriate regulations for the handling and disposal of chemicals.

4.3 Ergonomic design of the machine

The X-ray machine should be designed in such a way that it is easy to use by the radiographer and non-threatening to women.

The ergonomics of the X-ray machine play a role with respect to positioning. All radiographers, whatever their height, should find the X-ray machine easy to operate, knobs and buttons should be within easy reach. All movements should be quiet and smooth and the machine light in handling. It is essential that the X-ray machine is fitted with a foot-pedal operated compression plate in order to allow the radiographer to use both hands when positioning the breast. The breast support table should be easy to clean. It should not have any sharp edges, which may cause discomfort during positioning.

4.4 Mammographic examination

The colour, size and placement of the machine are important in order to create an atmosphere of calm and confidence in the mammography room. Ideally the room should be designated for breast imaging only.
The temperature and the lighting in the X-ray room should be conducive to a satisfactory examination.

4.4.1 Introduction to the examination

The radiographer greets the woman, introduces herself and establishes eye-contact. Wearing a name badge helps to create a more personal relationship with the woman.

The radiographer should determine the woman's previous mammographic experience and past breast problems. Any current breast symptoms or information, which may be of importance to the radiologist, should be recorded on the appropriate sheets.

In addition the radiographer should note any skin abrasions, skin tears or soreness particularly on the underside of the breast. If these are present, having the mammogram may aggravate the condition or make taking the mammogram more uncomfortable than might normally be expected. In that case the woman should be given the opportunity to make an informed decision regarding the possible consequences of undergoing mammography. (In some units local protocol may require the woman to sign a consent form before continuing with the examination.)

During the introductory talk, the information to the woman should include:
• the examination procedure, including the number of views to be taken and an outline of the positioning
• explanation of the importance of compression
• the procedure for notifying the results

4.4.2 Starting the examination

• select size of breast support table and compression paddle
• clean the X-ray machine
• decide which view to begin with and position X-ray machine accordingly
• select chamber position
• place cassette in cassette holder
• ensure correct identifications of the woman are in place
• position the breast
• ensure the woman is comfortable
• remove any overlying artefacts e.g. spectacles, shoulders and skin folds
• apply the compression slowly and carefully until the breast is firmly held
• make the exposure
• release the compression immediately
• remove and replace the cassette
• proceed to the next view

4.4.3 Compression

The radiographer should understand the need for compression in mammography. It is essential that the breast is properly compressed in order to achieve a good quality mammogram.

Compression is used for the following reasons:
• scattered radiation diminishes, thus improving the contrast of the images
• compression reduces the thickness of the breast, separates the various structures in the breast, thus reducing the overlapping of tissue shadows and giving better visualisation of the breast tissue
• radiation dose is reduced
• blurring due to movement is reduced

The importance of proper compression should be explained to the woman, before the breast is compressed. Most women find compression uncomfortable and for a few it might even be painful. The radiographer must emphasise that compression only lasts a few seconds but that it is necessary in order to obtain good images and does not harm the breast. The amount of compression women can tolerate varies. If a woman has extremely sensitive breasts it may be recommended that the examination is postponed and a suitable appointment can be made, when the breasts are less sensitive. The breast should be properly compressed, but no more than is necessary to achieve a good image quality. More compression will only cause the woman pain.

It has been shown that women will tolerate the compression better if they have a full understanding of the need. Experience has shown that compression is better accepted if the woman can feel in control and indicate when the pressure is starting to become unpleasant. Care should be taken to apply the compression slowly and carefully with encouragement throughout. During compression, the radiographer should constantly observe the woman.

The radiographer must never assume that the woman is putting on an act. Every woman is different and experiences mammography in a different way. Putting the woman and her feelings at the centre of the examination is conducive to a satisfactory experience.

4.4.4 Positioning

Breast positioning is an art. When evaluating a mammogram, incorrect positioning is the most common problem. The skills required to perform optimal mammographic positioning are high. It is important that the radiographer has sufficient time to carry out the investigation and pay sufficient attention to the woman in order to produce optimal images.

4.4.5 Standard views

• the cranio-caudal view
• the mediolateral oblique view

Common criteria for image quality assessment are:
• correct positioning of automatic exposure device
• appropriate compression
• absence of
  - skin folds
  - overlying artefacts such as shoulders, breast tissue
  - movement
  - post-development artefacts e.g. dust on the screens, pick-off from rollers
• correct identifications
• correct exposure
• correct development technique
• symmetrical images

4.4.5.1 Cranio-caudal view

The cranio-caudal (cc) view should show as much of the breast as possible. A correctly performed cc view will show virtually all the breast except the most lateral and axillary part.

The criteria for the image assessment of the cc view are:
• the medial border of the breast is shown
• as much as possible of the lateral aspect of the breast is shown
• if possible, the pectoral muscle shadow is shown on the posterior edge of the breast
• the nipple should be in profile
• symmetrical images

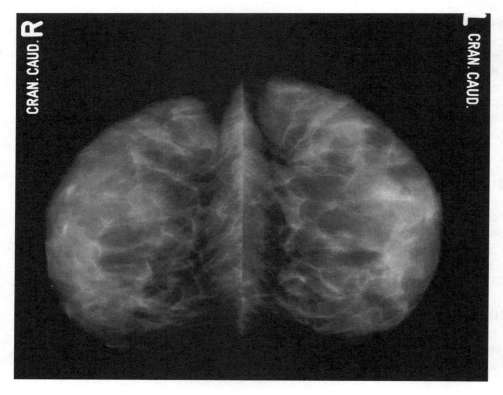

Cranio-caudal views, right and left

A key aspect to achieve a high quality cranio-caudal image is to adjust the film support table to the correct height for the woman. The height of the breast support table can be best determined when observed from the medial side of the breast. Once the height of the breast support table has been set, the radiographer lifts the breast and gently pulls the breast tissue forward away from the chest wall and places it on top of the breast support table. The breast should be in the centre of the breast support table. The breast should be held in place and the breast tissue smoothed out, while applying compression. It may occasionally be necessary to take an additional view in order to more fully visualise the lateral aspect of the breast.

To summarise:
• the breast is centrally positioned with the nipple in profile
• as much of the breast tissue as possible is visualised

Common errors leading to poor quality images:
• breast support table too low (this is also more uncomfortable for the woman)
• poor compression leading to pale images and movement blur
• skin folds in the lateral part of the breast
• breast tissue not pulled forward as much as possible
• nipple not in profile

4.4.5.2 Mediolateral oblique view
The criteria for the image assessment of the mediolateral oblique view:
• all the breast tissue clearly shown
• pectoral muscle to nipple level
• symmetrical images
• nipple in profile
• inframammary angle clearly demonstrated

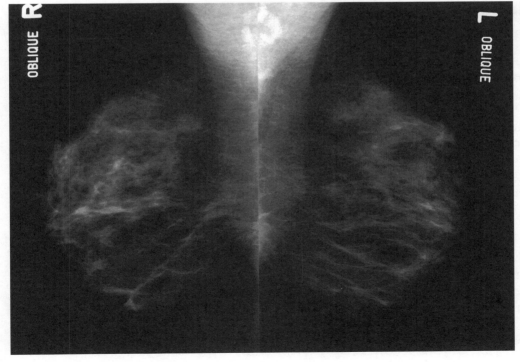

Mediolateral oblique views, right and left

Key aspects to achieve a high quality mediolateral oblique view are the height of the breast support table, the angle being used, the lift, spread and compression of the breast and the comfort of the woman.

To summarise:
• whole breast is imaged with the nipple in profile
• pectoral muscle shadow shown down the back of the breast at the correct angle
• the inframmary angle clearly demonstrated without overlying tissue

Common errors:
• breast support table too high or too low
• breast support table not correctly angled in order to follow the line of the woman's pectoral muscle
• inframammary angle not clearly shown
• insufficient lift and poor compression, resulting in a droopy breast

4.4.6 Other additional views

Other additional projections the radiographer should be aware of and should be able to perform include the lateral view (lateromedial/mediolateral) and the extended cranio-caudal view.

Techniques which are used in assessment include localised compression views and magnification views. Other specialised views may be required from time to time.

4.5 Social skills

In the context of a screening programme the radiographer is usually the only health professional the woman will meet. Communication between the radiographer and the woman is one of the most important aspects of the examination.

Radiographers play a key role in optimising the woman's experience, satisfaction and continued acceptance and uptake of the service. The acceptability of a breast screening programme is of the utmost importance to its success. The individual woman's needs and circumstances must be recognised in order to ensure a satisfactory and positive experience.

The radiographer must be friendly, caring and generate confidence in the woman, although she may have seen a great number of women on any day. When a pleasant, calm and informative atmosphere is created, the woman is more likely to relax. The radiographer should answer enquiries and explain the procedure carefully and emphasise the importance of proper compression in order to get understanding and cooperation from the woman. The woman should understand the process and timing for receiving her results. Women must feel at ease and feel they are being treated as important individuals. The radiographer should treat the woman the way she would like to be treated herself.

4.6 Consent

The woman should feel confident she has the ability to stop the procedure at any point. The radiographer should respect that right and recognise when consent is withdrawn.

4.7 Teamwork

It is recognised that good teamwork is required to produce optimal mammograms. Good communication including feedback is essential between radiographers, radiologists and physicists in setting, monitoring and evaluating standards for image quality.

The radiographers' responsibilities within the team are:
• to produce an optimum image with respect to positioning and technical aspects
• to produce the image in a manner which is acceptable to the woman to ensure a positive experience and therefore encourage future attendance
• to implement and carry out quality control procedures for equipment monitoring
• to assess the examinations she has performed

The radiographer should participate in multidisciplinary team meetings. Feedback is essential to maintain a high standard or to improve. In particular, regular communication with the radiologist is vital.

4.8 Radiographic quality standards

The radiographic quality objectives are:
• More than 97% of the women will have an acceptable examination, whether this is single view or double view mammography. A good diagnostic image meets the criteria laid down in the previous paragraphs.
• Less than 3% of the women will have a repeated examination, either a repeated mediolateral or cranio-caudal view. Audit must be carried out to monitor this.
• More than 97% of the women will feel satisfied with their screening visit and feel the radiographer has met their needs.
• 100% of the women will be informed by the radiographer of the method and time scale for receiving their results.

Audit on client satisfaction should be carried out to monitor standards 3 and 4. Information on verbal and/or written complaints or compliments should be taken into account.

In addition:
• Radiographers should have their skills, expertise and time allocated appropriately to facilitate high quality mammography and enhance personal and client satisfaction.

• Radiographers should have allocated sessions for quality assurance in order to audit the quality standards and carry out comprehensive daily quality control.
• Radiographers should be involved in self appraisal, peer group discussions and discussions with the radiologists on the radiographic quality of the images produced in the department.
• Every effort should be made by the radiographers to constantly improve the quality of the images and the service to the women.

It is desirable that:
• Radiographers participate in the assessment clinics and are familiar with investigative procedures.
• Radiographers understand the concept and value of the multidisciplinary approach to breast screening and are active members of the breast care multidisciplinary team.
• Radiographers should have up to date information and knowledge about issues on which the women may require further details relating to breast screening, for example, breast imaging and silicone breast implants, the impact of hormone replacement therapy on the breast and breast pain and tenderness.

4.9 Training

In order to achieve the radiographic standards required for high quality mammographic breast screening, all radiographers participating in the breast screening programme are expected to undergo a programme of training. This should be carried out by a recognised training centre.

The training programme should consist of two parts:
a.   academic   3 days to one week
b.   clinical   depending on the experience and existing skills of the radiographer two to six weeks

4.9.1 Academic component

A theoretical course to develop knowledge and understanding on all aspects of mammographic breast cancer screening and breast care that may include lectures, tutorials, demonstrations and reading.

Contents to include:
• anatomy and physiology
• pathology
• radiographic-pathologic correlation
• technical quality control
• communication and social skills
• organisation of the breast screening programme
• epidemiological aspects

• the management of breast cancer and treatment options
• health promotion

4.9.2 Clinical component

At the end of the clinical training the radiographer will be able to:
• make consistently good quality mediolateral oblique and cranio-caudal images
• decide if the images are acceptable from the positioning as well as the technical point of view
• carry out daily and/or weekly technical quality control procedures
• work with the woman in a satisfactory, friendly, caring way
• compare the mammogram with the previous one in order to achieve an optimum quality
• obtain satisfactory knowledge of X-ray equipment, film-screen combination and film processor
• carry out relevant administrative procedures

The radiographer will be familiar with:
• other imaging projections used to aid diagnosis e.g. magnification, stereotaxis
• other imaging techniques used to aid diagnosis e.g. ultrasound, MRI
• biopsy techniques e.g. fine needle aspiration cytology, needle core biopsy

4.9.3 Certification

It is desirable that the theoretical and practical knowledge, social skills, motivation and interest of the radiographer in training are tested. When the result is satisfactory the trainee should receive a certificate.

4.9.4 Continuing education

Every two to three years there should be at least a one-day refresher course in a recognised training centre for every radiographer involved in the screening programme. Subjects to be dealt with are positioning technique, physical quality control and the latest developments concerning equipment.

Radiographers are expected to update their knowledge and develop their skills in line with continuing professional development, for which participation in conferences and symposia can be a valuable contribution.

4.10 Staffing levels and working practices

Radiographic staffing levels are expected to reflect the workload. Working practices should not place undue pressure on the individual radiographer which may adversely effect quality.

Experience and research in the U.K. and the Netherlands have lead to recommended staffing levels for breast screening. When inviting the women it is important to take into account their expected participation rate. With 3 radiographers working together 10-12 women per hour can be examined. Each radiographer should be able to perform approximately 22 good quality sets of mammograms during a six-hour screening day. One may choose to work with two or three radiographers, with or without involving an administrative worker as receptionist.

Adjustment needs to be made for women with special needs who may take longer to examine.

The minimum requirement with regard to participation for radiographers involved in a population based breast screening programme is two days per week. This is in order to maintain and develop the skills required to carry out optimum mammography and to be an active and useful member of the multidisciplinary team.

Similarly in a diagnostic breast care facility, for the same reasons as stated above, radiographers should carry out a minimum of 20 mammographic examinations per week.

4.11 Summary

4.11.1 Skills

- To achieve high quality mammograms radiographers need good technical skills to position the woman and her breasts.
- Radiographers should have an understanding of the anxieties and fears of women attending for breast screening and assessment. They need to have the skills to address those and meet the expectations of the women in order to obtain an optimum mammogram and a satisfactory screening experience.
- Radiographers need the knowledge to critically appraise the mammograms to determine if optimum images are achieved.

4.11.2 Technical quality control

Radiographers should have a clear understanding of the requirements of technical quality control on a day-to-day basis. They should be familiar with the techniques required to this end and have knowledge of the recording, monitoring, evaluation and corrective actions required.

4.11.3 Multidisciplinary teamwork

Radiographers should understand the concept and value of the multidisciplinary approach to breast cancer diagnosis.

They should have up-to-date information and knowledge on topics which the woman may inquire about in relation to her screening experience.

4.11.4 Training

Training in the various aspects of the radiographic standards related to high quality screening is required. Radiographers carrying out breast screening mammography should attend a recognised training facility and ensure they are participating in continuing professional development.

4.12 Conclusion

Radiographers play a key role in a high quality breast screening programme aiming for a significant reduction in mortality of breast cancer.

4.13 Bibliography

1. NHSBSP Publication No 21. A radiographic quality control manual for mammography. Revised August 1993.

2. NHSBSP Publication No 30. Quality assurance guidelines for radiographers. February 1994.

3. NHSBSP Publication No 31. Messages about screening. April 1995.

4. NHSBSP Publication. Information and advice for radiographers. April 1993.

5. Wentz G. Mammography for radiologic technologists. McGraw-Hill 1992. ISBN 0-07-105387.

6. American College of Radiology. Mammography Quality Control Manual. Revised Edition 1994. ISBN 1-55903-136-0.

7. Lee L, Stickland V, Wilson ARM, Roebuck EJ. Fundamentals of mammography. W.B. Saunders Company Ltd 1995. ISBN 0-7020-1797-3.

8. Rickard MT, Wilson EA, Ferris A, Blackett KH. Positioning and quality control. Mammography today for radiographers. 1992. ISBN 0-646-08728-2.

9. Rijken H, Positionerungstechnik in der Mammographie. Georg Thieme Verlag 2000. ISBN 3-13-126911-1.

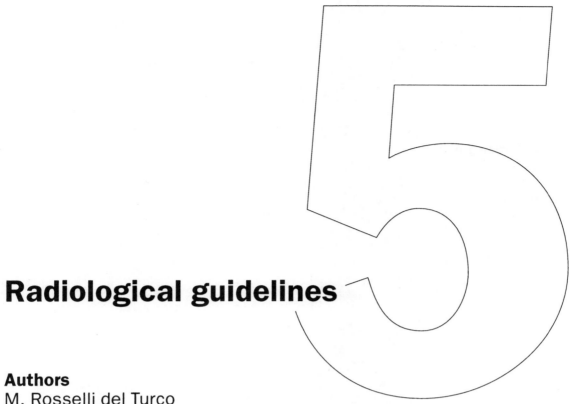

Radiological guidelines

Authors
M. Rosselli del Turco
J. Hendriks
N. Perry

Consultation group
A. Kirkpatrick
S. Ciatto
A. Frigerio

5.1 Introduction

The purpose of a breast screening programme is to reduce mortality from breast cancer in the invited population. The key factors necessary to achieve this are a high acceptance by the target population, and a high level of quality of the entire screening process.

The radiologist has a role of primary importance, taking the greatest overall responsibility for mammographic image quality, and diagnostic interpretation. A thorough knowledge and understanding of the risks and benefits of breast cancer screening, and the dangers of the use of inadequately trained staff and sub-optimal equipment is necessary.

The radiologist must ensure that protocols are in place for satisfactory and complete assessment (work-up) of women with screen-detected abnormalities. Women referred for assessment must be examined in fully equipped centres, staffed by properly qualified personnel, in collaboration with a radiologist experienced in and involved with the screening process. This is to ensure that adequate imaging assessment is not denied on the basis of a negative clinical examination.

The radiologist must encourage the formation of a skilled multi-disciplinary professional team incorporating clinical and non-clinical specialists involved in the entire process of screening and diagnosis. This team should include radiographers, pathologists, surgeons and nurses with additional input from oncologists, physicists and epidemiologists as appropriate. The radiologist must be intimately associated with the organisation of the screening programme, and where possible should act as Clinical Director.

The major responsibilities of the radiologist are to ensure that:

- a satisfactory quality assurance system is in place with sufficient quality control mechanisms to provide a high level of image quality

- radiological performance levels are sufficient to achieve the goals of the programme by effectively advancing the time of diagnosis of cancers arising in the screened population (and lowering the rate of advanced cancers)

- the adverse effects of screening are minimised

In order to reach these objectives it is necessary to accept the need for the setting of target standards and performance indicators, to comply with these wherever possible, and to take part in both internal and external audit procedures, with remedial action being undertaken where parameters are consistently breached. Standards in this document will frequently be defined at both minimum and desirable levels to acknowledge variation of expertise, but should never fall below those required to achieve mortality reduction, either in a centralised or decentralised setting. All standards should be regularly reviewed and if necessary revised in the light of experience and technological advances. It is accepted that certain standards may vary according to external factors such as geographical situation and background incidence of breast cancer.

These guidelines will outline some of the more important standards for radiologists and will describe methods to best achieve them. Essential prerequisites for screening units will be described in conjunction with other chapters, as will the importance of evaluating certain indicators (such as the interval cancer rate) and the organisation of optimal operating procedures.

The radiologist should constantly be aware of how the screening programme is performing and should encourage a process of continual quality improvement with performance feedback to team members. As digital techniques become more sophisticated and widespread, it is likely they will have a significant impact on practice, analysis and performance of screening programmes.

In planning the screening programme and implementing its organisation, sufficient resources must be identified and allocated in order to facilitate the achievement of desired standards. Particular attention should be paid to adequate levels of staffing and equipment.

5.2 Image quality

It is the responsibility of the radiologist to ensure that all necessary physico-technical and professional quality control processes have been satisfactorily carried out so that the resultant image quality is high.

Knowledge of adequate positioning techniques used by the radiographer is necessary and the radiologist should assess these factors first before reporting on the mammogram. The key criteria are for the whole breast to be imaged, the outline of the pectoral muscle to be demonstrated down to nipple level, the nipple to be in profile and the inframammary angle shown (see radiography chapter). To visualise the skin is no longer a primary requirement – this may in any case be achieved using a bright light – as penetration of breast tissue is more important for the detection of small cancers.

The radiologist must also be conversant with the important aspects of processing techniques and exposure which play a vital role in final image quality. The basic inter-relationship of kV, film-screen type, contrast, resolution, processing time and temperature must be understood, likewise the importance of sufficiently high optical density for the detection of small invasive cancers. Adequate compression and lack of motion artefact are also important diagnostically. Film artefacts such as scratches and skin folds indicate sub-optimal technique, but may not be sufficient to interfere with diagnosis. Further details of these issues may be found in the physico-technical chapter.

Ultimately, having analysed the image quality with regard to all these features, the radiologist must be resolute in refusing to accept mammograms not meeting sufficient criteria for adequate diagnosis. These films should be repeated, and the numbers of women subject to technical recall must be recorded. All repeat examinations should be recorded whether at the time of screening, due to a technical problem being identified by the radiographer, or at a later date if the radiologist judges the films to be inadequate for diagnostic purposes.

In a decentralised screening programme it is the responsibility of the lead programme radiologist/Clinical Director to suspend unsatisfactory clinics or offices where image quality in terms of radiographic positioning or adequate penetration of breast tissue remains unsatisfactory despite repeated attempts at quality improvement. It is the direct responsibility of the radiologist to ensure that individual films are not reported if they are of insufficient quality. Although this is not popular either with radiographers or with recalled women, it is a necessity in a small proportion of cases, acting as a safeguard for the quality of the screening process, and as a quality improvement feedback for radiographers.

Where there are problems with equipment or technique, the radiologist must discuss these matters with the relevant professional e.g. radiographer, physicist or equipment service engineer. High image quality is a key factor in the success of a screening programme, but the achievement of it is a complex issue and best managed with a multi-disciplinary input.

5.3 Radiologist performance issues

Good team work will enhance the screening process and is likely to improve outcomes, so it is important that the radiologist should work closely with other professional colleagues as part of a multidisciplinary team. In order to maintain radiological performance standards it is vital that the radiologist has direct access to key performance indicators, not only screening and assessment results, but also cytological and pathological records.

Feedback of results at all stages is an important learning and quality enhancing process and mechanisms should be in place to achieve this. Records must be kept of results and outcomes of all women in the programme. Regular multidisciplinary review meetings must be held to discuss cases both pre-operatively and postoperatively. This is benefical for feedback purposes as well as providing an ideal mechanism for refining case management decisions. The review of interval cancers by radiologists should be regarded as mandatory, being an excellent feedback and educational process.

5.3.1 Advancement of the time of diagnosis

Table 1 lists the principal performance standards necessary to bring forward the time of diagnosis. The ratio of detection rates at initial and subsequent examinations to the expected incidence gives a good indication. The detection rate of cancers 'per se' is influenced by the wide variation in European regions of the underlying base incidence of breast cancer in the age group of the target population. The ratio between detection rate and expected incidence can be influenced by possible overdiagnosis.

The proportion of invasive cancers ≤ 10 mm in diameter detected at screening is an important indicator reflecting both radiological performance and image quality. A substantial proportion of cancers at this stage will provide a positive impact from screening. This parameter is also relatively easy to calculate if the pathological form includes pTNM staging and the criteria for measurement of small cancers are well established as described in the pathology chapter.

The proportion of screen-detected ductal carcinoma in situ (DCIS) is also a good parameter for evaluating performance. It is believed that removal of DCIS, particularly of the high grade type, contributes to long term mortality reduction. Its detection is also an indicator of image quality, radiologist prediction and assessment adequacy. On the other hand, a high proportion of low grade DCIS may indicate an aggressive policy with adverse effects, alternatively a problem with pathological classification. Based on screening experience acquired mainly in national programmes from Northern Europe (UK, S, NL) we set the desirable standard value between 10 and 20% of cancers detected. Possible variation across Europe in incidence and pathological classification may be taken in account.

Table 1: Radiological performance: standards to advance the time of diagnosis in screened women age ≥ 50 years

Indicator	Minimum standard	Desirable standard
Detection rate in women at initial examination/ expected incidence rate	3	> 3
Detection rate in women at subsequent examination/ expected incidence rate	1.5	> 1.5
Proportion of invasive cancers detected at initial screening ≤ 10 mm	≥ 20%	≥ 25%
Proportion of invasive cancers detected at subsequent screening ≤ 10 mm	≥ 25%	≥ 30%
DCIS as a proportion of all screen-detected cancers	10%	10-20%

5.3.2 Reduction of adverse effects

Any recall for a mammographic abnormality that turns out to be normal or benign must be regarded as unnecessary and represents a negative effect of screening. Unnecessary recalls are costly, cause psychological discomfort to the woman and, due to the limited specificity of assessment, may result in unnecessary open biopsies. This, in turn, may cause further expense, anxiety and diagnostic problems at subsequent screening. A low specificity in the screening programme is likely to lead to sub-optimal acceptance.

Recall rate

Unfortunately the specificity of mammography is limited, especially for small preclinical cancers, which are the main target of screening. The positive predictive value of mammography for preclinical cancer varies according to the radiological appearance of non-palpable lesions, but, with the exception of spiculate opacities and linear-branching microcalcifications, is usually below 50%. Asymmetries, well defined opacities and punctate microcalcifications have a predictive value for cancer of well below 10%. Knowing the limited specificity of mammography and concerned not to miss a cancer, radiologists will call for assessment even in the presence of radiological abnormalities of intermediate predictivity, and some unnecessary recalls are unavoidable.

Recalled cases should be reviewed and the positive predictive value for malignancy determined for each category of mammographic abnormality. This will allow the identification at each unit of poorly predictive patterns and the adoption of refined recall criteria in order to optimise sensitivity and specificity.

For audit purposes, it is suggested that radiological findings are categorised as follows:
R1 - Normal/ benign
R2 - A discrete lesion having benign characteristics
R3 - An abnormality present of indeterminate significance
R4 - Features suspicious of malignancy
R5 - Malignant features

Double reading increases the recall rate by approximately a further 10% of the single reading figure. This number will be influenced by the training and experience of the radiologist, also the image quality of the mammogram. Another factor that might increase the recall rate is the use of the oblique view only as the screening test. It is well known that many asymmetric densities or parenchymal distortions may be false images created by superimposition and can be easily recognised as such if the cranio-caudal view is available.

Provided that the reference standards referred to in table 1 are achieved, recall rates should be kept to the lowest possible level, and as shown in table 2, should be below 5% at initial screening. At subsequent screening, the availability of previous films for review will enable many questionable findings to be ruled out as negative or benign. Recall rates at subsequent screening should therefore be consistently lower, ideally below 3%.

Repeated films for technical reasons should be kept to a minimum, ideally below 1 per 100 examined women. In some programmes the radiographer may repeat the examination on site before the radiologist has seen the films and without officially recalling the woman. This procedure decreases anxiety and organisational costs, but the numbers should also be recorded and monitored.

Early recall

Early recall may be defined as the recommendation for a woman to undergo a short term re-screen at an interval less than the routine round length of the programme. This practice creates anxiety and increases morbidity by promoting benign biopsies as well as having the potential to falsely reassure the woman. There is a low predictive value for malignancy with the use of early recall, and it should be avoided altogether or its use restricted to an absolute minimum (target < 1% of screened women). Early recall should never be used to mask insufficient or inadequate assessment procedures, or as a means of avoiding a skilled radiological decision.

If early recall is used in occasional cases, the time interval should be no less than 1 year as subtle changes in mammographic features may not become apparent in less than this time. It is not regarded as good practice to subject a woman to an early recall following the screening process alone. She should first have been completely assessed and the circumstances fully explained to her. Neither is it acceptable for a woman to undergo more than one early recall in a screening round, the only possible outcomes from this process being a decision to operate, or a return to routine screening.
Cancers detected in women placed on early recall are regarded by some programmes as interval cancers. They should in all cases be separately counted from other screen-detected cancers as they represent a delayed diagnosis for women and a failure of the screening and assessment process.

Benign biopsy and pre-operative diagnosis

The number of benign biopsies (open surgical excision) performed as a result of screening should be as low as possible. This can be achieved with adequate use of pre-operative techniques such as fine needle aspiration cytology (FNAC), core biopsy (CB) or mammotomy. Some benign biopsies are inevitable due to patient choice or diagnostic difficulties with imaging, clinical and pathological features.

The benign to malignant ratio is a simple indicator to express the predictivity of a referral for open (surgical) biopsy. This ratio is higher in the first round of screening as previous films are often not available for comparison. Some benign lesions will be removed in the first round allowing greater specificity in subsequent rounds, also the experience of the radiologist increases with time. The B/M ratio can be significantly lowered by accurate use of cytological or histological pre-operative investigations as described above. For this reason the proportion of such image-guided procedures with an inadequate or inconclusive result should be carefully monitored.

The proportion of women with a pre-operative diagnosis of malignancy, i.e. with a result of FNAC and/or CB conclusive for malignancy (see chapter 6) is a valid indicator of quality of assessment, related to a high predictive value for malignancy in referral for open biopsy. This facilitates treatment planning and allows more adequate and complete counselling for women, minimising delays and uncertainty.

Delay

Delay in communicating results, performing assessment or surgery is likely to cause distress and anxiety. It is bad practice, inconsiderate and must be avoided. Targets should be set for all stages as detailed in table 2.

Table 2: Standards to minimize adverse effects in screened women

Indicator	Minimum standard	Desirable standard
Recall for assessment rate in women at initial examination	< 7%	< 5%
Recall for assessment rate in women at subsequent examination	< 5%	< 3%
Technical repeat rate	< 3%	< 1%
Benign to malignant biopsy ratio in women at initial examination	≤ 1:1	≤ 0.5:1
Benign to malignant biopsy ratio in women at subsequent screening	≤ 1:1	≤ 0.2:1
Proportion of screen-detected breast cancer with a pre-operative diagnosis of malignancy (FNAC or core biopsy reported as definitely malignant)	> 70%	> 90%
Proportion of image-guided FNAC procedures with an insufficient result	< 25%	< 15%
Proportion of image-guided FNAC procedures from lesions subsequently proven to be malignant, with an insufficient result	< 10%	
Proportion of screened women subjected to early recall following diagnostic assessment	< 1 %	0

Indicator	Minimum standard	Desirable standard
Proportion of localised impalpable lesions successfully excised at the first operation	95%	> 95%
Proportion of wires placed within 1 cm of an impalpable lesion prior to excision	90%	> 90%
Delay between screening and result	15 wd	10 wd
Delay between result and offered assessment	5 wd	3 wd

wd= working days

5.4 Operating procedures

5.4.1 Viewing conditions

It is important to refer to the technical aspects of film viewing as referred to in the physico-technical chapter. Reading of screening mammograms requires a high degree of mental and visual concentration, and it is believed that performance may start to deteriorate after 30 - 40 minutes. It should only be done in a suitably undisturbed environment with control of background room light and care taken to reduce unnecessary light glare from the film viewer.

Unless a digital and computerised fully integrated viewing system is used, removal of films from an individual light box will result in excessive light glare prior to replacement with the next set of mammograms. This is likely to result in a diminution of visual acuity. The use of a pre-loaded multiviewer/roller viewer is recommended to avoid this problem, also to facilitate faster and more efficient film reading, allowing more prolonged maintenance of concentration. This technique also provides greater logistical ease and speed for double reading of screening mammograms.

Previous mammograms should either be displayed at the time of screen reading or be available for review. This has the dual purpose of increasing cancer detection by the ability to perceive changes in appearance between examinations, and of reducing unnecessary recall to assessment for long standing benign lesions. Where previous films are displayed with the current screening examination, it is a matter of personal choice whether these films are from the immediately previous screening round, or a prior screening round in order to enable easier assessment of subtle changes that have occurred over a longer period of time than one round. However it is often the case that mammograms from earlier rounds are not of equivalent image quality to the current examination and this in itself may be counter productive for comparison purposes.

5.4.2 Single/double reading

Double reading increases sensitivity and decreases specificity of the screening test, according to the methodology used and the skill of the reading radiologist.

In centralised programmes with well trained radiologists fully dedicated to breast cancer screening and diagnosis, double reading is not mandatory but related to cost-effectiveness issues. If double reading is adopted it should be independent i.e. the woman is recalled if the test is positive for either of the two readers in order to gain the maximum possible increase in sensitivity, provided the decrease of specificity is not too high. Excellent results have been obtained using the practice of arbitration from a third screening radiologist in cases of discordant double reading. Double reading is recommended in centralised programmes for the first screening round and until the performance of the radiologists can be fully assessed.

In decentralised programmes, or in programmes where the radiologists are not yet sufficiently experienced in breast cancer screening and diagnosis, double reading is mandatory and should be performed at a centralised level. Second reading should be performed by radiologists who read a minimum 5,000 mammograms per year. In order to avoid an excessive decrease in specificity, cases recalled by one or both radiologists should be reviewed by an expert radiologist who can arbitrate. Overall recall rates should be kept to the standard values reported in table 2.

5.4.3 Assessment of screen-detected abnormalities

An abnormal finding on a screening mammogram requires recall to an assessment process where further investigations are undertaken, in order to confirm the presence of a malignant, benign or normal condition. This process should be led by a radiologist fully trained and experienced in breast screening. Adequate protocols must be in place either in a centralised or decentralised programme to ensure that assessment procedures are robust and complete. A decision on further management, or a return to routine rescreen may then be made. Radiologist sensitivity and specificity should be optimal so that women are not subjected to unnecessary anxiety from this process. The assessment facilities available should include further diagnostic mammography with specialist radiographic techniques such as microfocus magnification, ultrasound and a multidisciplinary input including clinical examination. Image guided cytological or core biopsy sampling must be available.

It is advisable that documented assessment protocols be devised and followed. For example it is not necessary to drain a cyst detected at assessment unless it is symptomatic, causing diagnostic problems, or if the woman requests it. Microfocus magnification techniques for microcalcification should be performed in orthogonal planes, e.g. cranio-caudal and lateral. It is most effective to sample a lesion under ultrasound control if it can be demonstrated sonographically. Where there is doubt in the mind of the assessing radiologist, it is safest to sample under X-ray guidance. Unless the radiologist is very experienced, it is advisable that all solid lesions on ultrasound should be sampled as it is often not possible to reliably differentiate benign from malignant solid lesions on sonographic appearances alone.

Ideally, for quality loop purposes, the radiologist performing the screen reading should also be involved at assessment. Where this is not possible it is vital to ensure that a complete feedback system is in place for exchange of follow up information and outcomes. All unnecessary intervention and creation of anxiety must be avoided. It is the radiologists' responsibility to ensure that all necessary investigations are carried out at assessment, preferably at the same visit, so that a decision is reached and information provided to the woman.

5.4.4 Quality assurance organisation

In any population based screening programme it is vital to balance the risks and benefits, ensuring the emphasis is placed firmly on the latter. This is best achieved with the formation of an extensive quality assurance organisation and programme. Preferably this should be introduced at or before the commencement of screening activities so that adequate working arrangements can be established at the outset of a programme and not require changing at a later and more difficult time.

Local quality assurance manuals should be in use, which should be based upon this document. Regional and local organisations for QA should exist, working at individual discipline level as well in a multidisciplinary setting.

The organisation should ensure that all professionals participating in the screening programme are fully trained and comply with performance and working guidelines that should be approved by relevant national bodies and organisations. A central committee should decide policy. Results at local, regional and national levels must be produced in a complete and timely manner, available to political as well as professional groups, also being offered within the public domain.

Each screening unit should have a Quality Assurance Manager - one nominated person responsible for the overall quality of the programme who can be the focal point for all quality activities within that programme. Each programme must review its own results in order to understand its own performance and the Quality Assurance Manager must ensure that all results are collated for the programme and should act as a liaison between the local programme and the wider regional and national quality assurance organisations.

5.4.5 Number of views

Screening mammography using two views of each breast (medio lateral oblique plus cranio-caudal) has been shown to be more effective than single oblique view screening, particularly in the woman's first round. The use of two views provides a higher sensitivity and specificity as the second view may provide additional information by detecting abnormalities not seen on the oblique view only, and by avoiding unnecessary assessment for a woman with an apparent abnormality shown to be due to superimposition on the second view. The oblique projection gives the maximum possible visualisation of breast tissue. The cranio-caudal view does not demonstrate the axillary tail region so well, but provides a different projection of the breast tissue and the technique allows for better compression.

Disadvantages of two view screening are related to slightly increased costs, time of examination and additional radiation exposure for women. If films are double read, the overall beneficial effect of the second view may be lower at subsequent screening rounds.

In conclusion we recommend that a two view examination be performed for the woman's initial screening, and either one or two views at subsequent screening according to local resources and the density of the breast tissue as demonstrated initially.

5.4.6 Localisation of non-palpable lesions

A substantial proportion of screen-detected abnormalities will be impalpable and therefore require some form of localisation procedure prior to either diagnostic or therapeutic excision. It is the radiologist's responsibility to ensure that this process is carried out as effectively and accurately as possible so that lesions are satisfactorily excised in over 95% of cases at first operation.

Where abnormalities have been worked up as malignant and segmental mastectomy or wide local excision is planned, it may be adequate to skin mark such lesions prior to surgery.

In other cases especially for diagnostic excision purposes, more finite accuracy of localisation is required and use of a wire marker is recommended. For all practical purposes this wire should be placed within one centimetre of the lesion and if necessary a second wire should be placed if the first wire is not sufficiently accurate. Radiologists must ensure that satisfactory specimen radiography facilities are available for the surgeon so that rapid confirmation of completeness of excision may be provided prior to skin closure.

5.5 Interval cancers

Definition

Interval cancers are defined as breast cancers arising after a negative screening episode (which may include assessment) and before the next scheduled screening round. It is important not only to register invasive but also in situ (DCIS) interval cancers. Sometimes an interval cancer is not a failure of the screening but a failure of the assessment process. In some programmes, cancers found from early recall may be classified as interval cancers (see 5.3.2).

Importance

Interval cancers are inevitable in a screening programme but their number should be kept as low as possible. A high proportion of interval cancers will reduce the effectiveness of screening and the potential mortality reduction will be lowered. The screening process should be optimised and any potential delay in diagnosis must be minimised whether it is due to a failure of the screening process or of assessment. Tracing interval cancers is complex but fundamental to monitor the performance of any screening programme. Mechanisms should be in place to identify all breast cancers arising in the target screened population. Interval cancer monitoring is also important to evaluate the chosen screening interval and radiological performance.

The good practice of performing mammography prior to surgery in all symptomatic cases suspicious for breast cancer will enable more adequate classification of interval cancers as well as demonstrating the extent of malignancy and the presence of contralateral disease.

Reviewing process

Radiologists must ensure that a suitable mechanism exists for the review and audit of all interval cancers. This review should be an essential part of routine radiological audit, and plays a key role in the continuing medical education of radiologists involved in the programme.

Screening radiologists in a region should establish a review panel of a minimum of three screening radiologists including one radiologist from the unit to be reviewed and one from outside.

The subclassification of interval cancers is the responsibility of the reviewing panel and is not part of routinely submitted information for screening evaluation.

Methodology

1. The screening films should first be reviewed without seeing the presentation mammograms taken at the time of diagnosis (blind review). This is in order to make a provisional classification in one of the following categories:

   True interval The screening mammogram is normal, no reason for assessment.

   Minimal signs There is a possible subtle abnormality on the screening film. This would not necessarily be regarded as warranting assessment. A brief description of the lesion and its position should be noted.

   False negative An abnormality is clearly visible and warrants assessment. Description and position should be given.

2. Following provisional classification, the screening mammogram is reviewed again together with the diagnostic mammogram. A new and definitive classification should now be made, which may be different to the provisional classification. For example it may be possible to retrospectively identify minimal signs that were not identified on

blind review. It is also important to confirm that minimal signs identified on blind review correlate exactly with the site of interval cancer, otherwise the case, instead of minimal signs, becomes a true interval.

If there is disagreement on classification by the reviewing panel, the opinion of the majority should decide.

If mammography was not performed at the time of the diagnosis it is not possible to classify the interval cancer in a proper way, and the case is categorised as 'unclassifiable'.

In true interval cancers it is important to check the positioning technique and the physico-technical quality of the original screening mammogram, in order to identify whether sub-optimal images could have contributed to the cancer not being identified.

Table 3: Classification of interval cancers*

Categories	Subtypes	Screening films	Diagnostic mammogram
True interval		Negative	Positive
Minimal signs		Minimal signs	Minimal signs or positive
False negative	Reading error Technical error	Positive Negative (for technical reasons)	Positive Positive
Unclassifiable		Any	Not available
Occult		Negative	Negative

* Based on the UK Quality Assurance Guidelines for Radiologists, NHSBSP May 1997, page 50.

The group of interval cancers with minimal signs present is very important. It may be possible to split this group into significant and non specific signs. False negative cases should not exceed 20% of the total number of interval cancers. Radiological review of false negatives and minimal signs will directly influence performance and may lead to better screening results. Cancers arising in lapsed attenders are not classified as interval cancers, although it is important to review them. Advanced and node positive screen-detected cancers at subsequent screening should be reviewed in a similar fashion for educational purposes.

5.6 Professional requirements

Each screening radiologist should:
- be medically qualified and registered to practice in his/her country
- have had specific training in both diagnostic (symptomatic) mammography and screening mammography
- participate in a continuing medical education programme and in any relevant external quality assessment scheme
- undertake to read a minimum of 5,000 screening cases per year in centralised programmes. This applies to the radiologist carrying out second reading in the non-centralised programmes

In addition each radiologist should:
- be involved with assessment as well as basic screening
- have access to pathology and surgical follow up data
- attend multidisciplinary review and clinical management meetings
- be involved with symptomatic breast work, ideally having skill in clinical examination of the breast
- be fully experienced in all assessment techniques including the ability to perform ultrasound, FNAC and/or core biopsy

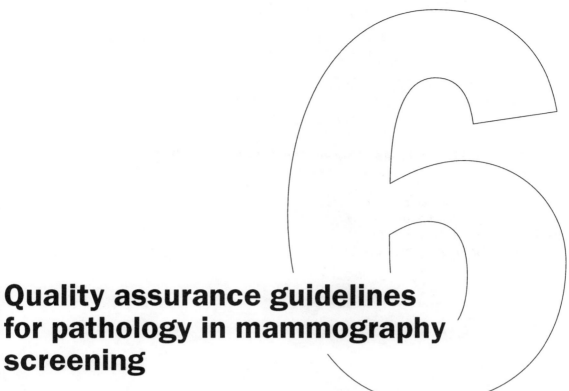

Quality assurance guidelines for pathology in mammography screening

Non-operative diagnosis

Editor
J. Sloane†

Produced by **the E.C. Working group on breast screening pathology**

*These guidelines are also
available in multimedia format
as part of the BreakIT project
(http://sos.ist.unige.it/breakit)*

6.1 Introduction

The decision about whether to operate on patients with screen-detected mammographic abnormalities involves the correlation of clinical and radiological data and findings from fine needle aspiration cytology (FNAC) or needle core biopsy (NCB; triple assessment). This is best achieved in multidisciplinary meetings where the clinician, radiologist and pathologist discuss these findings and reach a consensus on the appropriate management of each patient following pre-defined protocols.

Until recently, needle aspiration was the more widely used technique but core biopsy is being used increasingly. There has been much discussion about the relative merits and disadvantages of the two methods.

Core biopsy has several advantages. It is possible to distinguish in situ from invasive carcinomas although, not surprisingly, the technique has greater positive than negative predictive value as the invasive component of a tumour may not always be included in the biopsy. It is easier to diagnose carcinomas with low-grade cytological features (e.g. tubular, cribriform, lobular carcinomas) which are difficult to recognise without architectural interpretation. Specific benign diagnoses can be made and this allows better correlation of clinical, radiological and histological features. Another major advantage is that needle biopsies can be subjected to specimen radiography to ensure that the mammographic abnormality has been sampled. If the relevant calcification is included in the biopsy and is clearly associated with a benign process then an unnecessary operation is avoided.

On the other hand, fine needle aspiration is quicker to perform, does not require local anaesthetic and consequently uses less clinic time. Multiple passes with the needle can increase diagnostic accuracy with both techniques but this is easier to do with FNAC. Small and impalpable lesions are also generally easier to localise, particularly if imaging is used but localisation of lesions with needle core biopsy has improved significantly in recent years. As FNAC is a quicker technique cytopathologists can provide diagnoses in assessment clinics so that triple assessment can be completed in a single visit. Furthermore, if unequivocally malignant cells are identified, it is often possible to make a confident diagnosis of invasive carcinoma if the radiological and clinical appearances are typical.

Most pathologists, however, find it easier to interpret needle core specimens and consequently the standards of diagnosis are generally higher except where FNAC is performed in the major cytopathology centres. Pathologists should not provide fine needle aspiration cytopathology services unless they have sufficient experience and expertise.

It is thus clear that FNAC and needle core biopsy are complementary techniques in arriving at a non-operative diagnosis. The efficacy of both methods, however, is heavily dependent on the skill and experience of the operator who is rarely a pathologist, particularly in the case of needle biopsy.

6.2 Cytopathology

6.2.1 Registering basic cytopathology information

Information is registered using the standard registration form.

Registration form

Breast screening cytopathology

Surname _____ Forenames _____

Date of birth _____

Screening no. _____ Hospital no. _____

Centre _____ Report no. _____

Side
☐ Right   ☐ Left

Specimen type
☐ FNA (solid lesion)   ☐ FNA (cyst)   ☐ Nipple discharge   ☐ Nipple or
skin scrapings

Localisation technique
☐ Palpation   ☐ X-ray guided   ☐ Ultrasound guided

Opinion
☐ 1 Unsatisfactory   Comment _____
☐ 2 Benign   _____
☐ 3 Atypia probably benign   _____
☐ 4 Suspicious of malignancy   _____
☐ 5 Malignant   _____

Pathologist _____ Name of aspirator _____

Date _____

| **Centre/location** | Give the name of the assessment centre, clinic, department etc., where the specimen was obtained. |

Side   Indicate right or left. For specimens from both sides, use a separate form for each side.

Specimen type   Please choose one of the following terms:

FNA (solid lesion)	Fine needle aspiration of a solid lesion
FNA (cyst)	Fine needle aspiration of a cyst subjected to cytological examination
Nipple discharge	Cytological preparation of a nipple discharge
Nipple or skin	Cytological preparation of nipple or skin scrapings

Localisation technique Please choose one of the following terms:

Palpation	FNA guided by palpation
Ultrasound guided	FNA guided by ultrasound
X-ray guided	FNA guided by X-ray examination
	Stereotaxis is included in this category

Pathologist   The name of the pathologist giving the cytological opinion.

Aspirator   The name of the person performing the fine needle aspiration.

Recording the cytology opinion   See the reporting categories below. A comment field is included for any extra information to be recorded in free text.

6.2.2 Cytopathology reporting categories

A definitive diagnosis of malignancy or benignity should be made wherever possible. The proportion of definitive diagnoses will clearly increase with the experience of both pathologist and aspirator.

C1 Inadequate   Indicates a scanty or acellular specimen or poor preparation.

The designation of an aspirate as 'inadequate' is to a certain extent a subjective matter and may depend on the experience of the aspirator and/or the interpreter.
Poor cellularity (usually less than five clumps of epithelial cells) is sufficient to declare an aspirate inadequate. Preparative artefacts

or excessive blood may also be reasons for rejecting an aspirate as inadequate.

Preparative artefacts include:

1. Crush, when too much pressure is used during smearing.

2. Drying, when dry smears are allowed to dry too slowly or when wet-fixed smears have been allowed to dry out before fixation.

3. Thick smears, when an overlay of blood, protein-rich fluid or cells obscures the picture, making assessment impossible.

It is often helpful to make a comment as to the cause of the inadequate specimens in the Comment box on the form.

C2 Benign

Indicates an adequate sample showing no evidence of malignancy.

The aspirate in this situation is often poorly to moderately cellular and tends to consist mainly of regular duct epithelial cells. These are generally arranged as monolayers and the cells have the characteristic benign cytological features. The background is usually composed of dispersed individual and paired naked nuclei. Should cystic structures be a component of the aspirated breast, then a mixture of foamy macrophages and regular apocrine cells may be part of the picture. Fragments of fibrofatty and/or fatty tissue are common findings.

A positive diagnosis of specific conditions, for example: fibroadenoma, fat necrosis, granulomatous mastitis, lymph node, etc., may be suggested if sufficient features are present to establish the diagnosis with confidence.

C3 Atypia probably benign

All the characteristics of a benign aspirate may be seen as described above. In addition, there are certain features not commonly seen in benign aspirates, including any of the following, alone or in combination:
1. nuclear pleomorphism
2. some loss of cellular cohesion
3. nuclear and cytoplasmic changes resulting from hormonal influence (pregnancy, contraceptive pill, HRT) or treatment effects.
Increased cellularity may accompany the above features.

As thus defined, this group would be expected to contain approximately 20% of cases which were subsequently proven to be malignant.

C4 Suspicious of malignancy

The pathologist's opinion is that the material is suggestive but not diagnostic of malignancy. There are three main reasons:
1. the specimen is scanty, poorly preserved or poorly prepared, but some cells with features of malignancy are present.
2. the sample may show some malignant features without overt malignant cells present. The degree of abnormality should be more severe than in the previous category.
3. the sample has an overall benign pattern with large numbers of naked nuclei and/or cohesive sheets of cells, but with occasional cells showing distinct malignant features.

As thus defined, this group would be expected to contain approximately 80% of cases which were subsequently proven to be malignant.

C5 Malignant

Indicates an adequate sample containing cells characteristic of carcinoma, or other malignancy.

The interpreter should feel at ease in making such a diagnosis. Malignancy should not be diagnosed on the basis of a single criterion but on a combination of features.

Calcification

It is very useful for the radiologist if the pathologist reports the presence of calcification within specimens taken from stereotactic or perforated plate guided FNAC when the abnormality is one of mammographic microcalcification. If calcification is present in these circumstances, the radiologist or multidisciplinary team can be more certain that the lesion has been sampled accurately and that the likelihood of a false negative due to an aspiration miss is lower. This may allow the team to advise with greater confidence that the woman be routinely recalled or rescreened early rather than subjected to biopsy. It is desirable to specify the type of calcification (hydroxyapatite or weddellite).

Calcification alone does not discriminate between benign and malignant conditions.

6.2.3 Cytopathology quality assurance

Definitions

The following calculations are intended to reflect the quality of the FNAC service as a whole rather than the laboratory component alone. Inadequate FNAC results are not, therefore excluded from the calculations as in some publications. Cytologists wishing to evaluate purely their own accuracy in diagnosis may wish to calculate the figures differently.

Absolute sensitivity (C5)

The number of carcinomas diagnosed as such (C5) expressed as a percentage of the total number of carcinomas aspirated.

Complete sensitivity (C3, 4 and 5)

The number of carcinomas that were not definitely negative or inadequate on FNAC expressed as a percentage of the total number of carcinomas aspirated.

Specificity

The number of correctly identified benign lesions (the number of C2 results minus the number of false negatives) expressed as a percentage of the total number of benign lesions aspirated.

Positive predictive value of a C5 diagnosis

The number of correctly identified cancers (numbers of C5 results minus the number of false positive results) expressed as a percentage of the total number of positive results (C5).

Positive predictive value of a C4 diagnosis

The number of cancers identified as suspicious (number of C4 results minus the number of false suspicious results) expressed as a percentage of the total number of suspicious results (C4).

Positive predictive value of a C3 diagnosis

The number of cancers identified as atypia (number of C3 results minus the number of benign atypical results) expressed as a percentage of the total number of atypical results (C3).

Negative predictive value of a C2 diagnosis

The number of benign cases (including those with no histology) expressed as a percentage of the total number of C2 diagnoses.

False negative case

A case which subsequently turns out (over the next 2 years) to be carcinoma having had a negative cytology result. (This will by necessity include some cases where the cancer was missed rather than misinterpreted in the smears. Furthermore, the interval may vary from one programme to another depending on the screening interval.)

False positive case

A case which was given a C5 cytology result but which turns out at open surgery to have a benign lesion (including atypical hyperplasia).

False negative rate   The number of false negative results expressed as a percentage of the total number of carcinomas aspirated.

False positive rate   The number of false positive results expressed as a percentage of the total number of carcinomas aspirated.

Inadequate rate   The number of inadequate specimens expressed as a percentage of the total number of cases aspirated.

Suspicious rate   The number of C3 and C4 diagnoses expressed as a percentage of the total number of cytology results.

How to calculate these figures

It is intended that a computer system will be able to calculate these figures automatically from the data in the database cross-referencing with the histology or subsequent outcome and a report derived for quality assurance purposes.

Cytology QA standard report

Total cases screened in period _____
Total assessed   _____
Total FNAC performed   _____

Cytology

Histology	C5	C4	C3	C2	C1	Total
Total malignant	Box 1	Box 2	Box 3	Box 4	Box 5	Box 6
Invasive	Box 7	Box 8	Box 9	Box 10	Box 11	Box 12
Non-invasive	Box 13	Box 14	Box 15	Box 16	Box 17	Box 18
Total benign	Box 19	Box 20	Box 21	Box 22	Box 23	Box 24
No histology	Box 25	Box 26	Box 27	Box 28	Box 29	Box 30
Total C results	Box 31	Box 32	Box 33	Box 34	Box 35	Box 36

Each box (numbered 1 to 36) of the above table is calculated from the number of FNAC with a C code (C1, C2, etc.) cross-referenced with the worst histology diagnosis. The table and calculations (see below) should be produced for all FNAC tests (headed ALL TESTS) and also for all patients (headed ALL PATIENTS) where if two FNAC records are present the highest C number is taken. Only closed episodes should be used.

From the above table the sensitivity and specificity are then calculated in percentages for each of the categories in the cytology document. (The numbers correspond to BOX NUMBERS in the above table.)

1. Absolute sensitivity $\quad=\quad \dfrac{1 + 25}{6 + 25} \times 100$
(This assumes that all unbiopsied C5 results are carcinomas treated non surgically.)

2. Complete sensitivity $\quad=\quad \dfrac{1 + 2 + 3 + 25}{6 + 25} \times 100$

3. Specificity (biopsy cases only) $\quad=\quad \dfrac{22}{24} \times 100$

4. Specificity (full) $\quad=\quad \dfrac{22 + 28}{24 + 27 + 28 + 29} \times 100$
(This assumes that all cases of atypia (C3) which are not biopsied are benign.)

5. Positive predictive value (C5 diagnosis) $\quad=\quad \dfrac{31 - 19}{31} \times 100$

6. Positive predictive value (C4 diagnosis) $\quad=\quad \dfrac{2}{32 - 26} \times 100$

7. Positive predictive value (C3 diagnosis) $\quad=\quad \dfrac{3}{33} \times 100$

8. Negative predictive value (C2) $\quad=\quad \dfrac{34 - 4}{34} \times 100$

9. False negative rate $\quad=\quad \dfrac{4}{6 + 25} \times 100$
(This *excludes* inadequate results.)

10. False positive rate $\quad=\quad \dfrac{19}{6 + 25} \times 100$

11. Inadequate rate $\quad=\quad \dfrac{35}{36} \times 100$

12. Inadequate rate from cancers $\quad=\quad \dfrac{5}{6 + 25} \times 100$

13. Suspicious rate $\quad=\quad \dfrac{32 + 33}{36} \times 100$

It is recognised that the specificities are approximate and will be more accurate the longer the follow up.

Suggested minimum standards where therapy is partially based on FNAC

Absolute sensitivity (AS)	> 60%
Complete sensitivity (CS)	> 80%
Specificity (SPEC) (as calculated above)	> 60% (including non-biopsied cases)
Positive predictive value (C5) (+PV)	> 98%
False negative rate (F-)	< 5%
False positive rate (F+)	< 1%
Inadequate rate (INAD)	< 25%
Inadequate rate in samples taken from carcinomas	< 10%
Suspicious rate	< 20%

These figures will obviously depend on aspiration techniques and the experience and care of the aspirator and will vary widely between units. The figures are interrelated and strategy to improve one figure will affect others. Thus attempts to reduce the inadequate rate will often increase the number of suspicious reports and attempts to improve the specificity will increase the false negative rate and so on. Also, reducing the benign biopsy rate by not sampling the majority of lesions with benign cytology will reduce the specificity where this is based on cases with benign histology rather than on the total.

A high proportion of impalpable cases aspirated in any series is likely to make the figures worse as there is more chance of missing a small area of microcalcification leading to a false negative or inadequate result and more likelihood of aspirating atypical hyperplasia, radial scars and tubular carcinomas, leading to a high level of suspicious or atypical reports. In screening with aspiration of impalpable lesions the results are likely to reveal lower values than those achieved in the symptomatic setting.

6.3 Needle core biopsy

For the purposes of data recording and quality assurance in breast screening programmes, it is recommended that needle core biopsies be classified on a 5-point scale in a similar fashion to cytological specimens. Some units may wish to merge categories B3 and B4 as both indicate the need for further action.

It needs to be emphasised, however, that the categories are not the same as the five cytology categories and have different clinical inferences. It is essential that the histological appearances in needle core biopsies are compared with the clinical and radiological findings in order to ensure that the biopsy is representative.

Needle biopsy reporting categories

B1 Normal or uninterpretable

This may indicate an unsatisfactory biopsy which is: 1) uninterpretable because of artefact; 2) composed of stroma only, or 3) composed of normal breast tissue in cases where normal appearances are felt to be inconsistent with findings on imaging and clinical examination.

B2 Benign

Indicates that the sample contains a benign abnormality. The characteristics of the lesion can be described in an accompanying text report. Biopsies exhibiting normal appearances may be included in this category if they are felt to be consistent with the findings on imaging and clinical examination (e.g. hamartoma). Involutionary calcification should be classified as benign.

B3 Benign but of uncertain biological potential

Indicates a benign abnormality that is recognised to be associated with an increased risk of developing breast cancer, or is often associated with the presence of *in situ* or invasive carcinoma in the breast. Examples of such lesions include papillomas and radial scars/complex sclerosing lesions.

B4 Suspicious

Indicates that changes suggestive of *in situ* or invasive malignancy are present but a categorical diagnosis cannot be made because of artefact or because the appearances are borderline.

B5 Malignant

Indicates the presence of an unequivocal malignant process usually *in situ* or invasive carcinoma. Category a) indicates that *in situ* carcinoma only is present, b) that invasive carcinoma is seen and c) that it is not certain whether the carcinoma is invasive or not. If invasive malignancy other than a primary carcinoma is suspected, then use category 5b but enter a qualifying statement in the 'comment' section. It is important to remember that a lesion classified as 5a may be found to have an invasive component in later biopsy or resection specimens.

Calcification

Should a needle core biopsy be performed for investigation of suspicious microcalcification, the report should clearly indicate whether microcalcification has been identified in the biopsy and whether it is associated with a specific abnormality. Radiography of the specimen can assist in identifying microcalcification and confirming that its characteristics are the same as those of the mammographic abnormality.

Patient details, report number, side (right or left), localisation technique, names of pathologist and operator taking the biopsy are also included. In assessing performance it is essential to specify whether the performance indicators (e.g. sensitivity, specificity, positive predictive value) relate to the histological report alone or to the diagnosis reached after consideration of pathological, radiological and clinical findings.

Registration form

Breast screening wide bore needle biopsy

Surname _____ Forenames _____

Date of birth _____

Screening no. _____ Hospital no. _____

Centre _____ Report no. _____

Side

☐ Right ☐ Left Number of cores _____

Calcification present on specimen X-ray?

☐ Yes ☐ No ☐ Radiograph not seen

Histological calcification

☐ Absent ☐ Benign ☐ Malignant ☐ Both

Localisation technique

☐ Palpation ☐ X-ray guided ☐ Ultrasound guided ☐ Stereotaxis

Opinion

☐ B1 Unsatisfactory/Normal tissue only
☐ B2 Benign
☐ B3 Benign but of uncertain malignant potential
☐ B4 Suspicious of malignancy
☐ B5 Malignant   a. ☐ In situ
                  b. ☐ Invasive
                  c. ☐ Uncertain whether in situ or invasive

Pathologist _____ Operator taking biopsy _____

Date _____

Comment _____
_____
_____

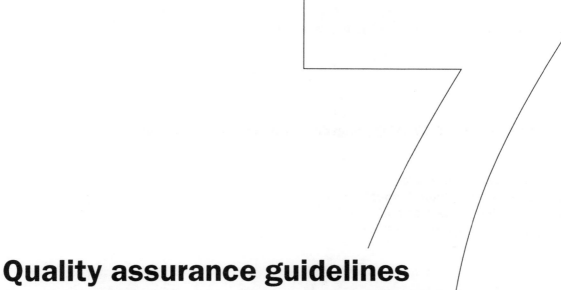

Quality assurance guidelines for pathology in mammography screening

Open biopsy and resection specimens

Editor
J. Sloane†

Produced by **the E.C. Working group on breast screening pathology**

These guidelines are also available in multimedia format as part of the BreakIT project (http://sos.ist.unige.it/breakit)

7.1 Introduction

The success of a breast screening programme depends heavily on the quality of the pathological service. Specimens from screened women provide pathologists with particular problems of macroscopic and histological examination; the former principally result from identifying impalpable radiological abnormalities and the latter from classifying borderline lesions which are encountered with disproportionate frequency. Accurate pathological diagnoses and the provision of prognostically significant information are important to ensure that patients are managed appropriately and that the programme is properly monitored and evaluated. A standard set of data from each patient, using the same terminology and diagnostic criteria is essential to achieve the latter objective. The opinions expressed represent the consensus view of the E.C. Working Group on Breast Screening Pathology and other pathologists who made written or verbal comments on this document and the United Kingdom document on which it is based. We hope that European pathologists involved in breast screening will find the guidance useful and the method of recording data convenient.

7.2 Macroscopic examination of biopsy and resection specimens

7.2.1 Biopsy specimens

Optimal handling

Biopsies of mammographically detected lesions may provide especial difficulty in histological interpretation and consequently require optimal fixation and careful handling. Sometimes a photographic record of the sliced specimen, with the guide wire in position may be necessary to maximize the value of case discussions with clinical and radiological colleagues. Provision for macroscopic photography must, therefore, be borne in mind, especially for difficult cases.

The surgeon should be discouraged from cutting the specimen before sending it to the pathologist and should ideally mark it with sutures in order to obtain proper orientation. Sutures are preferable to metal staples which often retract into the specimen, thus becoming impossible to recognize, and may obscure microcalcifications. A code of orientation for the sutures needs to be established and indicated on the request form.

Palpable lesions

Palpable lesions detected in the screening programme may be dealt with by conventional methods and there is no especial virtue in specimen radiography, assuming that there is no doubt that the radiological and palpable lesions are one and the same.

Confirming excision of radiological abnormality

After excision, the intact specimen - with guide wire in situ - must be X-rayed. Ideally this procedure is carried out by the staff of the radiological department, so that the radiologist or surgeon can determine whether the relevant lesion has been resected. It may be necessary on medico-legal grounds for centres to name consultants responsible for confirming that mammographic lesions have been removed. Ideally those consultants should be the radiologists who interpreted the clinical mammograms. A good working relationship between pathologists, surgeons and radiologists is essential. Two copies of the specimen radiograph at this time could be taken with benefit, one for the department of radiology and one for the pathologist.

If mammographic abnormality not identified

Clearly there will be a few occasions when the mammographic abnormality cannot be identified in the specimen. This may result from the excision of a lesion producing only architectural change in the clinical mammogram or from unsuccessful surgical localization. Detailed pathological examination should still be undertaken even in the latter case and the findings communicated to the surgeon. Clinical mammography can subsequently be repeated to determine if the lesion is still present in the breast.

Fresh specimens

Specimens should be examined within 2-3 hours if received fresh. Samples for oestrogen receptor determination should be snap frozen in liquid nitrogen within 30 minutes of excision if a ligand binding assay is used. Oestrogen receptor status is, however, increasingly being determined on standard formalin-fixed, paraffin-embedded sections (see 7.3.8.7).[1,2]

Frozen sections

Rapid frozen sectioning is generally inappropriate in the assessment of clinically impalpable lesions. Rarely, however, it may be justified to enable a firm diagnosis of invasive carcinoma to be made in order to allow definitive surgery to be carried out in one operation. Three essential criteria, however, must be fulfilled:
1) the mammographic abnormality must be clearly and unequivocally identified on macroscopic examination
2) it must be large enough (generally at least 10 mm) to allow an adequate proportion of the lesion to be fixed and processed without prior freezing
3) it must have proved impossible to make a definitive diagnosis pre-operatively

Fixation

The intact specimen may be examined in the fresh state or after fixation. Good fixation is very important to preserve the degree of morphological detail needed to diagnose borderline lesions and report features of prognostic significance, particularly grade and vascular invasion. Small specimens may be fixed whole but larger ones should be examined and sliced within 2-3 hours of excision, if possible, to allow adequate penetration of fixative.

Excision margins

In order to demonstrate adequacy of excision, the entire surface of the specimen should be painted with India ink, radiolucent pigments, dyed gelatin or other suitable material. An appropriate period of drying must be allowed if spread of the chosen reagent is to be avoided.

Naked eye examination

After determining its weight (and size if required), the specimen is then serially sliced at intervals of up to 4 mm. The cut surfaces are examined by careful visual inspection. Palpation may also be informative. The maximum diameter, contour, colour and consistency of any macroscopic lesion are recorded. The size of lesions measured macroscopically should be checked later on histological sections as the true extent of the abnormality is not always appreciated by macroscopic inspection alone. If different, the histological dimensions should be accepted as the true size. In the case of malignant lesions, adequacy of excision should be assessed by naked eye and later by microscopic examination.

Specimen radiography

Unless a lesion obviously accounting for the radiological abnormality is identified, a second radiograph of the sliced specimen should be performed. It is desirable for the pathologist to give a brief description of the abnormality in the specimen radiograph during macroscopic examination. Blocks should then be taken from the areas corresponding to the mammographic abnormalities and any other macroscopically suspicious zones. This method allows precise correlations to be made between the radiological and histological appearances and may serve as a reference map for orientation and reconstruction purposes. It is thus the favoured method of specimen radiography. It has been found, however, to be too time-consuming for some laboratories to undertake. A number of shorter, one stage, methods have been reported. For reviews see Anderson and Armstrong & Davies.[3,4]

Histological characterization of mammographic changes

Whichever method is adopted, pathologists must satisfy themselves that the pathological changes responsible for mammographic abnormalities have been identified in the histological sections; it may be necessary to consult with radiologiststo be certain of this. If not, the residual unblocked tissue and/or blocks should be re-X-rayed. Any residual tissue should be stored until the mammographic changes have been characterized histologically.

It is not recommended that tissue is simply taken from around a guide wire introduced pre-operatively which may not necessarily be very close to the mammographic abnormality.

Choice of specimen mammography equipment

Although it is possible to prepare adequate mammographs of specimens using a clinical mammography machine, this approach may present logistical difficulties. There are several dedicated specimen mammography cabinets on the market.

Extent of sampling

The precise number of blocks to be taken cannot be stated dogmatically and clearly depends on the size and number of lesions present. With small biopsies, all the tissue should be blocked and examined. For malignant tumours in excess of 20 mm, about 3 blocks of the tumour are desirable. Where possible, at least one block should include the edge of the tumour and the nearest excision margin to enable measurement of this distance, in mm, on the histological sections.

For larger biopsies which cannot be blocked in toto, some sampling of radiologically and macroscopically normal breast should be undertaken in order to increase the detection of small occult cancers (particularly in situ types) and atypical proliferative lesions. The frequency with which such lesions are detected incidentally in unscreened women depends on the number of blocks taken.[5] The extent of sampling of biopsies containing benign screen-detected mammographic abnormalities should be decided locally and will depend, amongst other things, on the extent of local resources. Additional sampling is more effective if restricted to fibrous parenchyma, ignoring the adipose tissue.

Large blocks

Large blocks and sections are used in some laboratories where they are found to be of value in identifying screen-detected lesions as well as in determining their size, extent of spread and adequacy of excision. They facilitate orientation by obviating the need for mental reconstruction of the overall picture from several separate sections. They also reduce the number of blocks required.[6] Other workers, however, have encountered problems in achieving adequate fixation and good cytological detail in addition to the technical difficulties of cutting large sections and the problems in storing them. These drawbacks can be overcome, but large blocks, although of value, are not regarded as essential for examining specimens from screened women and their use should depend on local preference.

7.2.2 Mastectomy specimens

Naked eye examination

Mastectomy specimens should be dealt with within 2 hours of removal and either examined in the fresh state or incised before fixation to allow adequate penetration of fixative. The favoured method of examination is by slicing the breast from the deep surface in the sagittal plane after measuring the dimensions or recording the weight. The slices should be about 10 mm thick and may be left joined by the skin or separated completely and arranged in order. The maximum diameter of the main lesion should be measured and the distance from the nearest margin of excision determined as for biopsies (see earlier).

Sampling

Blocks of tumour (the number depending on tumour size as above) should be taken to include the edges and should always be sufficient to represent the maximum extent of the lesion noted macroscopically. Blocks of the nearest excision margin should be taken. Painting with India ink or pigments may be helpful as in local excision specimens. If the tumour has been removed, then 3-4 blocks should be taken from the cavity wall. The breast slices should be examined by careful naked eye inspection and palpation. Blocks should be taken from any suspicious areas, noting the quadrant in which they are located. At least one block should be taken from each quadrant and ideally two from the nipple - one in the sagittal and one in the coronal plane through the junction with the areola.

Axillary dissection specimens

Axillary contents received with mastectomy or biopsy specimens should be examined carefully to maximize lymph node yield. This is usually achieved by cutting the specimen into thin slices which are then examined by careful inspection and palpation. The use of clearing agents or Bouin's solution may increase lymph node yield but are time-consuming and expensive of reagents and not regarded as essential. The axillary contents can be divided into three levels if the surgeon has marked the specimen appropriately.

Sampling

Pathological examination should be performed on all lymph nodes received and the report should state the total number and the number containing metastases. A representative complete section of any grossly involved lymph node is adequate. For nodes greater than 5 mm in maximum dimension, three slices should be taken and processed in a single block. Nodes less than 5 mm should be embedded in their entirety. They can be processed in groups and are ideally examined at two levels.

Histopathology reporting form

Surname _____ Forenames _____ Date of birth _____

Screening no. _____ Hospital no. _____ Side ☐ Right ☐ Left

Pathologist _____ Date of reporting _____ Report no. _____

Histological calcification ☐ Absent ☐ Benign ☐ Malignant ☐ Benign and malignant

Specimen radiograph seen? ☐ Yes ☐ No

Mammographic abnormality present in specimen ☐ Yes ☐ No

Specimen type ☐ Localisation biopsy ☐ Open biopsy ☐ Segmental excision

☐ Mastectomy ☐ Wide bore needle core

Specimen weight _____ g   Size _____ mm x _____ mm x _____ mm

---

Benign lesion present

☐ Complex sclerosing lesion/radial scar ☐ Fibroadenoma ☐ Multiple papilloma

☐ Periductal mastitis/duct ectasia ☐ Fibrocystic change ☐ Solitary papilloma

☐ Sclerosing adenosis ☐ Solitary cyst ☐ Other (please specify) _____

Epithelial proliferation ☐ Not present ☐ Present with atypia (ductal)

☐ Present without atypia ☐ Present with atypia (lobular)

Malignant lesions non-invasive ☐ Not present

☐ Ductal, high grade ☐ Ductal, other

  Growth pattern(s) _____   Cell type/pattern _____

☐ Lobular ☐ Paget's   Size (ductal only) _____

Microinvasion ☐ Not present ☐ Present ☐ Possible

Invasive ☐ Not present ☐ Mucinous carcinoma

☐ Ductal / no specific type (NST) ☐ Tubular carcinoma

☐ Lobular carcinoma ☐ Mixed (please tick component types present)

☐ Medullary carcinoma ☐ Not assessable

☐ Other primary carcinoma (please specify) _____

☐ Other malignant tumour (please specify) _____

Maximum diameter of invasive tumour _____ mm

Whole size of tumour (to include DCIS extending >1 mm beyond invasive area) _____ mm

Axillary nodes present ☐ Yes ☐ No   Number positive _____ Total number _____

Other nodes present ☐ Yes ☐ No   Number positive _____ Total number _____

  Site of other nodes _____

Excision margins ☐ Reaches margin ☐ Uncertain ☐ Does not reach margin (nearest _____ mm)

Grade ☐ I ☐ II ☐ III ☐ Not assessable

Disease extent ☐ Localised ☐ Multiple ☐ Not assessable

Vascular invasion (blood or lymphatic) ☐ Present ☐ Not seen

Oestrogen receptor status _____

Comments/additional information _____

Histological diagnosis ☐ Normal ☐ Benign ☐ Malignant

7.3 Using the histopathology reporting form

7.3.1 Introduction

This section gives guidance on how to use the histopathology form and provides definitions of the terms used. The aim is not to replace standard texts on breast histopathology but to focus on diagnostic criteria for including lesions in the various categories and therefore help to achieve maximum uniformity of reporting.

The guidance in this section is drawn from standard textbooks of breast pathology and other published data. Reporting forms can be obtained from, or may be computer-generated in, screening offices. It is not necessary to use the form as it appears in this document. It may be found desirable to undertake modifications locally, particularly if the form is also to function as the definitive pathology report to be entered in patients' notes and laboratory records. It is, of course, **essential** to record all the information requested by the form for submission to screening offices using exactly the same terminology. Evaluation of breast screening programmes depends upon provision of accurate pathology data.

7.3.2 Recording basic information

Side	Indicate left or right. For specimens from both sides, use one form for each side.
Pathologist	The pathologist should enter their name.
Date	Enter the date the specimen was reported.
Histological calcification	Indicate if calcification observed radiologically is seen in histological sections and, if so, whether it is present in benign or malignant changes or both.
Specimen radiograph seen?	Please indicate if you have seen a specimen radiograph.
Mammographic abnormality present in specimen?	Are you satisfied that the mammographic abnormality is present in the specimen? This may necessitate consultation with the radiologist responsible for examining the specimen radiograph. It is worth remembering that breast calcification is occasionally due to oxalate salts (Weddelite) which can only be detected satisfactorily in histological sections using polarized light.[7]

Specimen type	Please choose one of the following terms:
	- Localization biopsy Biopsy of impalpable lesion identified by radiologically guided marking.
	- Open biopsy Non-guided biopsy/excision, lumpectomy, tylectomy, dochectomy.
	- Segmental excision Include: wedge excisions, partial mastectomies and re-excision specimens for clearance of margins.
	- Mastectomy Where specimen includes all or nearly all of the breast parenchymal tissue. Include: subcutaneous mastectomy, total glandular mastectomy, simple mastectomy, extended simple mastectomy, modified radical mastectomy, radical mastectomy, Patey mastectomy, supra-radical mastectomy.
	- Wide bore needle core Pre-operative diagnostic needle biopsy, e.g. trucut, corescrew, etc.

Specimen weight   Please record the weight and/or size of all biopsy and segmental excision specimens. Weight is a more reproducible method of estimating the size of a specimen than threedimensional measurements to determine volume, even taking into account the different densities of fat and fibrous tissue, which form varying proportions of breast specimens.

7.3.3 Recording benign lesions

7.3.3.1 Fibroadenoma

A benign malformation composed of connective tissue and epithelium exhibiting a pericanalicular and/or intracanalicular growth pattern. The connective tissue is generally composed of spindle cells but may rarely also contain other mesenchymal elements such as fat, smooth muscle, osteoid or bone. The epithelium is usually double-layered but some multilayering is not uncommon. Changes identical to those found in lobular epithelium elsewhere in the breast (e.g. apocrine metaplasia, sclerosing adenosis, blunt duct adenosis, hyperplasia of usual type, etc.) may occur in fibroadenomas but need not be recorded separately unless they amount to atypical hyperplasia or **in situ** carcinoma.

Sometimes individual lobules may exhibit increased stroma producing a fibroadenomatous appearance and occasionally such lobules may be loosely coalescent. These changes are often called fibroadenomatoid hyperplasia or sclerosing lobular hyperplasia but may be recorded as fibroadenoma on the reporting form if they produce a macroscopically visible or palpable mass. Consequently, fibroadenomas need not be perfectly circumscribed.

Old lesions may show hyalinization and calcification (and less frequently ossification) of stroma and atrophy of epithelium. Fibroadenomas are occasionally multiple.

For the purposes of the screening form, tubular adenomas can be grouped under fibroadenomas.

Fibroadenomas should be distinguished from phyllodes tumours. The high grade or 'malignant' phyllodes tumours are easily identified by their sarcomatous stroma. The low grade variants are more difficult to distinguish but the main feature is the more cellular stroma. Phyllodes tumours may also exhibit an enhanced intracanalicular growth pattern with club-like projections into cystic spaces and there is often overgrowth of stroma at the expense of the epithelium. Adequate sampling is important as the characteristic stromal features may be seen only in parts of the lesion. Although phyllodes tumours are generally larger than fibroadenomas, size is not an acceptable criterion for diagnosis; fibroadenomas may be very large and phyllodes tumours small. For purposes of convenience, low grade phyllodes tumours should be specified under 'Other benign lesions' and high grade under 'Other malignant tumour' although it is recognized that histological appearance is often not a good predictor of behaviour.

7.3.3.2 Papilloma

A papilloma is defined as a tumour with an arborescent, fibrovascular stroma covered by epithelium generally arranged in an inner myoepithelial and outer epithelial layer. Epithelial hyperplasia without cytological atypia is often present and should not be recorded separately. Atypical hyperplasia is rarely seen and, when present, should be recorded separately under 'Epithelial proliferation'. Epithelial nuclei are usually vesicular with delicate nuclear membranes and inconspicuous nucleoli. Apocrine metaplasia is frequently observed but should not be recorded separately on the reporting form. Squamous metaplasia is sometimes seen, particularly near areas of infarction. Sclerosis and haemorrhage are not uncommon and where the former involves the periphery of the lesion, may give rise to epithelial entrapment with the false impression of invasion. The benign cytological features of such areas should enable the correct diagnosis to be made. The term '**intracystic papilloma**' is sometimes used to describe a papilloma in a widely dilated duct. These tumours should simply be classified as papilloma on the form. (For distinction from encysted papillary carcinoma, see table 1.)

Papillomas may be **solitary** or **multiple**. The former usually occur centrally in sub-areolar ducts whereas the latter are more likely to be peripheral and involve terminal duct lobular units. The distinction is important as the multiple form is more frequently associated with atypical hyperplasia and ductal carcinoma **in situ**, the latter usually of low grade type which should be recorded separately. This malignant change may be restricted to small foci and extensive sampling may be required to detect it. Some sub-areolar papillomas causing nipple discharge may be very small and extensive sampling may be required to detect them.

Lesions termed **ductal adenoma** exhibit a variable appearance which overlaps with other benign breast lesions. They may resemble papillomas except that they exhibit an adenomatous rather than a papillary growth pattern. These cases should be grouped under papilloma on the form. Indeed, some tumours may exhibit papillary and adenomatous features. Some ductal adenomas may show pronounced central and/or peripheral fibrosis and overlap with complex sclerosing lesions (see 7.3.3.4).

The condition of **adenoma of the nipple** (sub-areolar duct papillomatosis) should not be classified as papilloma in the screening form but specified under 'Benign lesions, Other'.

Diffuse microscopic papillary hyperplasia should be recorded under 'Epithelial proliferation' in the appropriate box depending on whether atypia is present or not.

Table 1: Distinguishing papilloma from encysted papillary carcinoma

Histological features	Papilloma	Encysted papillary carcinoma
1) Fibrovascular cores	Usually broad and extend throughout the lesion.	Very variable, usually fine and may be lacking in at least part of the lesion.
2) Cells covering papillae		
a) basal	Myoepithelial layer always present.	Myoepithelial cells usually absent but may form a discontinuous layer.
b) luminal	Single layer of regular luminal epithelium OR features of regular usual type hyperplasia.	Cells often taller and more monotonous with oval nuclei, the long axes of which lie perpendicular to stromal core of papillae. Nuclei may be hyper-chromatic. Epithelial multi-layering frequent, often producing cribriform and micropapillary patterns of DCIS overlying the papillae or lining the cyst wall.
3) Mitoses	Infrequent with no abnormal forms.	More frequent; abnormal forms may be seen.
4) Apocrine metaplasia	Common	Rare
5) Surrounding tissue	Benign changes may be present including regular epithelial hyperplasia.	Surrounding ducts may show ductal carcinoma in situ.
6) Necrosis and haemorrhage	May occur in either. Not a useful discriminating feature.	
7) Periductal and intratumoural fibrosis	May occur in either. Not a useful discriminating feature.	

NB: All the features of a lesion should be taken into account when making a diagnosis.
No criterion is reliable alone.

7.3.3.3 Sclerosing adenosis

Sclerosing adenosis is an organoid lobular enlargement in which increased numbers of acinar structures exhibit elongation and distortion. The normal two cell lining is retained but there is myoepithelial and stromal hyperplasia. The acinar structures may infiltrate adjacent connective tissue and occasionally nerves and blood vessels, which can lead to an erroneous diagnosis of malignancy. Early lesions of sclerosing adenosis are more cellular and later ones more sclerotic. Calcification may be present.

There may be coalescence of adjacent lobules of sclerosing adenosis to form a mass detectable by mammography or macroscopic examination. The term 'adenosis tumour' has been used to describe such lesions.[8] It is recommended that sclerosing adenosis is not entered on the screening form if it is a minor change detectable only on histological examination. Although sclerosing adenosis often accompanies fibrocystic change (see below), this is not always the case and the two changes should be recorded separately.

Occasionally apocrine metaplasia is seen in areas of sclerosing adenosis (apocrine adenosis). It can produce a worrying appearance and should not be mistaken for malignancy.[9]

Rarely, the epithelium in sclerosing adenosis may show atypical hyperplasia or **in situ** carcinoma. In such cases, please record these changes separately on the reporting form. The differential diagnosis of sclerosing adenosis includes tubular carcinoma, microglandular adenosis and radial scar. In tubular carcinoma, the infiltrating tubules lack basement membrane, myoepithelium, a lobular organoid growth pattern and exhibit cytological atypia. Ductal carcinoma **in situ** is a frequent accompaniment. Microglandular adenosis differs from sclerosing adenosis in lacking the lobular organoid growth pattern and being composed of rounded tubules lined by a single layer of cells lacking cytological atypia. The glandular distortion of sclerosing adenosis is lacking. Radial scar is distinguished from sclerosing adenosis by its characteristic floret-type growth pattern with ducto-lobular structures radiating out from a central zone of dense fibro-elastotic tissue. Furthermore, the compression of tubular structures associated with myoepithelial and stromal hyperplasia is lacking.

7.3.3.4 Complex sclerosing lesion/radial scar

Under this heading are included sclerosing lesions with a pseudoinfiltrative growth pattern which have been called various names including infiltrating epitheliosis, rosette-like lesions, sclerosing papillary proliferation, complex compound heteromorphic lesions, benign sclerosing ductal proliferation, non-encapsulated sclerosing lesion, indurative mastopathy and proliferation centre of Aschoff.

The radial scar is generally 10 mm or less in diameter and consists of a central fibro-elastotic zone from which radiate out tubular structures which may be two-layered or exhibit intra-luminal proliferation. Tubules entrapped within the central zone of fibro-elastosis exhibit a more random, non-organoid arrangement. Lesions greater than 10 mm are generally termed complex sclerosing lesions. They have all the features of radial scars and, in addition to their greater size, exhibit more disturbance of structure, often with nodular masses around the periphery. Changes such as papilloma formation, apocrine metaplasia and sclerosing adenosis may be superimposed on the main lesion. Some complex sclerosing lesions give the impression of being formed by coalescence of several adjacent sclerosing lesions. There is a degree of morphological overlap with some forms of ductal adenoma.

If the intra-luminal proliferation exhibits atypia or amounts to **in situ** carcinoma, it should be recorded separately under the appropriate heading on the screening form.

The main differential diagnosis is carcinoma of tubular or low grade 'ductal' type. The major distinguishing features are the presence of myoepithelium and basement membrane around the tubules of the sclerosing lesions. Cytological atypia is also lacking and any intra-tubular proliferation resembles hyperplasia of usual type unless atypical hyperplasia and/or **in situ** carcinoma are superimposed (see above). Tubular carcinomas generally lack the characteristic architecture of sclerosing lesions.

7.3.3.5 Fibrocystic change

This term is used for cases with several to numerous macroscopically visible cysts, the majority of which are usually lined by apocrine epithelium. The term is not intended for use with minimal alterations such as fibrosis, microscopic dilatation of acini or ducts, lobular involution, adenosis and minor degrees of blunt duct adenosis. These changes should be indexed as normal.

It is not intended that cystic change or apocrine metaplasia occurring within other lesions such as fibroadenomata, papillomata or sclerosing lesions should be coded here.

Apocrine metaplasia occurring in lobules without cystic change may produce a worrisome appearance, occasionally mistaken for carcinoma. This change should be specified as 'apocrine adenosis' under other benign lesions.

Papillary apocrine hyperplasia should be indexed separately under epithelial proliferation with or without atypia, depending on its appearance. It should be noted, however, that apocrine cells usually exhibit a greater degree of pleomorphism than is seen in normal breast cells. Hyperplasia should therefore be regarded as atypical only when the cytological changes are significantly more pronounced than usual.

7.3.3.6 Solitary cyst

This term should be used when the abnormality appears to be a solitary cyst. The size is usually greater than 10 mm and the lining attenuated or apocrine in type. The latter may show papillary change which should be indexed separately under epithelial proliferation of appropriate type. If multiple cysts are present, it is better to use the term 'fibrocystic change' as above. Intra-cystic papillomas and intra-cystic papillary carcinomas should not be entered here but under papilloma or carcinoma.

7.3.3.7 Periductal mastitis/ectasia (plasma cell mastitis)

This process involves larger and intermediate size ducts, generally in sub-duct areolar location. The ducts are lined by normal or attenuated epithelium, filled with amorphous, eosinophilic material and/or foam cells and exhibit marked periductal chronic inflammation, often with large numbers of plasma cells. There may be pronounced periductal fibrosis. The inflammatory infiltrate may contain large numbers of histiocytes giving a granulomatous appearance. Calcification may be present. The process may ultimately lead to obliteration of ducts leaving dense fibrous masses. Persistence of small tubules of epithelium around the periphery of an obliterated duct result in a characteristic garland pattern. Duct ectasia is often associated with nipple discharge or retraction.

Cysts are distinguished from duct ectasia by their rounded rather than elongated shape, tendency to cluster, lack of stromal elastin, frequent presence of apocrine metaplasia and less frequent presence of eosinophilic material or foam cells in the lumina.

Mammary duct fistula (recurring sub-areolar abscess) should be coded under 'Benign, Other'.

7.3.3.8 Other (specify)

This category is intended for use with less common conditions which form acceptable entities but cannot be entered into the categories above, e.g. fat necrosis, lipoma, adenoma of nipple, low grade phyllodes tumours. The index at the end of the chapter should help as a reference for lesions difficult to place in any of the above categories.

7.3.4 Classifying epithelial proliferation

This section is for recording intra-luminal epithelial proliferation in terminal duct lobular units or inter-lobular ducts.

7.3.4.1 Not present

This should be ticked if there is no epithelial multilayering (apart from that ascribed to cross-cutting) or if there is slight multilayering without atypia, not exceeding 4 cells in thickness.

7.3.4.2 Present without atypia

This term is used to describe all cases of intra-luminal proliferation showing no or only minor atypia where the epithelial cells are more than 4 thick. The change may involve terminal duct lobular units or inter-lobular ducts. The major features which distinguish hyperplasia from ductal carcinoma **in situ** of low nuclear grade are summarized in table 2.

7.3.4.3 Present with atypia (ductal)

Hyperplasia of usual type should be recorded if it occurs alone or in association with cystic change or other benign lesions, but not if it is confined to fibroadenomas, adenomas, papillomas or radial scars/complex sclerosing lesions. The term should be used for cases where there is no atypia or atypia of only minor degree, insufficient to raise the possibility of DCIS.

In the previous edition of these guidelines, the criteria of Page and Rogers[10] were recommended for diagnosing atypical ductal hyperplasia (ADH) but a subsequent study undertaken by the EC Working Group[11] has demonstrated a very low level of diagnostic consistency using these criteria. Poor diagnostic consistency is almost certainly a major factor contributing to the variable risks of developing breast cancer reported in association with this condition.[12, 13, 14, 15, 16, 17] The solution to the problem is not yet apparent but the category has been retained as a mechanism for expressing uncertainty and for communicating to clinicians that these patients are likely to have an increased risk of developing breast cancer, particularly if they have a family history of the disease.

If a diagnosis of ADH is contemplated then extensive sampling should be undertaken to search for evidence of unequivocal DCIS with which it frequently co-exists. ADH is a rare lesion. It may be detected by screening mammography as microcalcification or incidentally often in association with fibrocystic change or within a sclerosing lesion or papilloma. Its recognition rests on identification of some but not all the features of ductal carcinoma in situ. Most of the difficulties are encountered in distinguishing ADH from the low-grade variants of DCIS. Table 2 provides details of features that serve to distinguish ADH from usual type ductal hyperplasia and low nuclear grade DCIS.

Useful rules of thumb to distinguish atypical ductal hyperplasia from ductal carcinoma *in situ* are:

1) restrict the diagnosis of ADH to cases where the diagnosis of DCIS is seriously considered but in which the features are not sufficiently developed for a confident diagnosis.

2) DCIS usually extends to involve multiple duct spaces and is rarely under 2-3 mm in extent. A criterion that has been used for distinguishing ADH from DCIS is that lesions less than 2 mm in diameter are not regarded as DCIS unless they exhibit high grade cytology or necrosis.[18] In any lesion where the process with the above features extends widely, a diagnosis of DCIS is more likely to be correct.

In needle core biopsies, it is virtually impossible to make a definitive diagnosis of ADH. The presence of an atypical proliferation should be recorded with a recommendation to take more tissue.

Table 2: Comparison of histological features of ductal hyperplasia and DCIS*

Histological features	Usual type ductal hyperplasia	Atypical ductal hyperplasia	Low nuclear grade DCIS
Size	Variable size but rarely extensive unless associated with other benign processes such as papilloma or radial scar	Usually small (less than 2-3 mm) unless associated with other benign processes such as papilloma or radial scar	Rarely less than 2-3 mm and may be very extensive
Cellular composition	**Mixed. Epithelial cells and spindle-shaped cells** present. Lymphocytes and macrophages may also be present. Myoepithelial hyperplasia may occur around the periphery**	May be uniform single population but merges with areas of usual type hyperplasia within the same duct space. Spindle shaped cells may be intermingled with the proliferating cells	**Single cell population.** Spindle-shaped cells not seen. Myoepithelial cells usually in normal location around duct periphery but may be attenuated
Architecture	Variable	Micropapillary, cribriform or solid patterns but may be rudimentary	**Well developed micropapillary cribriform or solid patterns**
Lumina	**Irregular, often ill-defined peripheral slit-like spaces are common and a useful distinguishing feature**	May be distinct, well formed rounded spaces in cribriform type. Irregular, ill-defined lumina may also be present	**Well delineated, regular punched out lumina in cribriform type**
Cell orientation	**Often streaming pattern with long axes of nuclei arranged parallel to direction of cellular bridges which often have a 'tapering' appearance**	Cell nuclei may be at right angles to bridges in cribriform types, forming 'rigid' structures	**Micropapillary structures with indiscernible fibro-vascular cores or smooth, well-delineated geometric spaces. Cell bridges 'rigid' in cribriform type with nuclei orientated towards the luminal space**
Nuclear spacing	**Uneven**	May be even or uneven	**Even**
Epithelial/tumour cell character	Small ovoid but showing variation in shape	Small uniform or medium sized monotonous cell populations present at least focally	**Small uniform monotonous cell population**
Nucleoli	Indistinct	Single small	Single small
Mitoses	Infrequent with no abnormal forms	Infrequent, abnormal forms rare	Infrequent, abnormal forms rare
Necrosis	Rare	Rare	If present, confined to small particulate debris in cribriform and/or luminal spaces

Major diagnostic features are shown in bold type.

* See Page & Rogers[10]
** These cells are usually called myoepithelial cells but immunohistological studies have shown that they have characteristics of basal keratin type epithelial cells[19]

7.3.4.4 Present with atypia (lobular)

This change is characterized by proliferation within terminal duct lobular units of characteristic small rounded cells similar to those seen in lobular carcinoma **in situ**. The major points of distinction from the latter are summarized in table 3. Like the ductal variety, atypical lobular hyperplasia occurs in about 2% of non-cancer containing biopsies from unscreened women.

Table 3: Distinction of atypical lobular hyperplasia from lobular carcinoma in situ

Histological features	Atypical lobular hyperplasia	Lobular carcinoma in situ
Cellular composition	Polymorphic. Cells similar to those seen in LCIS accompanied by spindle-shaped cells, leucocytes and other epithelial cells.	Monomorphic proliferation of chracteristic small rounded cells with granular or hyperchromatic nuclei, inconspicuous nucleoli and high nucleo-cytoplasmic ratio.
Cell cohesion	Usually good	Often poor
Cell spacing	Irregular	Regular
Luminal occlusion	Partial	Complete
Lobular distension	Slight	Moderate to marked
Pagetoid spread into interlobular ducts	Very uncommon	Common

NB: All the features of a lesion should be taken into account when making a diagnosis.
No criterion is reliable alone.

7.3.5 Classifying malignant non-invasive lesions

7.3.5.1 Ductal carcinoma in situ

Ductal carcinoma **in situ** (DCIS) is defined as a proliferation of epithelial cells with cytological features of malignancy within parenchymal structures of the breast and is distinguished from invasive carcinoma by the absence of stromal invasion across the basement membrane.

DCIS varies in cell type, growth pattern and extent of disease and may thus represent a group or spectrum of related **in situ** neoplastic processes. Classification has traditionally been according to growth pattern but has been carried out with little enthusiasm given a perceived lack of clinical relevance. More recently, evidence has emerged that lesions composed of cells of high nuclear grade are more aggressive.[12,13] There is currently no generally accepted method of classifying DCIS but distinction between common histological subtypes is of value for correlating pathological and radiological appearances, improving diagnostic consistency, assessing the likelihood of invasion and determining the probability of recurrence after local excision. Despite the name, most DCIS is generally considered to arise from the terminal duct lobular units. The main points of distinction from lobular carcinoma **in situ** are summarized in table 4.

For measurement of size see 7.3.8.1. For assessment of excision margins see 7.3.8.3. The nuclear grading system adopted below is derived from that employed by Holland et al.[22]

7.3.5.2 High nuclear grade DCIS

This is composed of cells with pleomorphic, irregularly-spaced and usually large nuclei exhibiting marked variation in size, irregular nuclear contours, coarse chromatin and prominent nucleoli. Mitoses are frequently present and abnormal forms may be seen.

High nuclear grade DCIS may exhibit several different growth patterns. It is often **solid** with central, **comedo**-type necrosis which frequently contains deposits of amorphous calcification. This is the easiest pattern to recognize. Sometimes a **solid** proliferation of malignant cells fills the duct without necrosis but this is relatively rare and is usually confined to nipple ducts in cases presenting with Paget's disease. High nuclear grade DCIS may also exhibit **micropapillary** and **cribriform** patterns frequently associated with central, comedo-like necrosis. Unlike low nuclear grade DCIS, there is rarely any polarization of cells covering the micropapillae or lining the intercellular spaces.

7.3.5.3 Low nuclear grade DCIS

This is composed of monomorphic, evenly-spaced cells with roughly spherical, centrally-placed nuclei and inconspicuous nucleoli. The nuclei are usually, but not invariably, small. Mitoses are few and there is rarely individual cell necrosis.

The cells are generally arranged in **micropapillary** and **cribriform** patterns which are frequently present within the same lesion, although the latter is more common and tends to predominate. There is usually polarization of cells covering the micropapillae or lining the intercellular lumina. Less frequently, low nuclear grade DCIS has a **solid** growth pattern. When terminal duct lobular units are involved, the process can be very difficult to distinguish from lobular carcinoma in situ. Features in favour of DCIS are greater cellular cohesion and lack of intracytoplasmic lumina. Occasionally, however, there may be a combination of both processes.

7.3.5.4 Intermediate nuclear grade DCIS

Some cases of DCIS cannot be assigned easily to the high or low nuclear grade categories. The nuclei show mild to moderate pleomorphism which is less than that seen in high grade DCIS but they lack the monotony of the small cell type. The nucleus:cytoplasm ratio is often high and one or two nucleoli may be identified.

The growth pattern may be **solid, cribriform** or **micropapillary** and the cells usually exhibit some degree of polarization covering papillary processes or lining intercellular lumina although this is not as marked as in low nuclear grade DCIS.

7.3.5.5 Mixed types

A proportion of cases of DCIS exhibit features of more than one histological subtype. One of the advantages of classifying DCIS according to nuclear grade is that, although variations of growth pattern are frequent, there is usually a dominant cell type and the lesion is fairly easily classified into one of the above main groups.

Rarely, cells of different nuclear grade may be seen within a single lesion. This should be recorded but **the case should be classified according to the highest nuclear grade observed**.

7.3.5.6 Other histological types

The main features of **encysted papillary carcinoma** are listed in table 1 (see 7.3.3.2).

Ductal carcinoma **in situ** of **signet ring cell**, pure **apocrine cell**, **cystic hypersecretory** and **neuroendocrine** types have been described and may be classified separately. For further details of these rare variants, the reader is referred to recent standard textbooks of breast pathology.

Lobular carcinoma in situ

The histological features of lobular carcinoma **in situ** are compared with those of atypical lobular hyperplasia in table 3 and with ductal carcinoma in situ in table 4. To maximize consistency of diagnosis, it is recommended that the term lobular carcinoma **in situ** be used when the characteristic uniform cells comprise the entire population of the lobular units, that there are no residual lumina and that there is expansion and/or distortion of at least one half the acini in the lobule. Otherwise the lesion should be classified as atypical lobular hyperplasia.

7.3.5.7 Paget's disease

In this condition, there are adenocarcinoma cells within the epidermis of the nipple. Cases where there is direct epidermal invasion by tumour infiltrating the skin should be excluded. Paget's disease should be recorded regardless of whether or not an underlying **in situ** or invasive carcinoma is identified. The underlying carcinoma should be recorded separately.

Table 4: Distinction of ductal from lobular carcinoma in situ

Histological features	Ductal carcinoma in situ	Lobular carcinoma in situ
Cells	Variable, depending on nuclear grade (see 7.3.5)	Small, rounded with granular or hyperchromatic nuclei, inconspicuous nucleoli and high nucleo-cytoplasmic ratio
Intracytoplasmic lumina	Rare	Common
Growth pattern	Very variable, e.g. solid, comedo, papillary, cribriform	Diffuse monotonous with complete luminal obliteration
Cell cohesion	Usually good	Usually poor
Degree of distension of involved structures	Moderate to great	Slight to moderate
Pagetoid spread into inter-lobular ducts	Absent	Often present
Necrosis	Common with high nuclear grade, uncommon with low nuclear grade	Absent
Mitoses	Common with high nuclear grade, uncommon with low nuclear grade	Infrequent
Abnormal mitoses	Common with high nuclear grade, rare with low nuclear grade	Rare
Calcification	Common	Rare

NB: All the features of a lesion should be taken into account when making a diagnosis.
No criterion is reliable alone.

7.3.6 Diagnosing microinvasion

A microinvasive carcinoma is defined for the purposes of the reporting form as a tumour in which the dominant lesion is DCIS but in which there are one or more clearly separate foci of infiltration of non-specialized interlobular or interductal fibrous or adipose tissue, none measuring more than 1 mm (about 2 hpf - see later) in maximal diameter. This definition is very restrictive and tumours fulfilling the criteria are consequently very rare. If there is sufficient doubt about the presence of invasion, the case should be classified as DCIS. Where the evidence is equivocal, tick the 'Microinvasion - Possible' box on the reporting form. Possible microinvasion includes separate islands of appropriately abnormal epithelium which are embedded in periductal fibrosis or inflammation, where the true boundary of the specialized periductal or lobular stroma is not clear. The term 'possible' microinvasion completely excludes merely ultrastructural evidence of basement membrane breach, histochemical or immunohistochemically identified basement membrane discontinuities and lesions in which there is demonstrable continuity in a 5 µm section with the parent DCIS. Microinvasion is largely restricted to high nuclear grade variants of DCIS, mainly of comedo type.

Cases of apparently pure comedo DCIS should thus be extensively sampled to exclude invasion. Microinvasive carcinomas should likewise be extensively sampled in order to exclude the possibility of larger invasive foci. Where such foci are found, the lesion should be classified as an invasive carcinoma and the approximate number and size range of the invasive foci stated under 'Comments/additional information'. Small invasive carcinomas without an **in situ** component are classified as invasive.

7.3.7 Classifying invasive carcinoma

Typing invasive carcinomas has established prognostic value.[23, 24] Some caution should be exercised in typing carcinomas in inadequately fixed specimens or if they have been removed from patients who have been treated primarily by chemotherapy or radiotherapy. The more common types are described below.

'Ductal' - no specific type (ductal-NST)	This group contains infiltrating carcinomas which cannot be entered into any other category on the form, or classified as any of the less common variants of infiltrating breast carcinoma. Consequently, invasive ductal carcinomas exhibit great variation in appearance and are the most common carcinomas, accounting for about 75% in most series.
Infiltrating lobular carcinoma	Infiltrating lobular carcinoma is composed of small regular cells identical to those seen in the **in situ** form. In its classical form, the cells are dissociated from each other or form single files or targetoid patterns around uninvolved ducts. Several variants have been identified in addition to this classical form but in each case the cell type is the same: a) the **alveolar** variant exhibits small aggregates of 20 or more cells[25]

b) the **solid** variant consists of sheets of cells with little stroma[26]

c) the **tubulo-lobular** type exhibits microtubular formation as part of the classical pattern[27]

Tumours that show mixtures of typical tubular and classical lobular carcinoma should be classified as mixed (see below).

d) the **pleomorphic** variant is uncommon and exhibits the growth pattern of classical lobular carcinoma throughout but the cytological appearances are more pleomorphic

e) mixtures of above

At least 90% of the tumour should exhibit one or more of the above patterns to be classified as infiltrating lobular.

Tubular carcinoma (including cribriform carcinoma)

Tubular carcinomas are composed of round, ovoid, or angulated single layered tubules in a cellular fibrous or fibro-elastotic stroma. The neoplastic cells are small, uniform and may show cytoplasmic apical snouting. At least 90% of the tumour should exhibit the classical growth pattern to be classified as tubular. If the co-existent carcinoma is solely of the invasive cribriform type, however, then the tumour should be typed as tubular if the tubular pattern forms over 50% of the lesion.

7.3.7.1 Invasive cribriform carcinoma

Invasive cribriform carcinoma is composed of masses of small regular cells similar to those seen in tubular carcinoma. The invasive islands, however, exhibit a cribriform rather than a tubular appearance. Apical snouting is often present. More than 90% of the lesion should exhibit the cribriform appearance except in cases where the only co-existent pattern is tubular carcinoma when over 50% must be of the cribriform appearance in order to be so classified. If a diagnosis of cribriform carcinoma is preferred, then tick the 'Tubular' box and make the appropriate comment under 'Comments/additional information'.

7.3.7.2 Medullary carcinoma

These rare tumours are composed of syncytial interconnecting masses of large pleomorphic cells with vesicular nuclei and prominent nucleoli; they are usually of histological grade 3. The stroma may be sparse but always contains large numbers of lymphoid cells. The border of the tumour is well-defined. The whole tumour must exhibit these features to be typed as medullary. Surrounding **in situ** elements are very uncommon.

The term **atypical medullary carcinoma** may be specified under 'Other primary carcinoma' for lesions which do not fulfil all the criteria for medullary carcinoma. The atypical medullary group has been defined by both Fisher et al.[28] and Ridolfi et al.[29] These tumours show less lymphoid infiltration, less circumscription or areas of dense fibrosis while still having the other features of a medullary carcinoma. A well circumscribed tumour is also classified as atypical medullary if up to 25% is composed of 'ductal' type and the rest comprises classical medullary carcinoma. If in doubt, classify as 'Ductal-NST'.

7.3.7.3 Mucinous carcinoma

This type is also known as mucoid, gelatinous or colloid carcinoma. There are islands of uniform small cells in lakes of extracellular mucin. An **in situ** component is uncommon. At least 90% of the tumour must exhibit the mucinous appearance to be so classified.

7.3.7.4 Mixed tumours

Tubular or cribriform mixed carcinomas have a usually central tubular or cribriform zone, which amounts to 75-90% of the area, with a ductal-NST or infiltrating lobular component usually at the periphery accounting for the remainder.[30] Such tumours have a good prognosis but less so than the pure types. The **mixed NST** and mucinous carcinomas include any mixtures of mucinous with ductal NST where the former accounts for 10-90%. In **mixed NST and lobular carcinomas** distinct and separate ductal NST and lobular elements must be present; the former occupies between 10% and 90% of the tumour area. These tumours are regarded as biphasic and are distinct from mixed and pleomorphic lobular carcinomas (see above). Mixtures of NST and specific types not listed on the form should be classified as 'Other primary carcinoma'.

7.3.7.5 Other primary carcinoma

Other primary breast carcinomas should be entered under this heading and will include variants such as **atypical medullary, spindle cell, infiltrating papillary, argyrophil, secretory, apocrine**, etc.

7.3.7.6 Other malignant tumour

Please include non-epithelial tumours and secondary carcinomas in this category. For purposes of convenience, all high grade **phyllodes** tumours should be recorded here.

7.3.7.7 Not assessable

This category should be ticked only if an invasive carcinoma cannot be assigned to any of the previous groups for technical reasons, e.g. the specimen is too small or poorly preserved.

7.3.8 Recording prognostic data

7.3.8.1 Maximum diameter

All lesions should be measured in the fresh or fixed state and on the histological preparation. If the two measurements are discrepant then that obtained from histological examination should be recorded where tumours are small enough to be visualized in cross-section. This may give a small underestimation of size due to shrinkage of the tissue in processing. It is considered, however, that the slight but consistent underestimation in the size of all tumours is preferable to the larger and less predictable errors that may result from measuring poorly delineated tumours macroscopically. Clearly, sufficient blocks should be taken from the periphery of larger tumours to allow accurate estimates of their size to be made from combined histological and macroscopic examination. The largest dimension should be recorded to the nearest millimeter.

For non-invasive carcinomas, the maximum diameter should be entered in the 'Non-Invasive' section only where the tumour is of ductal type; lobular carcinoma **in situ** is not measured. For invasive carcinomas, the invasive component only needs to be recorded unless accompanying ductal carcinoma **in situ** extends more than 1 mm beyond the periphery of the infiltrative component, when the size of the infiltrative component and the overall size should be stated in the appropriate spaces of this section. This is to allow the identification of invasive carcinomas, where the **in situ** component forms a significant proportion of the lesion and may be important in determining the risk of recurrence after local excision. The largest dimension, to the nearest millimeter, is recorded in each case. The diagrams below illustrate whole and invasive tumour measurements in a variety of circumstances. Foci of lymphatic and blood vascular invasion are not included in the whole tumour measurement.

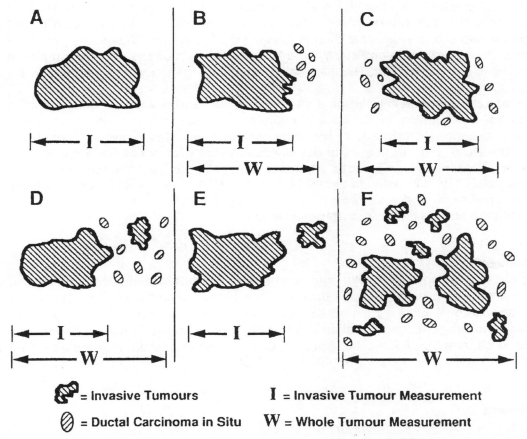

$\text{\raisebox{0pt}{\small\ding{...}}}$ = Invasive Tumours   I = Invasive Tumour Measurement

= Ductal Carcinoma in Situ   W = Whole Tumour Measurement

In E the satellite focus of invasive tumour is not included in the measurement

In F the best estimate of the total size of the invasive components is given

If a carcinoma (either infiltrative or ductal **in situ**) is insufficiently delineated to measure reliably, make an appropriate comment in the 'Comments/additional information' section and give an approximate estimate of the maximum dimension of the area over which the changes extend. It may be necessary to use combined histological, macroscopic and radiological information to make a reliable estimate.

7.3.8.2 Lymph nodes

All lymph nodes should be examined histologically. The use of immunohistology is most appropriate in cases where there is doubt about the presence of small metastases. The clinical relevance of metastases detected solely by this means remains controversial. Please record data from **axillary** nodes separately from nodes from other sites. The presence of extracapsular spread can be noted under 'Comments/additional information'.

7.3.8.3 Excision

For infiltrative tumours, the distance from the nearest resection margin should be recorded and checked from the histological sections. Other margins can be reported if required. This normally refers to the infiltrative component but, if associated ductal carcinoma **in situ** extends nearer to the margin than the infiltrative component, then enter its distance from the margin and state in the 'Comments' section that this measurement refers to the in situ component. The information should be related to orientation markers if used.

For pure ductal carcinoma **in situ**, the distance from the nearest excision margin should be recorded if the lesion is sufficiently delineated. If not, make a comment under 'Comments/additional information'. The presence of non-neoplastic breast parenchyma between the DCIS and the margin is usually associated with adequate excision. The specimen radiograph is also a useful adjunct in assessing surgical clearance. In cases where the adequacy of excision is uncertain, please tick the relevant box and state the reason for uncertainty under 'Comments/additional information'.

See earlier for guidance on macroscopic examination.

7.3.8.4 Grade

Grading can provide powerful prognostic information. It requires some commitment and strict adherence to a recommended protocol. The following protocol is based on that described by Elston & Ellis.[24] The method involves the assessment of three components of tumour morphology: tubule formation, nuclear pleomorphism and frequency of mitoses. Each is scored from 1-3. Adding the scores gives the overall histological grade as shown below.

Tubule formation

1) majority of tumour (greater than 75%)
2) moderate amount (10-75%)
3) little or none (less than 10%)

Nuclear pleomorphism

1) nuclei small, with little increase in size in comparison with normal breast epithelial cells, regular outlines, uniform nuclear chromatin, little variation in size
2) cells larger than normal with open vesicular nuclei, visible nucleoli and moderate variability in both size and shape

3) vesicular nuclei, often with prominent nucleoli, exhibiting marked variation in size and shape, occasionally with very large and bizarre forms

Mitoses

The size of high power fields is very variable and hence it is necessary to standardize the mitotic count using the graph below. In order to determine the mitotic count for an individual microscope, the following procedure should be adopted:

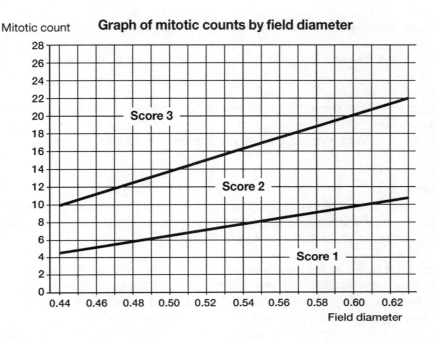

Graph of mitotic counts by field diameter

1) measure the field diameter of the microscope with a graticule
2) plot this value on the horizontal axis of the graph
3) draw a vertical line at this value
4) read off the value **a** on the horizontal axis where the line intersects the lower bold line
5) read off the value **b** on the horizontal axis where the line intersects the upper bold line
6) the count is then

Score	Count
3	>**b**
2	between **a**+1 and b
1	0 to **a**

For example, for a field diameter of 0.48, **a**=6, **b**=12 from the graph - therefore
Score 3 = >12 mitoses/10hpf
Score 2 = 7-12 mitoses/10hpf
Score 1 = 0-6 mitoses/10hpf
This needs to be done only once for each microscope.

Overall grade
The scores for tubule formation, nuclear pleomorphism and mitoses are then added together and assigned to grades as below:
Grade 1 = score 3-5
Grade 2 = score 6-7
Grade 3 = score 8-9

It is recommended that grading is not restricted to invasive carcinoma NST but is undertaken on all histological subtypes. There are two major reasons for this recommendation:
1) there are occasionally problems in deciding whether to classify a tumour as NST or some other type
2) there may be significant variation within certain subtypes, e.g. invasive lobular carcinoma

Tick '**Not assessable**' if for any reason the grade cannot be determined, e.g. specimen poorly preserved or too small.
It must be clearly stated if a grading system other than that described above is used.

7.3.8.5 Disease extent
The term '**localized**' is used to describe a single focus of tumour with defined borderlines of **any size**. It should also be used where the exent of the tumour cannot accurately be defined although all of it appears to be part of a single lesion.

The term '**multiple**' is used to describe multiple foci of **in situ** or infiltrating carcinoma which are widely separated (at least 40 mm) and present in quadrants or segments other than that of the main tumour. 'Multiple' is preferred to 'multifocal' or 'multicentric' as there is currently a lack of agreement on how these terms should be used.
Tick 'Not assessable' if the extent of the disease cannot be determined or if it is not clear whether the tumour is localized or multiple.

7.3.8.6 Vascular invasion
The presence of unequivocal tumour in vascular spaces should be recorded. If there is doubt about diagnosing vascular invasion, please tick the 'Not seen' box. The difficulty in identifying small blood vessels as blood or lymphatic precludes accurate recording of their type and specification of lymphatic or venous invasion is not required. Ideally, a clear rim of endothelium should be identified around the tumour before vascular invasion is recorded. The use of immunostaining for endothelial markers may be helpful in confirming vascular invasion in difficult cases but is not recommended on a routine basis. Morphological features which may be helpful when diagnosing vascular invasion are:
1) clumps of tumour in spaces outside the main tumour mass are more likely to indicate vascular invasion
2) nests of tumour separated from the stroma by shrinkage artefact usually conform better to the shape of the space in which they lie
3) the proximity of larger veins and arteries in the diagnosis of lymphatic invasion
4) the presence within the space of erythrocytes and/or thrombus

7.3.8.7 Oestrogen and progesterone receptor status

Many histopathology laboratories are now required to report oestrogen receptor status by immunohistochemistry. At the time of writing, there is no consensus on scoring methods or cut-off points, which in any case may vary according to the clinical setting. The features usually assessed are staining intensity and percentage of positive cells. In a study undertaken by the Working Group, the latter was reported with greater consistency. The following guidance is offered:

- Recommended fixatives are formal saline or neutral buffered formalin. Fixation should be rapid and even. In order to achieve this, tumours should be sliced immediately and immersed in adequate volumes of fixative.
- Sections should be heated onto slides coated with a suitable strong adhesive (e.g. APES, TESPA).
- Antigen retrieval is necessary and should be adapted to the method and duration of fixation. The following are usually used:
  a) 1-2 minutes in a pressure cooker in 0.01M citrate buffer, pH 6.0 or
  b) properly controlled microwaving
- Only antibodies validated in published work or EQA schemes should be used.
- Surfactants can reduce reactivity so caution is needed with some automated immunostainers.
- A sensitive detection system is needed e.g. ABC, Duet. Consequently, manual staining may be more reliable for cases with low levels of positivity.
- A composite block of tumours with high, low and negative reactivity is recommended. An internal control is normally provided by adjacent normal breast epithelium.
- It is essential to participate in an approved external quality assessment scheme.
- Only nuclear staining of the invasive component is counted.

7.3.8.8 Comments/additional information

Any relevant additional information may be entered here as free text. Please also state if any further special investigations have been undertaken, e.g. steroid hormone receptor determination, oncogene analysis, etc.

7.3.8.9 Histological diagnosis

If normal, tick the normal box and do not complete the rest of the form. 'Normal' includes minimal alterations such as fibrosis and microscopic dilatation of acini or ducts, lobular involution and enlargement and blunt duct adenosis. If malignant and benign changes are found, tick only the malignant box. Tick the benign box when the breast is neither normal nor exhibits malignancy.

7.4 References

1. Snead DRJ, Bell JA, Dixon AR, Nicholson RI, Elston CW, Blamey RW, Ellis IO. Methodology of immunohistological detection of oestrogen receptor in human breast carcinoma in formalin-fixed, paraffin-embedded tissue: a comparison with frozen section methodology. Histopathology 1993; **23**: 233-238.

2. Harvey JM, Clark GM, Osborne CK, Allred DC. Estrogen receptor status by immunohistochemistry is superior to the ligand binding assay for predicting response to adjuvant endocrine therapy in breast cancer. J Clin Oncol 1999; **17**: 1474-1481

3. Anderson TJ. Breast cancer screening: principles and practicalities for histopathologists. Recent Advances in Histopathology No. 14, 43-61, Churchill Livingstone 1989.

4. Armstrong JS, Davies JD. Laboratory handling of impalpable breast lesions: A review. J Clin Pathol 1991; **44**: 89-93.

5. Schnitt SJ, Wang HH. Histologic sampling of grossly benign breast biopsies: how much is enough? Am J Surg Pathol 1989; **13**: 505-512.

6. Gad A. Pathology in breast cancer screening: A 15-year experience from a Swedish programme. In: Breast Cancer Screening in Europe. A. Gad & M. Rosselli Del Turco (eds), Springer-Verlag 1993, 87-101.

7. Frappart L, Boudeulle M, Boumendil J et al. Structure and composition of microcalcifications in benign and malignant lesions of the breast. Human Pathol 1984; **15**: 880-889.

8. Nielsen BB. Adenosis tumour of the breast - a clinicopathological investigation of 27 cases. Histopathology 1987; **11**: 1259-1275.

9. Simpson JF, Page DL, Dupont WD. Apocrine adenosis: a mimic of mammary carcinoma. Surg Pathol 1990; **3**: 289-299.

10. Page DL, Rogers LW. Combined histologic and cytologic criteria for the diagnosis of mammary atypical ductal hyperplasia. Human Pathol 1992; **23**, 1095-1097.

11. Sloane JP, Amendoeira I, Apostolikas N, Bellocq JP, Bianchi S, Boecker W, Bussolati G, Coleman D, Connolly CE, Eusebi V, De Miguel C, Dervan P, Drijkoningen R, Elston CW, Faverly D, Gad A, Jacquemier J, Lacerda M, Martinez-Penuela J, Munt C, Peterse JL, Rank F, Sylvan M, Tsakraklides V, Zafrani B. Consistency achieved by 23 European pathologists from twelve countries in diagnosing breast disease and reporting prognostic features of carcinomas. Virchows Archiv 1999; **434**: 3-10.

12. Dupont WD, Page DL. Risk factors in women with proliferative breast disease. N Engl J Med 1985; **312**: 146-151.

13. Carter CL, Corle DK, Micozzi MS, Schatzkin A, Taylor PR. A prospective study of the development of breast cancer in 16,692 women with benign breast disease. Am J Epidemiol 1988; **128**: 467-77.

14. London SJ, Connolly JL, Schnitt SJ, Colditz G. A prospective study of benign breast disease and the risk of breast cancer. JAMA 1992; **267**: 941-944.

15. McDivitt RW, Stevens JA, Lee NC, Wingo PA, Rubin GL, Gersell D. Histologic types of benign breast disease and the risk for breast cancer. The Cancer and Steroid Hormone Study Group. Cancer 1992; **69**: 1408-1414.

16. Bodian CA, Perzin KH, Lattes R, Hoffman P, Abernathy TG. Prognostic significance of benign proliferative breast disease. Cancer 1993; **71**: 3896-3907.

17. Marshall LM, Hunter DJ, Connolly JL, Schnitt SJ, Byrne C, London SJ, Colditz GA. Risk of breast cancer associated with atypical hyperplasia of lobular and ductal types. Cancer Epidemiology, Biomarkers and Prevention 1997; **6**: 297-301.

18. Tavassoli FA. Ductal carcinoma *in situ*: introduction of the concept of ductal *in situ* neoplasia. Mod Pathol 1998; **11**: 140-154.

19. Böcker W, Bier B, Freytag G, Brömmelkamp B, Jarasch E-D, Edel G, Dockhorn-Dworniczak B, Schmid KW. An immunohistochemical study of the breast using antibodies to basal and luminal keratins, alpha-smooth muscle actin, vimentin, collagen IV and laminin. Part I: normal breast and benign proliferative lesions. Virchows Archiv A Pathol Anat 1992; **421**: 315-322.

20. Lagios MD. Duct carcinoma in situ. Surg Clin N Am 1990; **70**: 853-871.

21. Bellamy COC, McDonald C, Salter DM, Chetty U, Anderson TJ. Noninvasive ductal carcinoma of the breast: the relevance of histologic categorization. Human Pathol 1993; **24**: 16-23.

22. Holland R, Peterse JL, Millis RR, Eusebi V, Faverly D, van de Vijver MJ, Zafrani B. Ductal carcinoma in situ: a proposal for a new classification. Semin Diagn Pathol 1994; **11**: 167-180.

23. Page DL, Anderson TJ. Diagnostic Histopathology of the Breast, 1987, pp. 193-268. Churchill Livingstone, Edinburgh, London, Melbourne and New York.

24. Ellis IO, Galea M, Broughton N, Locker A, Blamey RW, Elston CW. Pathological prognostic factors in breast cancer. II. Histological type. Relationship with survival in a large study with long term follow-up. Histopathology 1992; **20**: 479-489.

25. Martinez V, Azzopardi JG. Invasive lobular carcinoma of the breast: incidence and variants. Histopathology 1979; **3**: 467-488.

26. Fechner RE. Histologic variants of infiltrating lobular carcinoma of the breast. Human Pathol 1975; **6**: 373-378.

27. Fisher ER, Gregorio RM, Redmond C, Fisher B. Tubulolobular invasive breast cancer: a variant of lobular invasive cancer. Human Pathol 1977; **8**: 679-683.

28. Fisher ER, Gregorio RM, Fisher B, Redmond C, Vellios F, Sommers SC and co-operating investigators. The pathology of invasive breast cancer: a syllabus derived from findings of the National Surgical Adjuvant Breast Project (Protocol No 4). Cancer 1975; **36**: 1-84.

29. Ridolfi RL, Rosen PP, Port A, Kinne D, Mike V. Medullary carcinoma of the breast: a clinicopathologic study with 10-year follow-up. Cancer 1977; **40**: 1365-1385.

30. Parl FF, Richardson LD. The histological and biological spectrum of tubular carcinoma of the breast. Human Pathol 1983; **14**: 694-698.

31. Elston CW, Ellis IO. Pathological prognostic factors in breast cancer. I. The value of histological grade in breast cancer: experience from a large study with long term follow up. Histopathology 1991; **19**: 403-410.

Appendix 1
Criteria for accrediting breast histopathology external quality assessment schemes in the European Union

1. The scheme should be educational. This is derived not only from the content of cases but also from feedback of other participants' diagnoses and from regional, national or international organising committees. This feedback, which may also include supplementary information such as lists of references, should allow individual participants to identify problems in their own performance.

2. Circulated cases on which individual or collective performance is assessed must be typical of routine practice and not rarities more suited to slide seminars. The latter can, however, be included for purely educational value.

3. To maximise the educational feedback to the individual, conferring with colleagues should not be permitted.

4. Responses must be assessed in a way that generates a numeric score for each response to each case. The method adopted must be clearly defined, understood and accepted by all participants.

5. Clear definitions of acceptable standards of performance are necessary. Schemes should have written operating procedures which are made available to all participants.

6. A scoring method to assess the level of consistency achieved by participants (e.g. kappa statistics) should be employed.

7. Confidentiality must be ensured.

8. Participants should have a defined complaints procedure if they are dissatisfied with the operation of the scheme.

9. Substandard performance in an EQA scheme can have many causes so it must not be assumed to equate to substandard work in routine practice unless there is other evidence. Conversely, good EQA performance cannot guarantee good routine work, so other audit measures are also necessary.

Appendix 2
Membership of working group

Chairman: **Prof. J.P. Sloane†,** Department of Pathology, University of Liverpool, Duncan Building, Daulby Street, Liverpool L69 3GA, United Kingdom

Dr. I. Amendoeira, Department of Pathology, Instituto de Patologia & Imunologia Molecular, da Universidade do Porto, Rua Roberto Frias s/n, 4200 Porto, Portugal

Dr. N. Apostolikas, Department of Pathology, Saint Savvas Hospital, 171 Alexandras Avenue, 115 22 Athens, Greece

Professor J.P. Bellocq, Service d'Anatomie Pathologique, Hopital de Hautepierre, Avenue Moliere, F-67098, Strasbourg cedex, France

Professor. S. Bianchi, Istituto di Anatomia e Istologia Patologica, Azienda Ospedaliera, Careggi, V. le Morgagni, 85, 50134 Firenze, Italy

Prof. Dr. med. W. Boecker, Gerhard-Domagk Institut fur Pathologie, Universitat et Munster, Domagkstr. 17, D-48129 Munster, Germany

Professor G. Bussolati, Istituto di Anatomia e Istologia Patologica, Via Santena 7, Torino, Italy

Professor C.E. Connolly, Department of Pathology, Clinical Sciences Institute, University College Hospital, Costello Road, Galway, Ireland

Professor P. Dervan, Pathology Department, Mater Hospital, Eccles Street, Dublin 7, Ireland

Professor M. Drijkoningen, Pathologische Ontleedkunde, University Hospital, Minderbroedersstr. 12, 3000 Leuven, Belgium

Dr. I.O. Ellis, Department of Histopathology, City Hospital, Hucknall Road, Nottingham. NG5 1PB, United Kingdom

Professor C.W. Elston, Department of Histopathology, City Hospital, Hucknall Road, Nottingham NG5 1PB, United Kingdom

Professor V. Eusebi, Sezione Anatomia Patologica M. Malpigni, Universita di Bologna, Ospedale Bellaria, Via Altura 3, 40139 Bologna, Italy

Dr. D. Faverly, CMP Laboratory, Av. Wybran, 45a, 1070 Bruxelles, Belgium

Dr. P. Heikkila, Haartman Institute, University of Helsinki, P.O. Box 21 FIN 00014, Helsinki, Finland

Professor R. Holland, National Expert & Training Centre for Breast Cancer Screening, Academisch Ziekenhuis Nijmegen, Geert Grooteplein 18, Postbus 9101, 6500 HB Nijmegen, The Netherlands

Dr. J. Jacquemier, Institut Paoli Calmettes, 232 Bd. Sainte Marguerite, 13273 Marseille cedex 9, France

Dr. M. Lacerda, Laboratorio De Histopatologica, Centro Regional De Oncologia De Coimbra, DO I.P.O.F.G., Avenida Bissaia Barreto, 3000 Coimbra, Portugal

Dr. J. Martinez-Penuela, Department of Pathology, Hospital de Navarra, Irunlarrea 3, 31008 Pamplona, Spain

Dr. C. De Miguel, Department of Pathology, Hospital Virgen del Camino, 31008 Pamplona, Spain

Dr. J.L. Peterse, Department of Pathology, The Netherlands Cancer Institute, Antoni van Leeuwenhoekziekenhuis, Plesmanlaan 121, 1066 CX Amsterdam, The Netherlands

Dr. F. Rank, Center of Laboratory Medicine and Pathology, Department of Pathology, Rigshospitalet, Copenhagen University Hospital, Blegdamsvej 9, 2100 Copenhagen, Denmark

Professor A. Reiner, Institute of Pathology, Donauspital, Langobardenstrasse 122, A-1220 Wien, Austria

Professor Eero Saksela, Haartman Institute, University of Helsinki, P.O. Box 21, FIN 00014, Helsinki, Finland

Dr. M. Sylvan, Department of Clinical Pathology & Cytology, F49 Huddinge University Hospital, S-141 86 Huddinge, Stockholm, Sweden

Dr. V. Tsakraklides, Department of Pathology, Hygeia Hospital, Vas. Logothetidi 15, Athens 11524, Greece

Dr. C.A. Wells, Department of Histopathology, St. Bartholomew's Hospital Medical School, West Smithfield, London EC1A 7BE, United Kingdom

Dr. B. Zafrani, Institut Curie, Section Medicale et Hospitaliere, 26 Rue d'Ulm, 75231 Paris cedex 05, France

7

Index
for screening office pathology system

Term	Place to classify on form
A	
Abscess	Other benign pathology (specify)
Adenocarcinoma (no special type)	Invasive ductal NST
Adenoid cystic carcinoma	Other primary carcinoma (specify)
Adenoma, apocrine	Other benign pathology (specify)
Adenoma intraduct	Enter as papilloma
Adenoma of nipple	Other benign pathology (specify)
Adenoma, pleomorphic	Other benign pathology (specify)
Adenoma, tubular	Fibroadenoma
'Adenomyoepithelioma'	Other primary carcinoma (specify) or Other benign pathology (specify)
Adenosis, NOS	Histology normal
Adenosis, apocrine	Other benign pathology (specify)
Adenosis, apocrine with atypia	Other benign pathology (specify) Epithelial proliferation-atypia (ductal)
Adenosis, blunt duct	Histology normal
Adenosis, microglandular	Other benign pathology (specify)
Adenosis, sclerosing with atypia	Sclerosing adenosis Epithelial proliferation atypia ductal or lobular
Adnexal tumours	Other benign pathology (specify)
Alveolar variant of lobular carcinoma	Invasive lobular
Aneurysm	Other benign pathology (specify)
Angiosarcoma	Other malignant tumour (specify)
Apocrine adenoma	Other benign pathology (specify)
Apocrine adenosis	Other benign pathology (specify)
Apocrine carcinoma (in situ)	Non-invasive malignant, ductal (specify type)
Apocrine carcinoma (invasive)	Other primary carcinoma (if pure) or ductal NST
Apocrine metaplasia multilayered/papillary	Fibrocystic change Epithelial proliferation present
Argyrophil carcinoma	Other primary carcinoma (specify)
Arteritis	Other benign pathology (specify)
Atypical blunt duct adenosis	Fibrocystic change Epithelial proliferation-atypia (ductal)
Atypical ductal hyperplasia	Epithelial proliferation-atypia (ductal)
Atypical epitheliosis (ductal)	Epithelial proliferation-atypia
Atypical lobular hyperplasia	Epithelial proliferation-atypia (lobular)
B	
B-cell lymphoma	Other malignant tumour (specify)
Benign phyllodes tumour	Other benign pathology (specify)
Blunt duct adenosis	Histology normal
Blunt duct adenosis (atypical)	Epithelial proliferation-atypia (ductal)
Breast abscess	Other benign pathology (specify)

Term	Place to classify on form
C	
Calcification (benign)	Calcification present, benign
Calcification (malignant)	Calcification present, malignant
Carcinoma, apocrine (in situ)	Non-invasive malignant, ductal (specify type)
Carcinoma, apocrine (invasive)	Other primary carcinoma (if pure) or ductal NST
Carcinoma, clear cell	Other primary carcinoma (specify)
Carcinoma, colloid	Invasive mucinous carcinoma
Carcinoma, comedo-in situ	Non-invasive malignant, ductal (specify type)
Carcinoma, cribriform (in situ)	Non-invasive malignant, ductal (specify type)
Carcinoma, cribriform (invasive)	Invasive tubular or cribriform
Carcinoma, ductal in situ	Non-invasive malignant, ductal (specify sub-type)
Carcinoma, lobular in situ	Non-invasive malignant, lobular
Carcinoma, lobular (invasive)	Invasive lobular
Carcinoma, lobular variant	Invasive lobular
Carcinoma, medullary	Invasive medullary
Carcinoma, metastatic	Other malignant tumour (specify)
Carcinoma, mixed	Other primary carcinoma (specify types)
Carcinoma, mucinous	Invasive mucinous carcinoma
Carcinoma, papillary	Other primary carcinoma (specify)
Carcinoma, signet ring	Other primary carcinoma (specify)
Carcinoma, spindle cell	Other primary carcinoma (specify)
Carcinoma, squamous	Other primary carcinoma (specify)
Carcinosarcoma	Other primary carcinoma (specify)
Cellular fibroadenoma	Fibroadenoma
Clear cell carcinoma	Other primary carcinoma (specify)
Clear cell hidradenoma	Other benign pathology (specify)
Clear cell metaplasia	Other benign pathology (specify)
Collagenous spherulosis	Other benign pathology (specify)
Comedocarcinoma	Non-invasive malignant, ductal
Comedocarcinoma invasive	Invasive ductal NST
Complex sclerosing lesion	Complex sclerosing lesion/radial scar
Cribriform carcinoma (in situ)	Non-invasive malignant, ductal (specify type)
Cribriform carcinoma (invasive)	Invasive tubular or cribriform
Cyclical menstrual changes	Histology normal
Cyst, epidermoid	Other benign pathology (specify)
Cyst, single	Solitary cyst
Cyst, multiple	Fibrocystic change
Cystic disease	Enter components
Cystic mastopathia	Enter components
Cystic hypersecretory hyperplasia	Other benign pathology (specify)
Cystic hypersecretory carcinoma	Non-invasive malignant, ductal
D	
Ductal carcinoma in situ	Non-invasive malignant, ductal
Ductal carcinoma invasive	Invasive ductal NST
Ductal hyperplasia (regular)	Epithelial proliferation present without atypia

Term	Place to classify on form
Ductal hyperplasia (atypical)	Epithelial proliferation, atypical (ductal)
Duct ectasia	Periductal mastitis/duct ectasia
Duct papilloma	Papilloma, single
Dysplasia, mammary	Enter components

E

Eccrine tumours	Other benign pathology (specify)
Epidermoid cyst	Other benign pathology (specify)
Epitheliosis (regular)	Epithelial proliferation present without atypia
Epitheliosis (atypical)	Epithelial proliferation, atypical (ductal)
Epitheliosis (infiltrating)	Complex sclerosing lesion/radial scar

F

Fat necrosis	Other benign pathology (specify)
Fibroadenoma	Fibroadenoma
Fibroadenoma, giant	Fibroadenoma
Fibroadenoma, juvenile	Fibroadenoma
Fibrocystic disease	Enter components
Fibromatosis	Other benign pathology (specify)
Fistula, mammillary	Other benign pathology (specify)
Focal lactational change	Histology normal
Foreign body reaction	Other benign pathology (specify)

G

Galactocoele	Other benign pathology (specify)
Giant fibroadenoma	Fibroadenoma
Glycogen-rich carcinoma	Other primary carcinoma (specify)
Grading of carcinomas	See 7.3.5
Granulomatous mastitis	Other benign pathology (specify)

H

Haematoma	Other benign pathology (specify)
Haemangioma	Other benign pathology (specify)
Hamartoma	Other benign pathology (specify)
Hyaline epithelial inclusions	Other benign pathology (specify)
Hyperplasia, ductal (regular)	Epithelial proliferation present without atypia
Hyperplasia, ductal (atypical)	Epithelial proliferation-atypia (ductal)
Hyperplasia, lobular (= adenosis)	Histology normal
Hyperplasia, lobular (atypical)	Epithelial proliferation-atypia (lobular)

I

Infarct	Other benign pathology (specify)
'Inflammatory carcinoma'	Specify by type (usually ductal NST)
Invasive carcinoma	Specify by type
Invasive comedocarcinoma	Invasive ductal NST
Invasive cribriform carcinoma	Invasive tubular or cribriform
Involution	Histology normal

Term	Place to classify on form
J	
Juvenile fibroadenoma	Fibroadenoma
Juvenile papillomatosis	Other benign pathology (specify)
L	
Lactation	Histology normal
Lactational change, focal	Histology normal
Lipoma	Other benign pathology (specify)
Lipid-rich carcinoma	Other primary carcinoma (specify)
Lobular carcinoma in situ	Non-invasive malignant, lobular
Lobular carcinoma invasive	Invasive lobular
Lobular hyperplasia (= adenosis)	Histology normal
Lobular hyperplasia (atypical)	Epithelial proliferation-atypia (lobular)
Lymphoma	Other malignant tumour (specify)
M	
Malignant phyllodes tumour	Other malignant tumour (specify)
Mammary duct ectasia	Periductal mastitis/duct ectasia
Mammillary fistula	Other benign pathology (specify)
Mastitis, acute	Other benign pathology (specify)
Mastitis, granulomatous	Other benign pathology (specify)
Mastitis, plasma cell	Periductal mastitis/duct ectasia
Mastopathia, cystic	Enter components
Medullary carcinoma	Invasive medullary
Menopausal changes	Histology normal
Metaplasia, apocrine (single layer)	Fibrocystic change
Metaplasia, apocrine multilayered/papillary	Fibrocystic change / Epithelial proliferation present
Metaplasia, clear cell	Other benign pathology (specify)
Metaplasia, mucoid	Other benign pathology (specify)
Metaplasia, squamous	Other benign pathology (specify)
Metastatic lesion	Other malignant tumour (specify)
Microcysts	Histology normal
Microglandular adenosis	Other benign pathology (specify)
Microinvasive carcinoma	Code by in situ component and specify microinvasion present
Micropapillary change	Epithelial proliferation present
Mixed carcinoma	Other primary carcinoma (specify types)
Mondar's disease	Other benign pathology (specify)
Mucinous carcinoma	Invasive mucinous carcinoma
Mucoele-like lesion	Other benign pathology (specify)
Mucoid metaplasia	Other benign pathology (specify)
Multiple papilloma syndrome	Papilloma, multiple
Multiple papilloma syndrome with atypia	Papilloma, multiple / Epithelial proliferation-atypia (ductal)
Myoepithelial hyperplasia	Other benign pathology (specify)

Term	Place to classify on form
N	
Necrosis, fat	Other benign pathology (specify)
Nipple adenoma	Other benign pathology (specify)
Nipple - Paget's disease	Non-invasive malignant Paget's disease
Normal breast	Histology normal
P	
Paget's disease of nipple Non-invasive malignant, Paget's disease	Non-invasive malignant, Paget's disease
Panniculitis	Other benign pathology (specify)
Papillary carcinoma (in situ)	Non-invasive malignant, ductal (specify type)
Papillary carcinoma (invasive)	Other primary carcinoma (specify)
Papilloma, duct	Papilloma
Papillomatosis	Epithelial proliferation (with or without atypia)
Papillomatosis, juvenile	Other benign pathology (specify)
Papillomatosis, sclerosing	Other benign pathology (specify)
Phyllodes tumour (low grade)	Other benign pathology (specify)
Phyllodes tumour (high grade)	Other malignant tumour (specify)
Pregnancy changes	Histology normal
R	
Radial scar	Complex sclerosing lesion/radial scar
Regular hyperplasia	Epithelial proliferation present without atypia
S	
Sarcoidosis	Other benign pathology (specify)
Sarcoma	Other malignant tumour (specify)
Sclerosing adenosis	Sclerosing adenosis
Sclerosing adenosis	Sclerosing adenosis
with atypia	Epithelial proliferation-atypia
Sclerosing subareolar proliferation	Specify under other benign pathology as adenoma of nipple
Squamous carcinoma	Invasive malignant, other (specify)
Squamous metaplasia	Other benign pathology (specify)
Spindle cell carcinoma	Invasive malignant, other (specify)
Scar, radial	Complex sclerosing lesion/radial scar
T	
Trauma	Other benign pathology (specify)
Tuberculosis	Other benign pathology (specify)
Tubular adenoma	Fibrodenoma
Tubular carcinoma	Invasive malignant, tubular or cribriform
W	
Wegener's granulomatosis	Other benign pathology (specify)

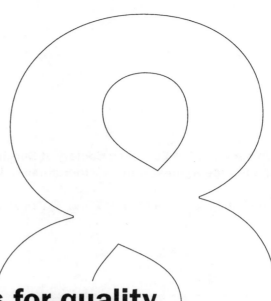

European guidelines for quality assurance in the surgical management of mammographically detected lesions

Authors
N. O'Higgins
D. Linos
M. Blichert-Toft
L. Cataliotti
C. de Wolf
F. Rochard
E. Rutgers
P. Roberts
W. Mattheiem
M. da Silva
L. Holmberg
K. Schulz
M. Smola
R. Mansel

**On behalf of the European Society of Surgical Oncology and
the Europe Against Cancer Programme of the European Commission**

Previously published in Eur J Surg Oncol 1998;24 (2):96-98

Preface

European Guidelines developed for mammography screening have contributed to the general discussion on quality assurance and on the important tasks of the health professionals dealing with breast cancer screening. The cooperation of each medical discipline is of utmost importance in order to achieve optimal results and eventually a mortality reduction. These guidelines are based on the British NHS quality assurance guidelines for surgeons in breast cancer screening. They are based on several meetings held during 1997 under the auspices and with the support of the Europe Against Cancer Programme of the European Commission and with the support and participation of representatives of the European Society of Surgical Oncology and the national surgical oncology groups in Europe.

8.1 Introduction

Mortality reduction for breast cancer is the ultimate endpoint of any screening programme. To meet this endpoint, it is essential that all elements of the screening service achieve and maintain high levels of quality if it is to be of significant benefit to women. The screening process can only be successful if followed by timely and appropriate management by surgeons.

These guidelines for surgeons are set out to identify outcome measures and targets, to suggest a framework for surgical quality assurance and to put forward ways in which the quality of performance of each surgical unit can be measured. They specify the delivery of surgical service and not the type of treatment. The choice of treatment remains within the competence of the surgical discipline and the jurisdiction of each centre. The delivery of service safeguards the rights of the patient to have adequate management and proficient follow up of her screen-detected breast lesion.

Some of the general quality assurance objectives and standards lie outside the influence of the surgeon alone, but the surgeon is a member of the multidisciplinary breast screening team responsible for achieving these objectives. The quality assurance standards achieved should be monitored by the responsible surgeon and one surgeon should be responsible for quality assurance audit in his/her centre.

These guidelines should be reviewed in three years time and modified in the light of new knowledge. The service should be consultant based. Assessment clinics and specialist operations e.g. marker guided biopsy, should not be delegated to unsupervised trainees.

The surgeon must have sufficient identified operating times for cases arising from the screening programme. This time depends on the population covered but should be at least one operating list per week for a screening population of 41,000. The surgeon should have access to cytology/histopathology services which conform to established quality assurance guidelines.

The surgeon should work with radiologists who can accurately localise lesions pre-operatively and who can carry out such diagnostic procedures on impalpable lesions which conform to established quality assurance guidelines.

8.2 General performance of a unit

The surgeon is a member of a multidisciplinary team. He/she expects the availability and close communication with professionals with specialist knowledge in imaging techniques, pathology, radiotherapy, medical oncology, specialist nursing and counselling. Conversely, the patients and the other members of the team expect specialist knowledge in the surgical management of screen-detected lesions from the surgeon. Regular multidisciplinary review meetings involving surgeons, radiologists and pathologists are essential for audit and represent a fundamental part of quality assurance guidelines for all disciplines involved in the screening process.

The desirable number of women accepting the invitation to be screened initially (prevalent round) should be more than 70%.

The desirable number of women recalled for further investigations (recall rate) should be less than 5% at the initial (prevalent) screening and less than 3% at the subsequent (incident) screening.

The interval from the screening mammogram to assessment should be minimised so that 90% of patients attend an assessment centre within one week of the decision that further investigation is necessary, and within three weeks of attendance for the screening mammogram.

Because of wide variations in breast cancer incidence among regions it is more appropriate to quote ratios rather than absolute numbers. The number of cancers detected at the initial (prevalent) screen should be at least 3 times the expected incidence rate in the absence of a screening programme and at the subsequent (incident) visit should be at least 1.5 times the expected incidence rate in the absence of screening, excluding ductal carcinoma in situ (DCIS) in both instances. It is expected that at subsequent visits the screening incidence rate should approach the incidence rate without screening.

The number of small (less than 15 mm in diameter) invasive cancers should be at a minimum of 50% of invasive cancers detected at screening.

The surgeon should be fully involved in the assessment of screen-detected cancers and he/she should always see the patient before accepting her for surgery. No more than one week should elapse between the first recall appointment and an appointment for surgical assessment.

8.3 Surgical diagnosis

The majority (more than 70%) of both palpable and impalpable cancers should receive a pre-operative diagnosis by fine needle cytology or core needle histology. Core needle histology can provide information about tumour invasiveness and grade in addition to other biological features, such as receptor status.

Unnecessary invasive procedures should be minimised. For open surgical biopsies the ratio of benign to malignant should not exceed 2 to 1 at the initial (prevalent) screening or 1 to 1 at the subsequent (incident) screening.

The operative identification (i.e. successful removal) of lesions producing mammographic abnormalities should be successful in more than 95% of impalpable lesions at the first localisation biopsy operation.

The correct identification and removal of the radiological lesion must be confirmed by the presence of the lesion on the specimen radiography. Preferably this procedure is carried out by the staff of the radiological department, so that the radiologist can determine whether the relevant lesion has been excised. The time between excision and the receipt of the specimen X-ray or report in the operating theatre should not exceed 10 minutes. There will be a few occasions when the mammographic abnormality cannot be identified in the specimen. This may result from the excision of a lesion producing only change in the clinical mammogram or from unsuccessful surgical localisation. Detailed pathological examination, including radiology of the sliced specimen, should still be undertaken and the findings communicated to the surgeon.

Clinical mammography must subsequently be repeated to determine if the lesion is still present in the breast.

When localisation biopsy is carried out, the positioning of marker wires or dye tracers should be within 10 mm of the lesion in any plane in at least 80% of cases.

Frozen sectioning is generally inappropriate in the assessment of clinically impalpable lesions. Rarely, however, it may be justified to enable a firm diagnosis of invasive carcinoma to be made in order to allow definitive surgery to be carried out in one operation. Three essential criteria, however, must be fulfilled:

1. The mammographic abnormality must be clearly and unequivocally identified on macroscopic examination.

2. It must be large enough (generally at least 10 mm) to allow an adequate proportion of the lesion to be fixed and processed without prior freezing.

3. It must have proved impossible to make a definitive diagnosis pre-operatively.

Palpable lesions detected in the screening programme may be dealt with by conventional methods and there is no need for specimen radiography, assuming that there is no doubt that the radiological and palpable lesions are one and the same.

The surgeon should be discouraged from cutting the specimen open after removal before sending it to the pathologist. The specimen should be marked according to local protocols.

The interval from the surgeon's decision to operate for diagnostic purposes and the first offered admission date should be minimised. Waiting time for operation should not exceed two weeks in 90% of patients in order to reduce patient anxiety.

To minimise the adverse cosmetic effects of operative biopsies carried out for diagnostic (not therapeutic) purposes placement and length of the incision should be considered. Eighty per cent of those biopsies which prove benign should weigh less than 30 grams fresh or fixed weight. It is recommended that the surgeon ensure that the weight is recorded.

8.4 Management

The surgical treatment of screen-detected cancers should follow the same guidelines for treating symptomatic breast cancer, that is total removal of the malignant lesion with clear margins*.

All surgeons involved in the treatment of screen-detected cancers must be aware that different treatment options are available for each woman, so that overtreatment or undertreatment is avoided. Breast conserving surgery is the treatment of choice for the majority of small sized screen-detected cancers.

Every woman should receive information on treatment options (breast conserving surgery versus total mastectomy). The patient, where appropriate, should be offered a choice of treatment, including immediate or delayed breast reconstruction. She may also be offered allocation of treatment within a clinical trial. A specialist breast care nurse should be present when the diagnosis of cancer is given to assist in the discussion and interpretation of the treatment options presented by the surgeon.

The surgeon should ensure completeness of excision. Specimens must be orientated by the surgeon and histological examination of the margins which could be done by frozen section should be made. Intra-operative assessment of margins may be improved by the use of two-plane specimen radiography. Surgeons should be aware of the histology report regarding the margins and if necessary re-excise the clear margins.

The number of repeat operations for therapeutic purposes should be minimised so that less than 10% of operations carried out with a proven pre-operative or intra-operative diagnosis of cancer (in situ and invasive) require a further operation for incomplete excision.

Information derived from the histopathological examination of the axillary lymph nodes is important for defining prognosis and further treatment selection for invasive tumours. The

---

* Radiologists involved in drawing up European Guidelines for Quality Assurance in Mammography Screening have pointed out that surgeons should be encouraged to carry out pre-operative mammography on all non-screen-detected cancers. This practice will reduce substantially the number of unclassifiable cases at interval cancer review meetings.

only method of evaluating lymph nodes with complete accuracy at the present time is histological examination of removed nodes. The surgeon should be aware of the likelihood of axillary nodal involvement, even with relatively small primary tumours. The most accurate information about axillary lymph nodes can be obtained by complete axillary dissection.

When breast conserving surgery is selected, radiation therapy to the conserved breast is indicated for most invasive tumours. Systemic treatment should be considered for all patients with factors indicating poor prognosis.

The appropriate treatment of ductal carcinoma in situ (DCIS) must be ensured. In this context, a local excision is not considered appropriate for extensive, multicentric or high grade DCIS lesions which cannot be excised with clear margins and cosmetically acceptable results. Axillary dissection is contraindicated after surgical excision. Radiotherapy to the breast may be given although its role in this situation is less clear than for invasive tumour.
The appropriate treatment of lobular carcinoma in situ (LCIS) must be ensured. The need for careful surveillance rather than further surgical intervention must be recognised.

Because of the uncertainty concerning the role of adjuvant therapy for in situ tumours surgeons should encourage women to participate in clinical trials for the treatment of screen-detected carcinoma in situ.

The interval from a surgical decision to operate for therapeutic purposes (i.e. where there is a pre-operative definitive diagnosis of cancer) and the first offered admission date should be minimised so that 90% of patients should be offered surgical treatment within three weeks of informing the patients who need surgical management.

8.5 Follow up

Adequate follow up of screen-detected cancers must be ensured, so that all women diagnosed with cancer and appropriately treated should be examined at least at annual intervals. The surgeon, as an active member of the screening unit, should be involved in the follow up process. Each screening centre must nominate a surgeon responsible for recording of the audit procedures for breast cancer screening, treatment and outcome, to generate reports on these issues and to report annually on results to the National Breast Cancer Screening Committee. The surgeon must be given clerical help as the collection of this data is mandatory. Mammography of the treated and/or contralateral breast to a radiological standard equivalent to that performed within the screening programme should be included.

Extensive laboratory investigation, including multiple tumour markers, is not necessary for asymptomatic patients.

Follow up should be audited according to an agreed standard.

8.6 Training

The management of cases coming to surgery from the screening programme should be carried out only by surgeons who have acquired the necessary specialist knowledge. The surgeon involved in breast screening should receive approved multidisciplinary training, including courses in communication and counselling.

8.7 References

1. European Guidelines for Quality Assurance in Mammography Screening-Second Edition. Editors: Dr. C.J.M. de Wolf and Dr. N.M. Perry, Luxembourg: Office for Official Publications of the European Communities, 1996.

2. Quality Assurance Guidelines for Surgeons in Breast Cancer Screening. NHSBSP Publication No. 20 (United Kingdom), 1996.

3. Guidelines for Surgeons in the Management of Symptomatic Breast Disease in the United Kingdom. European Journal of Surgical Oncology 1995;21 (Suppl.A):1-13.

4. Quality Indicators of Diagnosis, Treatment and Follow-Up in Breast Cancer Screening. EC Project 95/45303.

5. International Consensus Panel on the Treatment of Primary Breast Cancer. European Journal of Cancer 1995;31A (11):1754-1759.

6. Management of Non-palpable and Small Lesions Found in Mass Breast Screening. European School of Oncology. Commission of the European Communities - Europe Against Cancer Programme, September, 1992.

7. The Management of Early Breast Cancer. National Health and Medical Research Council (Australia), October 1995.

8. Irish Guidelines for Surgeons in the Management of Breast Cancer. Irish Medical Journal 1997;90:6-10.

9. Principles and Guidelines for Surgeons on Management of Symptomatic Breast Cancer. On behalf of the European Society of Surgical Oncology. European Journal of Surgical Oncology 1997;23:101-109.

10. Breast Cancer. Manual of Surgical Oncology of the Austrian Society of Surgical Oncology. Editors: M.G. Smola and M. Stierer; Springer Verlag, 1998; Wien - New York.

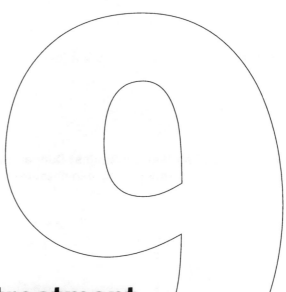

Data collection on treatment of screen-detected lesions

Authors
A. Ponti
N. Segnan
R. Blamey
R. Bordon
L. Cataliotti
M. Codd
V. Distante
D. Giorgi
T. Gorey
A. Linos
D. Linos
M. Mano
R. Sainsbury

Produced by **The 'Europe Against Cancer' project Working Group on monitoring surgical treatment of screen-detected breast cancer**

9.1 Background and aims

According to the 'Florence Statement on Breast Cancer' (1998) (1) 'quality assurance programmes should become mandatory for breast cancer services to qualify for funding from healthcare providers'. The surgical guidelines that precede this chapter make clear that the collection of data for auditing surgical treatment is mandatory for screening programmes and that a nominated surgeon should be given adequate resources and made responsible for the audit procedures. In the 2nd edition of the European Guidelines for Quality Assurance in Mammography Screening (1996) (2) for the first time a section, in the epidemiology chapter, dealt with data collection on treatment, suggesting a number of tables to be filled by screening programmes with grouped data. Since then a project sponsored by the European Commission within the 'Europe Against Cancer' (EAC) Breast Cancer Screening Network acquired experience in collecting individual data on treatment and produced a computerised audit system (Q.T.) on the management of screen-detected breast cancer. Even before, considerable and seminal work had been conducted in the United Kingdom, within the National Screening Programme (3) and the British Association of Surgical Oncology (BASO) (4), in devising surgical outcome measures that could be monitored on individual patients. One of the results of this work is another computer system, the BASO Breast Unit Database. The EAC study had the opportunity to cooperate with this experience with reciprocal advantage.

The aim of this section is to suggest how recommendations included in the European surgical guidelines can be monitored in practice by using relevant outcome measures and adopting one of the available audit systems. Based on the data collection experience of the Working Group, a minimum set of quality indicators for which monitoring has been proved feasible is included here.

9.2 Main available computerised audit systems on surgical treatment of breast cancer

The software named Q.T. (Audit System on Quality of Breast Cancer Treatment) was first issued in October 1995 and is available in English and Italian. Q.T. is designed to facilitate monitoring of screen-detected and clinical breast cancer diagnosis, treatment and follow up and allows users to easily analyse their own data and produce reports on about 40 quality outcome measures of treatment and several of the early indicators of effectiveness of breast cancer screening. A useful feature of this programme is the availability in the same package of data entry and data analysis facilities, ranging from free analysis with use of the main statistical procedures to the production of several standard reports. This audit system has been developed by a multidisciplinary team from the Italian Breast Cancer Screening Network, or *Gruppo Italiano per lo Screening Mammografico* (GISMa) and from the EAC Breast Screening Network.

The BASO Breast Unit Database v2 (copyright 1999 Clin IT, NHS Executive Northwest) 'is an attempt to work towards a common data set within the area of the management of symptomatic breast disease, providing a system to audit the BASO Guidelines for Surgeons in the Management of Symptomatic Breast Disease in the United Kingdom'. 25 reports are available to users to monitor the BASO guidelines. Moreover, the programme contains many patient management data items, enabling the production of additional reports (survival analysis, administration reports, patient lists) and the printing of letters, forms and patient referrals details.[1]

Both databases have been designed taking into account the fact that each patient can have more than one breast lesion diagnosed. All items in the data sets are associated with a specific lesion, and analyses can be performed by patient or by lesion. Both programmes can be customised, and can be used freely as they are not licensed. Registration is, however, required and *Microsoft Access* and *Epi Info* are not supplied with the programmes. Use of Q.T. is encouraged, as it has been produced with funding by the European Commission with specific reference to screen-detected lesions.

9.3 The data set

To allow uniform and precise monitoring of surgical treatment, it is necessary for data items to be defined and coded consistently. The list in appendix 1 includes data items used by the Q.T. Audit System to produce the minimum set of 12 surgical outcome measures described in the next paragraph. The other chapters in this document carry precise definitions of items of radiological, pathological and epidemiological interest. Many of these items are included in Q.T. and have been defined and coded accordingly.

9.4 Monitoring a minimum set of outcome measures from the European surgical guidelines

This section lists in table 1 the main performance parameters needed to monitor the application of the European surgical guidelines. Q.T. calculates each of the 12 indicators according to its operational definition, also included in the table. Only reports based on individual patient information are included. A specific report is not available for all indicators in the BASO database, as it has been designed for symptomatic breast cancer. This does not mean necessarily that such information cannot be derived from the database. Indicators about the general performance of a screening unit and about completeness of pathological data, described in other chapters of the European guidelines, are excluded. Reference to three national guidelines is also provided, with the suggested numerical target for each indicator. These are the Italian Guidelines from the GISMa and FONCaM[2] groups

---

[1] Members of the BASO Breast Unit Database team are H. Forbes (Clin IT Manager), M. Dowler, D. Jones, B. Callaghan, W. Smith and S. Still. The BASO Breast Unit Database v2 is a Microsoft Access Database produced by the Clinical Information Team, Clatterbridge Centre for Oncology, Bebington, Wirral L63 4JY, United Kingdom.

[2] FONCaM: Forza Operativa Nazionale sul Carcinoma Mammario, a national working group on breast cancer.

---

(5), the Guidelines for Surgical Units working within the National Health Service Breast Screening Programme (NHSBSP) in United Kingdom (3), and the Guidelines on Symptomatic Breast Cancer by the BASO Breast Surgeons Group (4). In any guideline, it is stated if no recommendation is given, while the expression 'no target specified' means that the recommendation does not include a numerical standard. As for the European guidelines, a target has been given or is suggested for all indicators in the minimum set. For the sake of simplicity, all targets are expressed as 'more than or equal to' the given standard.

Indicators have been devised keeping in mind the following ultimate outcomes:
1. Minimise mortality from breast cancer
2. Improve quality of life, or
   - minimise anxiety
   - minimise complications
   - minimise recurrences
   - minimise cosmetic disadvantages

According to the classical distinction proposed by Donabedian (6) three dimensions of quality can be measured: structure, process and outcome. Most of the performance parameters in the minimum set pertain to the domain of process. Some of those available from the audit systems relate to structure (patient seen by a trained breast surgeon, access to a specialist breast nurse) or directly measure outcomes (minimise recurrences and complications, improve survival). Process parameters included here are assumed to be a proxy measure of a relevant outcome or to indicate a high standard of care. They provide the opportunity of feasible and prompt monitoring, so that action can be taken quickly if the need arises.

Although most performance parameters concern surgical or postoperative procedures, one pre-operative indicator is also included (proportion of cases with pre-operative cytological or histological diagnosis). This is relevant to radiologists and pathologists in the first place, but surgeons must also be aware of it because it influences their performance concerning correct excision, weight of benign biopsies, number of operations and assurance of clear margins.

Table 1: Minimum set of performance parameters

Pre-operative indicators

1. Pre-operative cyto/histological diagnosis
The proportion of patients operated on for invasive or in situ cancer (palpable or impalpable) with a positive pre-operative cytological (C5) or histological (B5) diagnosis for cancer. The denominator is the total number of patients operated on for invasive or in situ breast cancer for whom information is available, whether or not they had a fine needle aspiration or core biopsy before surgery. Patients for whom the pre-operative diagnostic status is unknown are counted separately.

European surgical guidelines:	target ≥ **70%**

Italy, GISMa:	target ≥ 70%

UK, NHSBSP:	target > 70%; impalpable cancers > 60%

UK, BASO Breast Surgeons Group:	target for palpable cancers ≥ 90%

Surgical indicators

2. Correct excision at 1st surgical biopsy

The proportion of patients with benign or malignant impalpable lesions excised correctly at the first surgical biopsy, out of the total number of patients operated on for impalpable lesions. Patients are counted separately if it is not known whether their lesion was excised correctly. It should be noted that the issue here is not the state of the margins but the fact that there was a failed biopsy i.e. a post-biopsy mammogram shows the same lesion that was identified on the pre-operative films, or the histology is entirely incompatible with the pre-operative diagnostic features.

European surgical guidelines:	target ≥ **95%**

Italy, GISMa:	target ≥ 95%

UK, NHSBSP:	no target specified

UK, BASO Breast Surgeons Group:	no recommendation

3. No frozen section if tumour diameter < 10 mm

The proportion of patients operated on for invasive breast carcinoma (excluding microinvasive cancer) with a pathological size less than 10 mm for which there was no frozen section, out of the total number of patients with the same diagnosis. The number of patients with the same diagnosis for whom there is no information for this parameter is indicated separately.

European surgical guidelines:	no target; suggested ≥ **95%**

Italy, GISMa:	target ≥ 95%

UK, NHSBSP:	no target specified

UK, BASO Breast Surgeons Group:	without size indication, >90%

4. Benign biopsy specimen weight ≤ 30 grams

The proportion of patients with diagnostic open biopsies weighing less than or equal to 30 grams (fresh or fixed weight), out of the total number of patients operated on for impalpable lesions which were benign. Open diagnostic biopsies on benign palpable lesions are also included in the denominator if clinical/instrumental size is ≤ 10 mm. The number of patients with benign biopsies for whom there is no information on biopsy weight is indicated separately.

European surgical guidelines:	target ≥ **90%**
Italy, GISMa:	target ≥ 80%
UK, NHSBSP:	target ≥ 80%, weight < 20 grams
UK, BASO Breast Surgeons Group:	target for impalpable breast lesions ≥ 90%

5. Clear margins after last operation

The proportion of breast conservation operations (last operation if more than one) for invasive or in situ cancer which ensured clear margins (results for different cut-offs are shown: distance > 0 mm, > 1 mm, > 2 mm, > 5 mm from the lesion), out of the total of conservation operations done. The number of patients who had conservation surgery and for whom the state of the margins is unknown is indicated separately. If the distance is not specified, but according to the pathologist's report, margins are clear, this assessment is used. Lists of cases with 'not clear' margins are also provided, with the following information: whether the cancer is in situ or invasive, the nearest component, the distance, and whether the tumour reaches the margins focally or extensively. The suggested target is not intended to represent a guideline but is given as an indicator to distinguish cases less likely to have been appropriately treated. It is recommended that local recurrences are monitored.

European surgical guidelines:	no target; suggested ≥ **95% for distance > 1 mm**
Italy, GISMa:	no target specified
UK, NHSBSP:	no target specified
UK, BASO Breast Surgeons Group:	no target specified

6. Breast conservation surgery in pT1 cases

The proportion of patients who were given breast conservation surgery among those diagnosed with:
- pT1 invasive breast carcinoma without a ductal carcinoma in situ (DCIS) component, **or**
- invasive breast carcinoma, with a DCIS component, of whole pathological size equal to or less than 20 mm.

Multiple tumours are excluded. Microinvasive cancers (ductal carcinoma in situ where an invasive component measuring less than 1 mm has been seen and reported) are included. Whole pathological size includes accompanying DCIS extending more than 1 mm beyond the periphery of the invasive component (see chapter 7). The denominator is the total number of women operated on for unifocal invasive or microinvasive breast carcinoma of whole pathological size equal to or less than 20 mm. The number of patients with the same diagnosis for whom there is no information on the type of operation carried out is indicated separately.

European surgical guidelines:	**'majority of small sized screen-detected cancers'**
Italy, GISMa:	target ≥ 80%
UK, NHSBSP:	no target specified
UK, BASO Breast Surgeons Group:	no recommendation

7. Breast conservation surgery in carcinoma in situ ≤ 20 mm

The proportion of patients diagnosed with breast carcinoma in situ of pathological diameter equal to or less than 20 mm who were given breast conservation surgery. Multiple tumours are excluded. The denominator is the total number of women operated on with the same diagnosis. The number of patients with the same diagnosis for whom there is no information on the type of operation carried out is indicated separately.

European surgical guidelines:	**'majority of small sized screen-detected cancers'**
Italy, GISMa:	no target specified
UK, NHSBSP:	no target specified
UK, BASO Breast Surgeons Group:	no recommendation

8. Single operation following pre-operative diagnosis of cancer

The proportion of patients whose first operation was not followed by further local surgery due to incomplete excision (excluding failed biopsies), out of the total number of patients with invasive or in situ breast cancer who were operated on following positive or suspicious pre-operative cytological or histological diagnosis of cancer. The number of patients where this information is incomplete is indicated separately.

European surgical guidelines:	target ≥ **90%**
Italy, GISMa:	target ≥ 95%
UK, NHSBSP:	target > 90%
UK, BASO Breast Surgeons Group:	no recommendation

9. Number of lymph nodes removed > 9

The proportion of patients operated on for invasive breast carcinoma and who had an axillary dissection (I-III level) from whom at least 10 lymph nodes were excised, out of the total number of patients operated for invasive breast carcinoma and who had an axillary dissection. The number of patients for whom there is no information on the number of lymph nodes excised is indicated separately.

European surgical guidelines:	no target; suggested ≥ **95%**
Italy, GISMa:	target ≥ 95%
UK, NHSBSP:	sampling: at least 4 lymph nodes if sampling is performed, no target
UK, BASO Breast Surgeons Group:	at least 4 lymph nodes if sampling is performed, no target

10. Ductal carcinoma in situ (DCIS) without axillary dissection

The proportion of patients diagnosed with DCIS or not otherwise specified carcinoma in situ (microinvasive cancers excluded) on whom no axillary dissection, not even level 1, has been carried out. The sentinel lymph node procedure however is excluded. The number of patients for whom there is no information on axillary dissection is indicated separately.

European surgical guidelines:	no target; suggested ≥ **95%**
Italy, GISMa:	target ≥ 95%
UK, NHSBSP:	no target specified
UK, BASO Breast Surgeons Group:	no target specified

Waiting times

11. Operation within 21 days after decision to operate

The proportion of patients operated on for the first time for suspicious breast lesions (whatever the diagnosis) within 21 days of surgical referral, out of the total number of similar patients for whom information is available. This only applies to patients for whom the first treatment is surgical. The number of patients for whom information on operation or surgical referral date is not available is indicated separately.

European surgical guidelines:	target ≥ **90%**
Italy, GISMa:	target ≥ 80%
UK, NHSBSP:	target ≥ 90% (within 2 / 3 weeks if diagnostic / therapeutic operation)
UK, BASO Breast Surgeons Group:	target ≥ 90% (as above)

Radiotherapy

12. Radiotherapy (RT) done after breast conservation surgery

The proportion of patients who had breast conservation surgery for invasive or in situ carcinoma and for whom RT followed, out of the total number of patients who had conservation surgery. The number of patients for whom there is no information on RT is indicated separately. Given the greater uncertainties concerning radiotherapy for DCIS, this target applies to invasive cancers only.

European surgical guidelines:	'most invasive tumours'; suggested ≥ **95% (invasive cancers)**
Italy, GISMa:	target ≥ 95% (invasive cancers)
UK, NHSBSP:	no target specified
UK, BASO Breast Surgeons Group:	no target specified

The European surgical guidelines include a few recommendations not sufficiently covered by available reports from computerised audit systems. Reports on these issues are under evaluation and will be included in the next version of Q.T.:

• perform specimen X-ray and minimise time between excision and receipt of the report in the operating theatre
• minimise the adverse cosmetic effects
• local excision is not considered appropriate for extensive, multicentric or high grade DCIS
• systemic treatment should be considered for all patients with factors indicating poor prognosis

Additional reports beyond the described minimum set (some of which are being evaluated for feasibility and validity) are available in the audit systems and are listed in table 2.

Table 2: Other reports available in the audit systems

	Q.T. 2.3	BASO Breast Unit Database v2
Minimum number of diagnostic visits	Not available	Reports 4,5
Rapid referrals and communication of results	Not available	Report 3
Patient seen by specially trained surgeon	Not available	Report 6
Access to a specialist breast care nurse	Not available	Report 16
Time b/t screening mammogram and assessment	Report 21C	Not available
Time b/t screening mammogram and operation	Report 21B	Not available
Specimen unopened and orientated by surgeon	Reports 17A/C	Not available
Weight of specimen for small cancers	Report 12B	Not available
Benign to malignant biopsy ratio	B/M Report	Not available
Grade and hormone receptors available	Reports 18C/D	Not available
Serial section of excised specimen	Report 18B	Not available
Avoid unnecessary RT on axilla	Not available	Report 21
Immediate reconstruction done	Report 12C	Not available
Minimise surgical complications	Reports 3,4,20	Not available
Time b/t operation and histology	Reports 22,24,25	Not available
Time b/t biopsy and therapeutic operation	Report 23	Not available
Time b/t operation and start of RT or CT	Reports 26A/C	Not available
Mammographic and clinical follow up	Reports 37,38	Not available
Clinical trial participation	Report 19	Not available
Recurrences	Reports 4,5,6,7	Reports 22,23
Survival	Reports 2A, 2B	Survival report

9.5 Organisation of the audit procedures and resources required

As appropriately underscored by the European surgical guidelines auditing requires resources, particularly data managers with some clinical expertise, that should be available for this activity in the screening programme organisation unit or in surgical units caring for patients with screen-detected lesions. For auditing to produce change, feedback and careful analysis of emerging problems is of course necessary, and the best setting for these activities is multidisciplinary meetings. In fact, although many of the indicators relate to individual surgical skill or to knowledge of recommendations by individual surgeons, most involve the team as well. Discussion of data analysis reports during multidisciplinary meetings often prompts improvement of quality of data itself, like reduction of missing values and more accurate item definition, classification and coding. Typical examples of surgical indicators that need discussion in the team include margins of excision and number of excised lymph nodes, the role that pathological procedures play in these measures, and the assessment of correct excision at surgical biopsy compared to radiological features. The feedback process is likely to be easier in a centralised screening programme with nominated surgical staff. However, whatever the organisation of the screening programme, efforts should be made to perform surgical audit and to do this in connection with radiologists and cytopathologists from the programme.

While the recommended minimum set of indicators should be permanently monitored, this should not necessarily be the case for all other indicators available in the audit systems. Many, in fact, concern recommendations (e.g. not opening the operation specimen) that, once correct practice has come in use, do not need continuous quantitative measurement. The minimum set of indicators can be monitored 'by hand' collecting items described in appendix 1, but the use of an audit system is highly recommended for practical reasons and because it facilitates homogeneous data recording. Q.T. calculates some performance parameters that are relevant to other chapters of this document e.g. 'pre-operative diagnosis', 'correct excision at first biopsy', and waiting times.

The potential benefits of audit are unlikely to be accomplished unless surgeons take responsibility for it and see it as an opportunity for permanent education and professional improvement rather than an attempt to control their activity.

9.6 References

1. Cataliotti L., Costa A., Daly P.A., Fallowfield L., Freilich G., Holmberg L., Piccart A., van de Velde C.J.H., Veronesi U. Florence Statement on Breast Cancer, 1998. Forging the way ahead for more research on and better care in breast cancer. European Journal of Cancer, 35,1:14-15, 1999.
2. Broeders M.J.M., Codd M.B., Ascunce N., Linos A., Verbeek A.L.M. Quality Assurance in the Epidemiology of Breast Cancer Screening. In: C.J.M. de Wolf and N.M.Perry (Editors), European Guidelines for Quality Assurance in Mammography Screening, 2nd Edition. European Commission - Public Health, Europe Against Cancer Programme, Radiation Protection Actions, Luxembourg, 1996.
3. National Co-ordination Group for Surgeons working in Breast Cancer Screening. Quality Assurance Guidelines for Surgeons in Breast Cancer Screening. NHSBSP, Publication no. 20, 1996 (first edition 1992, revision 1996).
4. The Breast Surgeons Group of the British Association of Surgical Oncology. Guidelines for Surgeons in the Management of Symptomatic Breast Disease in the United Kingdom. Europ J Surg Onc, 21 (Supplement A): 1-13, 1995 (revision 1998).
5. Forza Operativa Nazionale sul Tumore Mammario. Controllo di qualità nel trattamento. In: I Tumori della Mammella: protocollo di diagnosi, trattamento e riabilitazione. Progetto finalizzato CNR-ACRO. Milan, March 1997, pp. 252-259.
6. Donabedian A. Explorations in Quality Assessment and Monitoring. Volume I: The Definition of Quality and Approaches to its Assessment. Health Administration Press, Ann Arbor, Michigan, USA, 1980.

Membership of Working Group and acknowledgements
The following members of the 'Europe Against Cancer' Working Group on monitoring surgical treatment of screen-detected breast cancer served as writing committee and are authors of this section:

Dr. A. Ponti, CPO-Piemonte, Turin, Italy
Dr. N. Segnan (Project Manager), CPO-Piemonte, Turin, Italy
Prof. R. Blamey, Professorial Unit of Surgery, Nottingham City Hospital, United Kingdom
Dr. R. Bordon, Breast Unit, S. Anna Hospital, Turin, Italy
Prof. L. Cataliotti, Inst. of *Clinica Chirurgica I*, University of Florence, Italy
Dr. M. Codd, Dept. of Epidemiology, *Mater Misericordiae* Hospital, Dublin, Ireland
Dr. V. Distante, Inst. of *Clinica Chirurgica I*, University of Florence, Italy
Dr. D. Giorgi, Unit of Epidemiology, CSPO, Florence, Italy
Mr. T. Gorey, Dept. of Surgery, *Mater Misericordiae* Hospital, Dublin, Ireland
Dr. A. Linos, Inst. of Preventive Medicine, Kifissia, Athens, Greece
Dr. D. A. Linos, Dept. of Surgery, Athens Medical School, Athens, Greece
Dr. M. P. Mano, Breast Unit, S. Anna Hospital, Turin, Italy
Mr. R. Sainsbury, Dept. of General Surgery, Huddersfield Royal Infirmary, United Kingdom

The contribution of all surgeons, epidemiologists, radiologists, pathologists, oncologists, radiotherapists from each centre participating in the Working Group is gratefully acknowledged. Special thanks go to Dr. R. Arisio, Dr. E. Berardengo, Prof. S. Bianchi, Dr. C. Coluccia, Prof. P. Dervan, Dr. A. Frigerio, Dr. R. Giani, Dr. E. Paci, Dr. G. Peppas, Dr. E. Riza, Dr. M. Rosselli Del Turco, Prof. A. Sapino, Dr. C. Senore, Dr. R. Simoncini, to Q.T. developers M. Dalmasso, G. Delmastro, A. Tomatis, M. Tomatis and to all members of the G.I.S.Ma. (Italian Network of Breast Cancer Screening) Group on Treatment. Recognition for financial support is given to the **European Commission** ('Europe Against Cancer Programme': SOC 95/200596, 96/200974, 97/200967, 98/200444, 99/CVF2-033) and to the **Italian Association for Cancer Research** ('AIRC Breast Cancer Project', 1995-1997).

Contact details
The Q.T. Audit System operates under *Epi Info*, a public domain programme produced by CDC - Centres for Disease Control and Prevention of Atlanta, USA - in conjunction with the World Health Organisation. Q.T. incorporates as well a module for data entry and printing patient medical records which operates under *Microsoft Access,* which can be used by owners of *MS-Access 95, 97* and *2000.* Data entry in Q.T. under *Access* has so far been tested successfully in data sets with over 3,000 cases. To register and order or download the current version of Q.T. (2.3 as for May 2000) with the user's manual contact the address below:
CPO Piemonte
Cancer Epidemiology Unit ASL 1
via S. Francesco da Paola 31
10123 Torino, Italy
Fax + 39 011 5664561
Tel. + 39 011 5664566
www.cpo.it

Appendix 1

Definition and coding of data items used by the Q.T. 2.3 Audit System for producing the minimum set of indicators devised to monitor the European surgical guidelines[3]

Item	Meaning	Coding	Description
Other lesions	Classification of this lesion with respect to any other lesions recorded in the database for the same patient	0=single lesion 1=main lesion 2=double, contralateral 3=double, ipsilateral 4=metachronous, contralateral 5=metachronous, ipsilateral 9=unknown	Only use value 1 when there are two or more lesions. Main lesion refers to the worst lesion (invasive cancer, CIS, benign; within each category use preferably diameter). Update each time a new lesion appears and is recorded in the database.
Disease extent		0=localised 1=multifocal 2=multicentric 9=unknown	Assessed clinically or by imaging. 1=more foci in same quadrant; 2=synchronous lesions in different quadrants: fill a report for each lesion.
Palpable lesion		0=no 1=yes 9=unknown	Assessed clinically pre-operatively.
Imaging/clinical size	Lesion size by imaging or clinical examination		In millimeters. If available, use size determined by ultrasound. Otherwise, use mammographic (preferable) or clinical size.
Date of referral for first therapy	Date of surgical decision to operate or first therapy referral		Write in date as DD/MM/YYYY. Date when the patient is informed of treatment referral (surgical or other).

[3] The following additional items, required for the minimum set of surgical indicators, are described in the chapters 6 and 7 of this document:
- fine needle aspiration and core biopsy findings
- pathological diagnosis, pT, in situ type
- maximum pathological diameter and total size
- specimen margin status and distance of nearest margin to tumour
- number of lymph nodes recovered

In order to analyse surgical indicators in relation to screening, at least the following items described in the epidemiological evaluation chapter are also needed:
- source of referral
- screening status (screen-detected, interval case, etc.)
- date of last screening mammogram
- screening round and screening examination (first, second, etc.)

Appropriate identification of patient, hospital and physicians is also included in the Q.T. data set.
The Q.T. manual includes the description of the coding of all the above listed items.

Item	Meaning	Coding	Description
Type of first therapy		1=surgery 2=radiotherapy 3=chemotherapy 4=radio+chemotherapy 9=unknown	
Surgery	Surgical operation performed	0=no 1=yes 9=unknown	Update with each significant change.
Date of operation(s)	Date of the 1st, 2nd, 3rd breast operation		Write in dates as DD/MM/YYYY.
Breast procedure type	Type of conclusive operation performed during surgical session, for each operation	1=excision biopsy 2=lumpectomy 3=wide excision 4=quadrantectomy 5=mastectomy - subcutaneous 6=mastectomy - simple 7=mastectomy - NOS 8=other 9=unknown	Indicate the most extensive operation of those performed in the same session. Any failed biopsy must not be considered in this section. Use value 4 for **segmentectomies**, value 5 for **adenomammectomies**, value 6 for **total mastectomies** and value 8 for **incisional biopsies**. 'NOS' means 'Not Otherwise Specified'.
Frozen section - lesion	Result of frozen section of the lesion	0=not done 1=yes, negative 2=yes, dubious 3=yes, positive for CIS 4=yes, positive for inv. ca. 5=yes, result unknown 9=unknown	
Frozen section - margins	Result of frozen section of the lesion (specimen margins)	0=not done 1=T does not reach margin 2=CIS in proximity 3=inv. ca. in proximity 4=CIS reaches margin 5=inv. ca. reaches margin 6=done, result unknown 9=unknown	

Item	Meaning	Coding	Description
Weight of specimen	Fresh or fixed weight of specimen removed (in grams)		As stated in the histology report (preferable) or measured in theatre. Biopsies or conservation surgery only, any diagnosis. Enter 999 for weight unknown.
Axillary operation		0=no 1=yes 9=unknown	
Date of operation	Date of axillary operation		Write in date as DD/MM/YYYY.
Lymph node procedure	Type of axillary operation (level)	1=level I 2=levels I+II 3=levels I+II+III 4=other 9=unknown	If value 4 is used (for example in the case of sampling), enter description in the following field.
Pectoral muscles	Total or partial excision of pectoral muscles	1=both intact 2=minor removed 3=both removed 9=unknown	
Number of operations	Number of surgical operations on the same lesion	1=one 2=two 3=more than two 9=unknown	Number of operations for the same lesion at different surgical sessions, on breast and/or axilla. Do not count failed biopsies.
Reasons for > 1 operation	Reasons for more than one surgical operation	1=axillary operation 2=clearance of margins 3=margins and axilla 4=neoadjuvant therapy 5=other 9=unknown	State the main reason.
Failed biopsy		0=no 1=yes 9=unknown	It means failure in removing the lesion at a biopsy previous to surgery recorded in QT as first intervention.
Radiotherapy	Radiotherapy performed	0=no 1=yes 2=patient refusal 9=unknown	

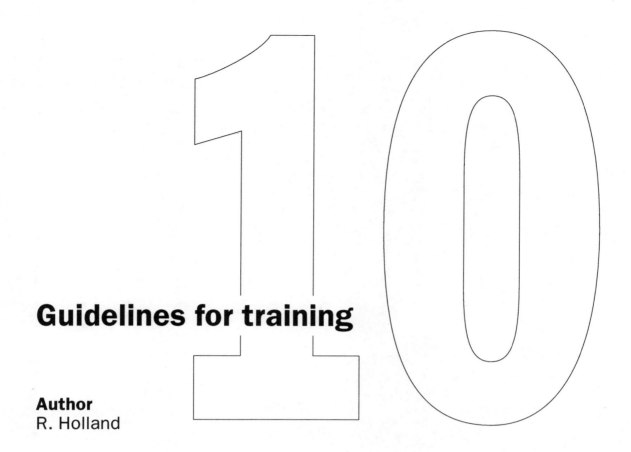

Guidelines for training

Author
R. Holland

10.1 Introduction

The success of a screening programme is largely dependent on the availability of specially trained staff committed to providing a high quality, efficient service. All staff involved in a programme should attend a course of instruction at an approved training centre prior to the commencement of the programme. High quality screening performance is based on a multidisciplinary approach, therefore both unidisciplinary and multidisciplinary training packages should be offered. Updating of knowledge within the framework of Continuing Medical Education should be encouraged.

In the EUREF certification system specific training requirements are set both in terms of quality and volumes, to determine eligibility for certification. Only centres that employ sufficiently skilled personnel are eligible for certification. The Certification Protocol is included in the annexes. The EUREF organisation can be contacted for advice on sources of training and coordination (www.EUREF.org).

10.2 General requirements

A There is general agreement at present based on research evidence that **multidisciplinary services** provide better patient care. Effective communication between the various professionals of a Breast Care Team is essential. Therefore, training courses should also focus on the good interprofessional communication. Joint courses given for the multidisciplinary team may facilitate this goal.

B **Continuing education**, including refresher courses at various intervals are essential to gain information on new developments and to improve the quality of the diagnostic and therapeutic process.

It is important to keep records of training activities as they are useful indicators of the quality of a given centre. They will be part of a certification review process.

C All medical staff involved in a screening programme should acquire a basic knowledge of the **epidemiological aspects** of such a programme.

Relevant topics are:
- breast cancer epidemiology (incidence, prognosis, mortality)
- introduction to screening philosophy (concept of secondary prevention),
- breast cancer screening terminology (sensitivity, specificity, predictive value)
- evaluation of screening effectiveness (performance parameters, mortality reduction)
- current screening practices (centralised and decentralised programmes, population based programmes)

10.3 Epidemiologists

A breast cancer screening programme is, of necessity, a multidisciplinary undertaking. Many disciplines will contribute to monitoring and evaluating the programme. It is essential therefore that directly from the start of the programme, a designated individual with relevant epidemiological knowledge, is given the task of overlooking the data generation process which should be designed to facilitate evaluation. Assessing the programme's impact on breast cancer mortality is only possible if adequate provision has been made in the planning process for the complete and accurate recording of the data required. The protocol for quality assurance of the epidemiological aspects of screening for breast cancer (see chapter 2) gives more detailed guidance for this effort.

Basic training:
The person overseeing data generation and evaluation should have attended a basic training course in clinical epidemiology.

The training programme for epidemiologists to be involved in breast cancer screening should give specific emphasis to:
• breast cancer epidemiology: incidence, prevalence, mortality, trends
• screening philosophy: preclinical lesions, lead time
• breast cancer screening terminology: sources of bias, current screening practices
• breast cancer screening programme: sensitivity, specificity, predictive value
• ethical and confidentiality issues
• setting up a mammography screening programme: identification and invitation of target population, call-recall system, follow up system
• strategies for data collection and management: use of appropriate databases, individual files, computerised archives, linkage to appropriate registries, classification of screening outcomes, quality control procedures in data collection
• statistical analysis and interpretation of results: performance indicators for process evaluation, predictors of screening impact, assessing screening impact and effectiveness, basic cost-effectiveness calculations, sources of bias, outcomes, adherence to the programme, side-effects of screening
• presentation of data and report writing

The training programme should preferably be organised as secondments for a period of at least one week to one or two established screening centres running population-based screening programmes. In addition, international courses on relevant aspects of the work involved should be attended if appropriate.

10.4 Physicists

Involvement of a qualified physicist is required within any breast cancer screening programme. The physicist should be able to set up and maintain a quality assurance system. The physicist should be able to advise on the purchase and use of mammography equipment in general, and must be able to communicate the current standards of practice in a concise way to radiologists, radiographers and manufacturers alike. He or she must have a broad knowledge of imaging techniques in general but be an expert in the imaging of breast tissue.

The physicist must be able to build up and maintain a network of professionals in order to keep these skills in touch with the current technology. In some of the tasks (e.g. solving conflicting interests) management skills are necessary. With an eye on the (near) future it is also necessary to be a skilled computer user for e.g. digital mammography, building databases and developing specific local software.

Each physicist should have a degree in physics (or physics engineering, biomedical engineering or technical physics) and have undergone further postgraduate training.

Ongoing education and training is indispensable for achieving professional standards. As a guide, the physicist should spend about 5% of working time undergoing training.

The theoretical and practical training in the physics of breast screening should cover at least the following topics:
- organisation of quality assurance
- physics of mammography (including digital mammography systems)
- quality assurance measurements on mammography X-ray sets, stereotactic accessories, specimen cabinets
- principles of film processing (including film artefacts and their causes)
- quality assurance testing of processors films and screens (including sensitometric techniques)
- measurement of image quality in mammography
- measurement of radiation dose in mammography
- the risks of radiation associated with mammography

Specific training in the physics of mammography in both theoretical and practical matters at an established institute or training centre is obligatory. Practical training should be arranged by secondment in a centre experienced in this work for a period of about 1 week.

In order to maintain skill levels it is desirable that each physicist has a fairly substantial involvement in breast imaging systems. If for practical reasons some physicists look after relatively small numbers of systems e.g. 1 or 2, then additional steps must be taken to coordinate and compare their work with other more experienced physicists.

10.5 Radiographers

Radiographers have a key role in obtaining and maintaining recognised targets for the success of a mammography screening programme. Training in the various aspects of their work is mandatory.

Outlines of the radiographic quality objectives are summarised in chapter 4. In order to achieve these objectives, all radiographers participating in a breast screening programme are expected to undergo a programme of training which should consist of two parts:
- academic: three days to one week
- clinical: two to six weeks depending on the experience and skills of the radiographer

The academic component should include:
- the normal breast, anatomy and physiology
- radiology and pathology of benign and malignant lesions
- the management of breast cancer
- organisation of a breast screening programme
- epidemiological aspects
- technical quality control
- communication and social skills

The course may include lectures, tutorials, demonstrations and reading.

The clinical component should include:
- standard and additional views e.g. magnification, coned views and specimen radiography
- daily and weekly technical quality control procedures
- technical aspects of X-ray equipment, film-screen combination and film-processor
- the assessment of the quality of the images from the positioning as well as the technical point of view
- relevant administrative procedures
- additional imaging techniques e.g. ultrasound and MRI
- localisation and biopsy techniques for impalpable lesions

10.6 Radiologists

Radiologists responsible for the radiological aspects of breast screening must have undergone formal training and have experience in mammography and in the radiological assessment of women with screen-detected abnormalities.

Training programmes should include at least the following subjects:
- physical principles of mammography, grid techniques, film-screen combinations, processing options, radiation dose, quality control and quality assurance
- radiographic positioning, standard views, additional views, magnification, coned views and specimen radiography
- radiology of the normal breast and variants of normal
- the radiology and pathology of benign lesions, especially those which simulate malignancy
- the radiology and pathology of malignant breast disease
- the differential diagnosis of mass lesions, microcalcifications, parenchymal distortion and asymmetrical density
- the importance of radiologic-pathologic correlation in cases where there is an extensive intraductal disease component, and the implications for management and treatment
- the use and place of ultrasound in the diagnosis and management of breast lesions
- localisation and biopsy techniques for impalpable lesions, fine needle aspiration cytology, and needle core biopsy

- involvement in the daily reading of screening and clinical mammograms
- self-assessment procedures, review of interval cancers,
- the epidemiological aspects of breast screening
- participation in multidisciplinary pre-operative and postoperative meetings
- additional imaging techniques including MRI and digital mammography
- current issues of breast diagnosis and treatment

The training programme should preferably have a tutorial structure with direct interaction between the participants and the experts.
Before undertaking screen film reading or screening assessment radiologists should be seconded to a screening and assessment centre. This should be an approved training centre with a throughput of at least 10,000 screens per year, for a period of time which, depending on experience and aptitude, could vary from some days to some weeks.

10.7 Pathologists

The quality of the pathology service is crucial in order to provide the definitive diagnosis of a mammographically detected lesion and to give information on its prognostic significance. In addition, the pathology data, e.g. tumour size, grade and axillary node status, are essential indicators of screening performance. Each screening programme should have access to high quality pathology services provided by pathologists with special expertise in breast pathology. Pathologists involved in a screening programme should have undergone specialist training for at least one to two weeks in an approved training centre.

Such a training programme should include:
- optimal handling of biopsy specimens, the use of specimen radiography and the extent of sampling of the specimen for histological examination
- the classification of malignant invasive and non-invasive lesions
- recording prognostic data: tumour size, malignancy grade, axillary node status
- radiologic-pathologic correlation of benign and malignant lesions: mass lesions, microcalcifications, parenchymal distortions and asymmetrical densities
- the importance of radiologic-pathologic correlation in cases where there is an extensive intraductal disease component, and the implications for management and treatment
- common pitfalls in histological diagnosis, e.g. atypical ductal hyperplasia vs. ductal carcinoma in situ, florid adenosis vs. tubular carcinoma, "microinvasion", benign vs. malignant papillary lesions
- the interpretation of fine needle aspiration cytology and needle core biopsy samples, and the associated pitfalls in diagnosis
- the pathologist's role in the sentinel-node biopsy technique
- the assessment of margins and consequences for treatment modalities
- participation in multidisciplinary pre-operative and postoperative meetings
- the epidemiological aspects of breast screening

10.8 Surgeons

The management of cases coming to surgery from the screening programme should be carried out *only* by surgeons who have undergone specific training and have acquired the necessary specialist knowledge. Attendance at an approved multi-disciplinary training course is mandatory.

Such a training programme should include:
- the diagnosis and treatment of invasive and *in situ* breast cancer
- the diagnosis and management of benign breast disease
- the management of screen-detected breast disease
- psychological evaluation, communication and counselling
- breast reconstruction
- radiotherapy relating to breast cancer
- the use of chemotherapy for breast cancer in the adjuvant setting and for advanced disease
- breast pathology: histopathology, cytology and immunohistochemistry
- breast radiology/ ultrasound/ stereotaxis
- epidemiology and genetics of breast cancer and screening
- clinical trials and statistics
- principles and practice of audit procedures

10.9 Bibliography

- BASO Breast Speciality Group. The British Association of Surgical Oncology Guidelines for Surgeons in the Management of Symptomatic Breast Disease in the U. K. (1998 revision), *Eur J Surg Oncol 1998*; 24: 464-467
- BASO Breast Surgeons Group. The Training of a Surgeon with an Interest in Breast Disease, *Eur J Surg Oncol 1996*; 22 (suppl. A): 2-4
- Blichert-Toft M., Smola M. G., Cataliotti L. and O'Higgins N. on behalf of European Society of Surgical Oncology. Principles and Guidelines for Surgeons in the Management of Symptomatic Breast Cancer, *Eur J Surg Oncol 1997*; 23: 101-9
- Clinical Outcomes Group. Guidelines for Purchasers - Improving Outcomes in Breast Cancer, NHS Executive, Leeds, 1996; Cat 96 CC 0021
- European Commission. European Guidelines for Quality Assurance in Mammography Screening, De Wolf C and Perry N, eds, Office for Official Publications of the European Communities, Luxembourg, 1996
- Health Insurance and Executive Board (the Netherlands). Regeling van Taken en Verantwoordelijkheden Bevolkingsonderzoek naar Borstkanker (*Regulation of Tasks and Authorities Breast Cancer Screening*), Health Insurance and Executive Board, 1998
- National Accreditation Committee of the National Programme for the Early Detection of Breast Cancer. National Accreditation Requirements, Commonwealth Department of Human Services and Health, Canberra, 1994
- The National Committee of the Canadian Breast Cancer Screening Initiative. Quality Determinants of Organized Breast Cancer Screening Programs, Minister of Public Works and Government Services Canada, 1997
- NHSBSP Radiographers Quality Assurance Coordination Committee. Quality Assurance Guidelines for Radiographers, NHSBSP Publications, 1994
- The Royal College of Pathologists Working Group. Pathology Reporting in Breast Cancer Screening (2nd edn.), NHSBSP Publications, 1997

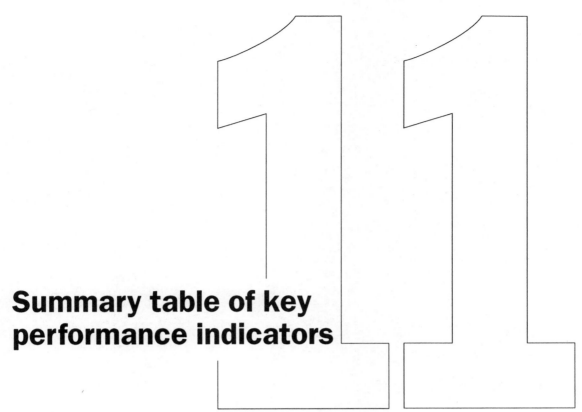

Summary table of key performance indicators

Authors
M. Broeders
A. Ponti
N. Perry

Introduction

For ease of reference we have included a summary table of key performance indicators from these guidelines. For more complete information regarding definition and context, further reference should be made to the source of each parameter within the text as listed. On occasions we have had to accept that different disciplines, and different Member States show some variation of priorities and target levels. In all cases we have attempted to list what we regard as the most widely used and generally appropriate professionally agreed levels for usage in a Pan-European setting. In any case, all targets, should be constantly reviewed in the light of experience and revised accordingly with regard to results achieved and best clinical practice. As far as possible, targets given refer to women over 50 years of age attending a screening programme.

Abbreviations used for reference to the chapters, e.g.:
3T1 Chapter 3, table 1
4.7 Chapter 4, paragraph 7

Summary table of key performance indicators

Performance indicator	Acceptable level	Desirable level
Target optical density [3.2.1.3]	1.3 - 1.8 OD	1.3 - 1.8 OD
Spatial resolution [3T1]	> 10 lp/mm	> 13 lp/mm
Reference dose (surface entrance dose) [3T1]	< 15 mGy	< 14 mGy
Threshold contrast visibility [3T1]	< 1.5%	
Proportion of women invited that attend for screening [2T33]	> 70%	> 75%
Proportion of women with a radiographically acceptable screening examination [4.8]	97%	> 97%
Proportion of women that are satisfied with the screening service [4.8]	97%	> 97%
Proportion of women informed of procedure and time scale of receiving results [4.8]	100%	100%
Proportion of women undergoing a technical repeat screening examination [4.8, 5T2]	< 3%	< 1%
Proportion of women undergoing additional imaging at the time of the screening examination in order to further clarify the mammographic appearances [2T33]	< 5%	< 1%

Performance indicator	Acceptable level	Desirable level
Proportion of women recalled for further assessment [2T33, 5T2]		
• initial screening examinations	< 7%	< 5%
• subsequent screening examinations	< 5%	< 3%
Proportion of women screened who are subjected to early recall following assessment [5T2]	< 1%	0%
Breast cancer detection rate, expressed as a multiple of the underlying, expected, breast cancer incidence rate in the absence of screening (IR) [2T34, 5T1]		
• initial screening examinations	3 x IR	> 3 x IR
• subsequent screening examinations	1.5 x IR	> 1.5 x IR
Interval cancer rate as a proportion of the underlying, expected, breast cancer incidence rate in the absence of screening [2T34]		
• within the first year (0-11 months)	30%	< 30%
• within the second year (12-23 months)	50%	< 50%
Proportion of screen-detected cancers that are ductal carcinoma in situ [5T1]	10%	10-20%
Proportion of screen-detected cancers that are stage II+ [2T34]		
• initial screening examinations	25%	< 25%
• subsequent screening examinations	20%	< 20%
Proportion of screen-detected cancers that are node-negative [2T34]		
• initial screening examinations	70%	> 70%
• subsequent screening examinations	75%	> 75%
Proportion of invasive screen-detected cancers that are ≤ 10 mm in size [2T34, 5T1]		
• initial screening examinations	≥ 20%	≥ 25%
• subsequent screening examinations	≥ 25%	≥ 30%
Proportion of invasive screen-detected cancers that are < 15 mm in size [8.2]	50%	> 50%
Proportion of invasive screen-detected cancers < 10 mm in size for which there was no frozen section [9T1]	95%	> 95%
Proportion of screen-detected cancers, both palpable and impalpable, with a pre-operative diagnosis of malignancy [2T33, 5T2, 8.3, 9T1]	> 70%	> 90%

Performance indicator	Acceptable level	Desirable level
Proportion of impalpable lesions producing mammographic abnormalities successfully removed at the first localisation biopsy operation [5T2, 8.3, 9T1]	95%	> 95%
Proportion of image-guided FNAC procedures with insufficient result [5T2, 6.2.3]	< 25%	< 15%
Proportion of image-guided FNAC procedures from lesions subsequently proven to be malignant, with insufficient result [5T2, 6.2.3]	< 10%	
Benign to malignant open surgical biopsy ratio [2T33, 5T2] • initial screening examinations • subsequent screening examinations	≤ 1 : 1 ≤ 1 : 1	≤ 0.5 : 1 ≤ 0.2 : 1
Proportion of wires placed within 1 cm of an impalpable lesion prior to excision [5T2]	90%	> 90%
Proportion of benign biopsies weighing less than 30 grams fresh weight [9T1]	90%	> 90%
Proportion of women whose first operation was not followed by further local surgery due to incomplete excision following a pre-operative diagnosis of cancer [8.4, 9T1]	90%	> 90%
Proportion of women operated on for invasive cancer, including axillary dissection, for whom at least 10 lymph nodes were excised [9T1]	95%	> 95%
Proportion of ductal carcinoma in situ where no axillary dissection was carried out [9T1]	95%	> 95%
Proportion of women who have a waiting time: • between screening examination and result of the screening examination of ≤ 2 weeks [5T2] • between result and offered assessment of ≤ 1 week [5T2] • between surgical decision to operate and first offered admission date of ≤ 3 weeks [8.4, 9T1]	90% 90% 90%	> 90% > 90% > 90%

Position paper

Recommendations on cancer screening in the European Union

Reprinted from European Journal of Cancer, vol. 36, Advisory Committee on Cancer Prevention, Position paper. Recommendations on cancer screening in the European Union, pp. 1473-1478, ©2000, with permission from Elsevier Science.

Authors
E. Lynge
J. Patnick
S. Törnberg
J. Faivre
F. Schröder

Acknowledgement:
The document was finalised after discussion at the Conference on Screening and early Detection of Cancer, Vienna 18-19 November 1999.

Correspondence to:
Elsebeth Lynge,
Institute of Public Health, University of Copenhagen,
Blegdamsvej 3, DK-2200 København N, Denmark.
Tel: + 45 35 32 76 35, Fax: + 45 35 35 11 81,
e-mail: elsebeth@pubhealth.ku.dk

1 Introduction

Screening allows the detection of cancers at an early stage of invasiveness or even before they become invasive. Some lesions can then be treated more effectively and the patients can expect to live longer. The key indicator for the effectiveness of screening is decrease in disease-specific mortality or incidence.

Screening is, however, testing of healthy people for diseases which have so far not given rise to symptoms. Aside from its beneficial effect on disease-specific mortality or incidence, screening might therefore also have some negative side-effects for the screened population.

Healthcare providers should know all the potential benefits and risks of screening for a given cancer site before embarking on new cancer screening programmes. Furthermore, for the informed public of today, it is necessary to present these benefits and risks in a way that allows the individual citizen to decide on whether to participate in the screening programmes.

The purpose of this document is to give recommendations on cancer screening in the European Union. These recommendations address the people, the politicians and the health administrations of the Member States, the European Commission and the European Parliament.

Principles for screening as a tool for the prevention of chronic non-communicable diseases were published by the World Health Organisation in 1968 (1) and by the Council of Europe in 1994 (2). These two documents form, together with the present state of art in each of the cancer screening fields, the basis for the present recommendations.

All data on incidence and mortality are quoted from the recently published EUCAN data covering 1995. An estimated number of 1,488,000 new cancer cases, excluding non-melanoma skin cancer, occurred in the European Union in 1995. Of these, 2% were cervical cancers, 13% breast cancers, 13% colorectal cancers and 8% prostate cancers. Cervical and breast cancer constituted 4% and 29%, respectively, of new cancers in women, and prostate cancer constituted 14% of new cancers in men. All rates presented here are age standardised with the European Standard Population (3).

2 General principles

Screening is only one method of controlling cancer. Whenever possible primary cancer prevention should be given first priority. When cancer screening is undertaken it should be offered only in organised programmes with quality assurance at all levels, and good information about benefits and risks. The benefits of a screening programme are achieved only if the coverage is high. When organised screening is offered high compliance should, therefore, be sought. Opportunistic screening activities are normally not acceptable as they may not achieve the potential benefits and may cause unnecessary negative side-effects.

New cancer screening tests should be evaluated in randomised trials before being implemented in routine healthcare.

The reduction in the disease-specific mortality achieved in trials depends on the sensitivity of the screening test, the compliance amongst the invited, the screening frequency, the number of screens each person has, the completeness of the follow-up and the benefit of early treatment. The negative side-effects in the screened population depend on the sensitivity and the specificity of the test, and on the possible side effects of early treatment. The findings from trials can be extrapolated to the general population only if the conditions in the trials can be reproduced in the routine healthcare system. This requires an organisation with a call-recall system and with quality assurance at all levels, and it requires an effective and appropriate treatment service.

Centralised data systems are needed for the running of organised screening programmes. This includes a computerised list of all persons to be targeted by the screening programme. It includes also computerised data on all screening tests, assessment and final diagnoses. Organised screening also implies scientific analysis of the outcome of the screening and quick reporting of these results to the population and screen providers. This analysis is facilitated if the screening database is linked to cancer register data.

High quality screening is possible only if the personnel at all levels are adequately trained for their tasks. Performance indicators should be monitored regularly.

Ethical, legal, social, medical, organisational and economic aspects have to be considered before decisions can be made on the implementation of cancer screening. Resources, human as well as economic, must be available in order to assure the appropriate organisation and quality control. Actions have to be taken to ensure different socio-economic groups equal access to screening. The implementation of a cancer screening programme is therefore a decision to be made locally, depending on the disease burden and the healthcare resources.

Cancer is a leading disease and cause of death throughout Europe. European collaboration should facilitate high quality cancer screening programmes and protect the population from poor quality screening.

3 Cervical cancer screening

3.1 Epidemiology

In an unscreened population, the incidence of cervical cancer reaches its maximum around the age of 50 years. In screened populations the incidence tends to be highest for women above the age of 60 years. The incidence of cervical cancer reflects both background risk and screening activity during the previous decades. The highest incidence of cervical cancer is now observed in Portugal with 19 per 100,000 and the lowest in

Luxembourg with 4 per 100,000. Mortality rates are highest in Denmark, Austria and Portugal with 6-7 per 100,000 and lowest in Luxembourg and Finland with about 1 per 100,000.

3.2 Present situation

Whilst no randomised trials on cervical screening with Pap smears were ever carried out, the effectiveness of cervical screening programmes has been demonstrated in several countries (4-6). It is estimated that cervical smears every three years can prevent 90% of cervical cancers in a population if all women attend and all detected lesions are adequately followed-up (7). High compliance is thus vital and a high degree of organisation is needed to achieve this.

Nationally organised cervical screening programmes exist in Sweden, Finland, Denmark, The Netherlands and the UK. A European set of guidelines for cervical screening was developed in 1993. It provides targets for quality assurance of organised screening programmes (8). Ten centres with cervical screening have, in the past, been financially supported by the Europe Against Cancer programme. These 10 programmes have recently formed a network focussing on quality assurance, epidemiology and new technologies.

The limited screening resources should be concentrated in the age range of 30-60 years. A large proportion of cervical abnormalities will regress to normal if left untreated. Screening should therefore definitely not start before the age of 20 years and in many countries probably not before the age of 30 years. The protective effect of screening of women older than 60 years is limited, especially if these women previously had negative tests.

Screening should be undertaken with a 3-5 year interval. Prolonged intervals may be considered in women with a history of negative tests. The benefit of more frequent screening is very limited and, in addition, it increases the risk of overtreatment of otherwise regressing lesions.

3.3 Recommendations

3.3.1 To the Member States

Pap smears should be the method used in cervical cancer screening.

When screening is offered it should start at the latest by the age of 30 years and definitely not before age 20 years. The upper age should depend on the available resources but should preferably not be lower than 60 years. Limited screening resources should be concentrated in the age range of 30-60 years.

Screening intervals should be between 3 and 5 years. Screening more often than every third year should be discouraged. Smear taking in healthy women should be undertaken only in organised screening programmes with quality assurance at all levels.

Cervical cancer screening programmes should be organised in accordance with the European guidelines.

3.3.2 To the European Commission and the European Parliament

A common terminology for histology and cytology should be implemented. For the laboratories, a detailed quality control programme should be defined based on the existing guidelines and implemented at the national level.

Recommendations for training and quality control could be proposed and tested in the network centres. As different treatment options are currently adopted, auditing of cases should be performed by a core group of clinicians. A concerted effort should be made to find the most effective methods for follow-up and treatment of cervical abnormalities.

Validation studies of liquid-based and automated screening methods with special attention to cost-effectiveness should be undertaken. Well-designed studies should be undertaken on the use of human papilloma virus (HPV) testing as a screening method and/or as a supplementary method in the follow-up of cervical abnormalities.

Studies should be undertaken of recent trends in the incidence of cervical cancer in Europe in order to optimise the lower and upper age limits for screening.

4 Breast cancer screening

4.1 Epidemiology

In countries with national population-based cancer statistics, such as the Nordic countries, the incidence of breast cancer has increased during the last four decades. The start of a mammography screening programme is associated with a temporary increase in the incidence of breast cancer, and the European differences in breast cancer incidence therefore at present reflect both background risks and screening activities. At present the incidence is highest with 120 per 100,000 in The Netherlands, where a screening programme started recently, and lowest in Spain and Greece with 61-63 per 100,000. Breast cancer is rare under the age of 30 years and the incidence increases with age. Breast cancer mortality is highest in Denmark 38 per 100,000 and lowest in Greece 23, per 100,000. Mortality rates have increased during the last decades in the majority of European countries, whereas they have been stable or decreased slightly in the Nordic countries and in the UK.

4.2 Present situation

Screening for breast cancer with mammography has been studied in a number of randomised trials. Data from five Swedish counties showed a 30% decrease in breast cancer mortality amongst women invited to screening at age 50-69 years (9). Updated data from Sweden also indicate a reduction in breast cancer mortality among women invited to screening at age 40-49 years (10). The cost-effectiveness is, however, not clear in this lower age group.

A European breast cancer screening network was established in 1989 with the aims to provide experience for countries with no breast screening service, to explore methods of implementation into the national health systems, to establish contact for exchange of information between Member States, and most importantly to develop guidelines for best practice related to breast screening. The desirable endpoint for each member of the network is to establish a co-ordination of the screening activities in their country and to operate a service and/or reference centre for these activities.

During its 10 years of existence the network has noted that population-based screening requires the full support of national or regional health authorities, and that the decision to start a programme needs to be taken by appropriate health authorities. Screening for breast cancer is multidisciplinary and the quality of the whole process (invitation, diagnosis, assessment of suspicious lesions, treatment and follow-up) needs to be ensured before initiating a programme. Initial and continuous training of all personnel involved is mandatory. Mechanisms are needed to monitor the quality of the screening programme.

The different healthcare systems in Europe have made it necessary to find different solutions to common problems. The network has demonstrated the importance of high quality radiological examination and the need for a centralised reading of mammograms taken in a decentralised setting. It has also demonstrated the need for standards on the minimal number of women to be examined in a centre in order to maintain the level of expertise.

European Guidelines for Quality Assurance in Mammography Screening is a document with minimal and optimal requirements for quality assurance of organised screening programmes (11). An updated version will be published in year 2000.

4.3 Recommendations

4.3.1 To the Members States

Mammography should be the method used in breast cancer screening. There is at present no convincing evidence for the effect of screening based on breast self-examination or clinical breast examination.

Women without symptoms of breast cancer should be offered mammography examination only in organised screening programmes with quality assurance at all levels. When mammography screening is offered, only women aged 50-69 years should be invited.

Screening intervals should be 2-3 years.

Breast cancer screening programmes should be organised in accordance with the European guidelines (11).

Adverse effects of mammography screening in women aged 40-49 years may not be negligible, due to the lower predictive value of mammography in this age group, the possible detection of non-progressive cancers and the higher radiation hazard.

Thus, if screening is offered to women aged 40-49 years in some centres or European regions, according to local resources and quality standards reached in screening offered to older women, the following requirements are needed: 1) women should be clearly informed about the possible benefits and adverse effects of screening; 2) organised programmes should be set up in order to discourage spontaneous screening in units without adequate quality control systems; 3) two-view mammography with double reading and 12-18 months of interval should be used; 4) data monitoring and proper evaluation should be mandatory.

4.3.2 To the European Commission and European Parliament

Efforts should be continued to improve breast cancer screening in Europe by promoting exchange of experience. This may best be achieved by continuation of the activities of the European breast cancer screening network.

Updated guidelines should be published at regular intervals. Quality management should be ensured, including training and education in business strategy, recruitment, training and retention of qualified staff, quality assurance providing consumer protection, and management of political, governmental, economic, social and technical aspects of a programme.

Research should be encouraged on the impact of screening on breast cancer mortality, progression of mammography-detected lesions, ethical questions, population acceptance, method of invitation, cost-effectiveness, and psychosocial effects. These research activities should address mammography screening both below the age of 50 years, in the age range of 50-69 years, and from the age of 70 years onwards. Support should be given to development of appropriate data registration systems.

A system should be set up for accreditation on a European level of screening programmes applying to become reference centres in the breast cancer screening network.

5 Colorectal cancer screening

5.1 Epidemiology

For men the highest incidence of colorectal cancer incidence is found in Ireland, Austria and Denmark with 58-61 per 100,000 and the lowest in Greece with 25 per 100,000. For women the highest incidence is found in Denmark, The Netherlands and Ireland with 40-43 per 100,000 and the lowest in Greece with 19 per 100,000. Mortality rates for men are highest in Denmark and Ireland with 35-36 per 100,000 and lowest in Greece with 13 per 100,000. For women the mortality is highest in Denmark with 27 per 100,000 and lowest in Greece with 9 per 100,000. Despite advances in diagnostic techniques and treatment the 5-year survival rates remain poor.

5.2 Present situation

Faecal occult blood test, sigmoidoscopy and colonoscopy have all been considered as screening tests for colorectal cancer.

The faecal occult blood test is the only test which has been extensively evaluated as a screening tool on the population level. Four European trials have been undertaken (12-16). There are three randomised trials from Funen, Nottingham, UK and Gothenburg, Sweden and one non-randomised trial from Burgundy, France. In the last trial people from small areas "cantons" were allocated to either the screening or the control group. Only two screening rounds were undertaken in Gothenburg. In Funen, Nottingham and Burgundy screening was offered five times. A recent meta-analysis of all randomised faecal occult blood test trials showed a 16% reduction in colorectal cancer mortality (17).

Pilot screening programmes with the faecal occult blood test will start in two areas in England and Scotland in the year 2000, and pilot projects are under consideration in one area in Austria and one in Spain. Annual faecal occult blood tests are offered as part of the German cancer screening activities.

More complex faecal occult blood tests, especially immunological tests, have been developed (18-19). They are more sensitive, but their specificity at the population level is not well established. The effectiveness of flexible sigmoidoscopy as a screening tool is currently being tested in randomised trials in England and Italy (20-21).

5.3 Recommendations

5.3.1 To the Member States

As colorectal cancer is a major health problem in many European countries faecal occult blood screening should be seriously considered as a preventive measure. The decision on whether or not to embark on these screening programmes must depend on the availability of the professional expertise and the priority setting for healthcare resources.

If screening programmes are implemented they should use the faecal occult blood screening test and colonoscopy should be used for the follow-up of test positive cases. Screening should be offered men and women aged 50 years to about 74 years. The screening interval should be 1-2 years.

Other screening methods such as immunological tests, flexible sigmoidoscopy and colonoscopy can at present not be recommended for population screening.

5.3.2 To the European Commission and Parliament

Guidelines should be developed both at the European and national levels on quality assurance of faecal occult blood screening programmes.

Efforts should be continued to improve faecal occult blood tests. They must be carefully evaluated at a population level before being proposed in organised screening programmes with a special attention to cost-effectiveness. The effectiveness of flexible sigmoidoscopy as a screening tool should be evaluated in randomised controlled studies.

6 Prostate cancer screening

6.1 Epidemiology

The highest incidence of prostate cancer is observed in Finland, 101 per 100,000 being four times higher than in Greece, 24 per 100,000. This pronounced difference between European countries may reflect differences in medical procedures, in addition to variation in exposure to risk factors. This is supported by a smaller variation in mortality, being highest in Sweden, 36 per 100,000 and lowest in Greece, 17 per 100,000.

Prostate cancer is predominantly a disease of older age, and due to increasing longevity the number of cases is expected to increase over the coming years (22). Part of the presently observed increase in incidence in some European countries is most likely due to opportunistic screening with the prostate specific antigen (PSA).

6.2 Present situation

The effect of screening on prostate cancer mortality has not been documented. Rectal examination has been part of the annual health check up offered in Germany since the 1970s, but apart from this prostate cancer screening has not been an accepted policy in Europe. Opportunistic screening is, however, increasing. In the USA, the incidence of prostate cancer has almost doubled from 1986 to 1992 to decline again from 1992. This is most likely due to PSA screening (23). A slight decline in prostate cancer mortality started in American men in 1992, but the decline is so far without a conclusive explanation (24-25).

The European Randomised Study of Screening for Prostate Cancer (ERSPC) was initiated in 1994 in two and later in seven EU countries. It is the purpose of the study to test a 20% reduction in prostate cancer mortality after two screens in men followed up for 10 years. The study aims at randomising 192,000 men to the screening or control groups. In November 1999, 170,000 men have been randomised. Final results are expected in 2008.

ERSPC has joined forces with the Prostate, Lung, Colon, Ovary (PLOC) screening study of the US National Cancer Institute (26). The US study will include 63,625 men. A common analysis has been planned. In the meantime, the collected data offer excellent opportunities for evaluation of the screening test (27-28), potential overdiagnosis (29), quality of life and interval cancers. An update of the international co-operation will be published soon. A comprehensive review on prostate cancer screening has been published recently (30).

6.3 Recommended Activities

6.3.1 To the Member States

As long as randomised studies have not shown an advantage on prostate cancer mortality or related quality of life, screening for prostate cancer is not recommended as a health care policy.

6.3.2 To the European Commission and European Parliament

The European randomised trial should be completed.

7 Conclusions

Decisions on implementation of cancer screening programmes should be made within the frame of the general priority setting on use of healthcare resources.

Cancer screening should only be offered to healthy people if the screening is proven to decrease the disease-specific mortality or incidence, if the benefits and risks are well-known, and if the cost-effectiveness of the screening is acceptable. At present, these screening methods are:

- Pap smear screening for cervical abnormalities starting at the latest by the age of 30 years and definitely not before the age of 20 years,
- Mammography screening for breast cancer in women aged 50-69 years,
- Faecal occult blood screening for colorectal cancer in men and women age 50-74 years.

No other screening test should be offered healthy people before these tests have been shown to decrease the disease-specific mortality or incidence. Once the effectiveness of a new screening test has been demonstrated, evaluation of modified tests (e.g. alternative tests to the faecal occult blood analysis or interpretation of cervical specimens) may be possible using surrogate endpoints.

Potentially promising screening tests should be evaluated in randomised controlled trials, as is currently the case for:

- PSA testing for prostate cancer,
- Mammography screening for women aged 40-49 years,
- Flexible sigmoidoscopy for colorectal cancer.

Pap smear screening for cervical abnormalities, mammography screening for women aged 50-69 years, and faecal occult blood screening for colorectal cancer in subjects aged 50-74 years should be offered only in organised screening programmes with quality assurance at all levels, and good information about benefits and risks.

References

1) Wilson JMG, Jungner G. Principles and practice of screening for disease. Public Health Papers 34. Geneva: World Health Organisation, 1968.

2) Council of Europe: Committee of Ministers. On screening as a tool of preventive medicine. Recommendation no. R (94) 11. Strasbourg: Council of Europe, 1994.

3) http://iarc.fr. International Agency for Research on Cancer. Cancer Incidence Data Bases. EUCAN 1995. (retrieved 13 October 1999).

4) Hakama M. Trends in the incidence of cervical cancer in the Nordic countries. In: Magnus K, ed. Trends in cancer incidence. Washington, Hemisphere, 982.

5) Läärä E, Day N, Hakama M. Trends in mortality from cervical cancer in the Nordic countries: association with organised screening programmes. Lancet 1987, i, 1247-1249.

6) Sasieni PD, Adams J. Effect of screening on cervical cancer mortality in England and Wales: Analysis of trends with an age period cohort model. Br Med J 1999, 318, 1244-1245.

7) IARC Working Group on Evaluation of Cervical Cancer Screening Programmes. Screening for squamous cervical cancer: duration of low risk after negative results of cervical cytology and its implication for screening policies. Br Med J 1986, 293, 659-664.

8) Coleman D, Day NE, Douglas G, et al. European Guidelines for Quality Assurance in Cervical Cancer Screening. Eur J Cancer 1993, 29A (supplement 4), 1-38

9) Nyström L, Rutqvist LE, Wall S, et al. Breast cancer screening with mammography: overview of Swedish randomised trials. Lancet 1993, 341, 973-978.

10) Larsson L-G, Andersson I, Bjurstam N, et al. Updated overview of the Swedish randomised trials on breast cancer screening with mammography: age group 40-49 at randomisation. Monogr Nat Cancer Inst 1997, 22, 57-61.

11) European Commission. European Guidelines for Quality Assurance in Mammography Screening, 2nd edn. Bruxelles, European Commission, 1996.

12) Hardcastle JD, Chamberlain JO, Robinson MHE, et al. Randomised controlled trial of faecal-occult-blood screening for colorectal cancer. Lancet 1996, 348, 1472-1477.

13) Kronborg O, Fenger C, Olsen J, Jørgensen OD, Søndergaard O. Randomised study as screening for colorectal cancer with faecal-occult blood test. Lancet 1996, 348, 1467-1471.

14) Kewenter J, Brevenge H, Engaras B, Haglind E, Ahren C. Results of screening, rescreening and follow-up in a prospective randomised study for detection of colorectal cancer by faecal occult blood testing. Results of 68,308 subjects. Scand J Gastroenterol 1994, 29, 468-473.

15) Tazi MA, Faivre J, Dassonville F, Lamour J, Milan C, Durand G. Participation in faecal occult blood screening for colorectal cancer in a well defined French population : results of five screening rounds from 1988 to 1996. J Med Screen 1997, 4, 147-151.

16) Faivre J, Tazi MA, Milan C, Lejeune C, Durand G, Lamour J. Controlled trial of faecal occult blood screening for colorectal cancer in Burgundy (France). Results of the first 9 years. Gastroenterology 1999, 116, A400.

17) Towler B, Irwig L, Glasziou P, Kewenter J, Weller D, Silagy C. A systematic review of the effects of screening for colorectal cancer using the faecal occult blood test, Hemoccult. Brit Med J 1998, 317, 559-565.

18) Saito H, Soma Y, Koeda J, et al. Reduction in risk of mortality from colorectal cancer by fecal occult blood screening with immunochemical hemagglutination test. A case-control study. Int J Cancer 1995, 61, 465-469.

19) Castiglione G, Zappa M, Grazzini G, et al. Immunochemical vs guaiac faecal occult blood tests in a population-based screening programme for colorectal cancer. Br J Cancer 1996, 74, 141-144.

20) Atkin W, Cuzick J, Northover JMA, Whynes D. Prevention of colorectal cancer by once-only sigmoidoscopy. Lancet 1993, 341, 736-740.

21) Senore C, Segnan N, Rossini FP, et al. Screening for colorectal cancer by once only sigmoidoscopy: a feasibility study in Turin, Italy. J Med Screen 1996, 3, 72-78.

22) Boyle P, Maisonneuve P, Napalkov P. Geographical and temporal patterns of incidence and mortality from prostate cancer. Urology 1999, 46 (Suppl. 3A), 47-55.

23) Hankey BF, Feuer EJ, Clegg LX, et al. Cancer surveillance series: interpreting trends in prostate cancer – part I: evidence of the effects of screening in recent prostate cancer incidence, mortality, and survival rates. J Natl Cancer Inst 1999, 91, 1017-1024.

24) Feuer EJ, Merrill RM, Hankey BF. Cancer surveillance series: interpreting trends in prostate cancer – part II: cause of death misclassification and the recent rise and fall in prostate cancer mortality. J Natl Cancer Inst 1999, 91, 1025-1032.

25) Etzioni R, Legler JM, Feuer EJ, Merrill RM, Cronin KA, Hankey BF. Cancer surveillance series: interpreting trends in prostate cancer – part III: quantifying the link between population prostate-specific antigen testing and recent declines in prostate cancer mortality. J Natl Cancer Inst 1999, 91, 1033-1039.

26) Auvinen A, Rietbergen JBW, Denis LJ, Schröder FH, Prorok PhC for the International Prostate Cancer Screening Trial Evaluation Group. Prospective evaluation plan for randomised trials of prostate cancer screening. J Med Screen 1996, 3, 97-104.

27) Beemsterboer PMM, Kranse R, Koning HJ de, Habbema JDF, Schröder FH. Changing role for 3 screening modalities in the European Randomised Study of Screening for Prostate Cancer (Rotterdam). Int J Cancer 1999, 84, 437-441.

28) Schröder FH, Van der Maas P, Beemsterboer PMM, et al. Digital rectal examination (DRE) – its value in the diagnosis of prostate cancer. J Natl Cancer Inst 1998, 90, 1817-1823.

29) Schröder FH, Cruijssen-Koeter I van der, Kranse R, et al. Prostate cancer detection at low values of prostate specific antigen (PSA). J Urol 2000, 163, 806-812.

30) Schröder FH. Prostate Cancer. In Kramer BS, Gohagan JK, Prorok PC, eds. ancer Screening: Therapy and Practice. New York, Marcel Dekker Inc, 1999, 461-514.

Council of Europe I Committee of Ministers

Recommendation No. R (94) 11

**Of the Committee of Ministers to Member States
on screening as a tool of preventive medicine**

*(Adopted by the Committee of Ministers on 10 October
1994 at the 518th meeting of the Ministers' Deputies)*

The Committee of Ministers,

Considering that the aim of the Council of Europe is to achieve a greater unity between its members and that this aim may be pursued, inter alia, by the adoption of common action in the public health field;

Noting that chronic diseases are the major causes of death and a high social and economic burden in developed countries;

Considering that screening for the early detection of some of these diseases could, in principle, provide a method for their control;

Considering that, as yet, there is no absolute proof of the value of screening and early treatment in most diseases;

Considering that few, if any, diseases can at the present time be regarded as fulfilling all the desirable criteria for screening, and that the recommended evaluative procedures are not often carried out in full;

Recognising that the implementation of widespread screening programmes raises major ethical, legal, social, medical, organisational and economic problems which require initial and ongoing evaluation;

Taking into account the provisions of the Europe an Convention on Human Rights and of the European Social Charter;

Bearing in mind the Convention for the protection of individuals with regard to automatic processing of personal data of 28 January 1981, as well as the provisions of Recommendation No. R (81) 1 on regulations for automated medical banks and Recommendation No. R (83) 10 on the protection of personal data used for purposes of scientific research and statistics;

Recommends to governments of member states that they take account in their national health planning regulations and legislation of the conclusions and recommendations set out in the appendix to this recommendation.

Appendix to Recommendation No. R (94) 11

1. Introduction

1.1. For the purposes of this recommendation, screening means applying a test to a defined group of persons in order to identify an early stage, a preliminary stage, a risk factor or a combination of risk factors of a disease. In any case it is a question of detecting phenomena, which can be identified prior to the outbreak of the disease.

1.2. The object of screening as a service is to identify a certain disease or risk factor for a disease before the affected person spontaneously seeks treatment, in order to cure the disease or prevent or delay its progression or onset by (early) intervention.

1.3. The value of existing forms of screening for infectious diseases is fully acknowledged but these established methods are not considered in detail in this recommendation. Emphasis is made on screening for chronic degenerative non-communicable disorders.

1.4. Screening is only one method of controlling disease. It should be viewed in the whole context of reducing the burden of ill health to the individual and the community by, for example, socio-economic, environmental measures, health education and improvement of existing health care and disease prevention systems.

1.5. Environmental factors are recognised as important contributors to disease, but inherited factors may also play an important role. With the advent of new genetic knowledge, an increasing number of genetic diseases and genetic risk factors for disease will be identified and offer the possibility for new screening procedures. As the procedures for genetic screening are not fully established nor fully evaluated, they have not been included in this recommendation.

1.6. The present position is that the implementation of screening in European countries is fragmentary, with few national screening programmes for the total population but many screening schemes restricted to population groups.

1.7. Because there are differences in health needs and health services, as well as in ethical values and in legal norms and rules between countries, the decision to implement a particular screening programme should be taken in cooperation with the medical profession by each country. Nevertheless there are common general principles and problems which are equally relevant to all systems.

1.8. Screening is a tool which is potentially capable of improving the health of the population but it also has adverse effects. Constant care should be taken to ensure that in any screening programme the advantages prevail over the disadvantages.

1.9. The general benefits of screening are often described. It is, however, also important to be aware of the adverse effects which can be:
- stigmatisation and/or discrimination of (non) participants;

- social pressure to participate in the screening and undergo the intended treatment/intervention;
- psychological distress where there is no cure for the disease or where the treatment and/or intervention is morally unacceptable to the individual concerned;
- exposure to physical and psychological risks with limited health gains;
- creation of expectations which probably cannot be fulfilled;
- individuals who are positively screened might experience difficulties such as access to insurance, employment, etc.;
- severe side effects of invasive clinical diagnosis of false positives;
- delay in diagnosing false negatives;
- unfavourable cost-benefit relationship of a screening programme.

1.10. The various problems which are encountered in the introduction and provision of screening interrelated. Nevertheless, a distinction may be made between those concerned with:
  I.   ethical and legal issues;
  II. selection of diseases (medically) suitable for screening;
  III. economic aspects and evaluation of screening;
  IV. quality assurance;
  V.   organisation of a screening programme;
  VI. scientific research.

2. Ethical and legal values

2.1. Effectiveness is a necessary prerequisite for the screening to be ethical. It should none the less be kept in mind that screening can be effective and still unethical.

2.2. Advantages and disadvantages of screening for the target population and the individual must be well balanced, taking into account social and economic costs, equity as well as individual rights and freedoms.

2.3. Failure to make known information on the positive and negative aspects of the screening is unethical and infringes the autonomy of the individual.

2.4. The decision to participate in a screening programme should be taken freely. The diagnoses and treatments which may follow the screening should also require a free and separate consent. No pressure should be used to lead somebody to undergo any of these procedures.

2.5. The right to privacy requires that the results of the tests as a general rule are not communicated to those who do not wish to be informed, are collected, stored, and handled confidentially, and adequately protected. It is preferable not to screen individuals who do not wish to be informed of the results of the screening.

2.6. Neonatal screening can only be justified if the intervention is of direct health benefit to the child. Otherwise screening should be postponed until the child can decide for itself.

2.7. No personal data derived from the screening should be communicated to third parties unless the data subject has given consent to it or in accordance with national law.

2.8. When a screening programme is provided as a service and conducted also for research purposes, the decision to make available personal medical data stemming from the screening programme for research purposes should be taken freely, without undue pressure.

The decision not to take part in the research should not in any way prevent the individual from participating in the screening programme.

3. Criteria for selecting diseases suitable for screening

3.1. The disease should be an obvious burden for the individual and/or the community in terms of death, suffering, economic or social costs.

3.2. The natural course of the disease should be well-known and the disease should go through an initial latent stage or be determined by risk factors, which can be detected by appropriate tests. An appropriate test is highly sensitive and specific for the disease as well as being acceptable to the person screened.

3.3. Adequate treatment or other intervention possibilities are indispensable. Adequacy is determined both by proven medical effect and ethical and legal acceptability.

3.4. Screening followed by diagnosis and intervention in an early stage of the disease should provide a better prognosis than intervention after spontaneously sought treatment.

4. Economic aspects

4.1. The increasing financial burden of health care makes it necessary to assess the economic aspects of screening. However these aspects should not be the overriding consideration. In all screening programmes human consideration regarding the value and quality of life, life expectancy as well as respect for individual rights are of prime importance.

4.2. Economic assessments are necessary to enable rational decisions to be made on the priority to be given to alternative ways of using health resources.

4.3. Measurement of the economic aspects of screening is not fully mastered. Early detection and treatment may be less expensive than late treatment. However, available studies relate only to present screening costs and further work is necessary to determine possible cost control in the long term.

4.4. Non systematic screening or spontaneous screening results in high marginal costs. Only systematic screening is able to provide means for controlling cost. Therefore, constant care should be taken to ensure that in any screening programme the allocated resources are used in an optimal way.

5. Quality assurance

5.1. Screening should aim at the highest possible standards of quality from the medical and organisational point of view.

5.2. Because of the expectations that screening creates as well as its adverse effects, screening should meet the highest quality assurance standards in all its aspects.

5.3. An assessment of the scientific evidence of the effectiveness of screening in the control of a disease should be made by experimental studies before introducing a screening programme as a service. The practical arrangements for a mass screening, which are directly linked to the health structures and systems, should obtain the same effectiveness as that obtained in the randomised trial.

5.4. Having implemented a screening programme, it should be subjected to continuous independent evaluation. Evaluation will facilitate adaptation of the programme, correction of deficiencies noted and verification of achievement of objectives. The adverse effects of the screening programme should not be ignored in the evaluation which should be carried out by independent public health experts.

5.5. If quality assurance standards are not met in the long term it should be possible for the screening programme to be corrected, and, if this is not possible, stopped.

5.6. The programme must evaluate participation, and the percentage of people screened in the target population, the technical quality of testing and the quality of diagnosis and treatment provided as a follow-up for persons with a positive test result. Severe side effects of false positives should be revealed and evaluated.

5.7. There is a need for more teaching of medical students in epidemiology and its application to measuring the effects of screening. Similarly post-graduate education in this field is also needed to enable practising doctors to understand the principles and evaluation of screening.

5.8. Provision of screening programmes requires that training in techniques and interpretation of screening tests is included in undergraduate and post-graduate medical teaching programmes.

5.9. A screening programme requires resources in both staff and technical facilities for carrying out the screening tests. In many instances tests can be performed by non medical staff. Provision should be made for initial and further training of the medical and technical staff who will be involved in performing the screening tests and interpreting their results. Technical methods, including automated techniques, are useful in screening for some diseases. Quality of screening methods should be monitored.

6. Organisation

6.1. The organising body of a screening programme should be held responsible throughout the programme. The organisation of a screening programme should comply with what is described in national guidelines and protocols.

6.2. Within the organisational framework the target population should be defined (by age or otherwise) as well as the frequency of screening tests and the general and specific objectives and quality assurance guidelines.

6.3. It must be stressed that screening cannot succeed without co-operation between preventive and curative systems. Organisation must be tailored to the structures of the health system. If appropriate structures in the curative health care system are lacking, screening should not be implemented until they are developed (pilot programmes, for example). There are various degrees to which screening services may be integrated with curative services or develop as a separate speciality. The advantages and disadvantages of these should be assessed separately in different health care systems.

6.4. Provisions should be made for the financing of the programme, the cost of organising and evaluating the structure, the cost of testing, the cost of quality assessment and monitoring, and the cost of the follow-up care of those people who screen positively.

6.5. Process and outcome indicators should be constantly evaluated.

6.6. Systematic collection of data is required in screening programmes to serve the needs of the individual and of the health service. To that end, data should be collected on the target population, on persons screened (with dates and the results of the test carried out), and on the results of eventual diagnostic examinations. Access to a morbidity register considerably facilitates evaluation.

6.7. Adequate protection of all data collected by means of a screening programme should be guaranteed.

6.8. Participation of the public in screening programmes is determined by personal factors (for example attitudes, motivation and anxiety) and by situational factors (waiting time and efficient organisation, for example). These can be influenced for instance by health education and by good organisation of the screening procedure.

6.9. In order to ensure optimal participation by the target population, the best possible information should be widely provided and awareness-raising and education programmes should be organised for both the target population and the health professionals.

6.10. Invitations should be accompanied by written information on the purposes and effectiveness of the programme, on the test, on potential advantages and disadvantages, on the voluntary nature of participation and on how data will be protected. An address should be provided for those who require further information.

6.11. Participants should be informed on how, when and where their test results will be available or will be communicated to them.

6.12. The positive results found at screening should always be confirmed by subsequent diagnostic tests before commencing a treatment/intervention, unless the screening test is a diagnostic test. It is absolutely essential that adequate diagnostic facilities are available to confirm or reject the screening finding as soon as possible. Similarly, treatment facilities must be available and easily accessible to the confirmed cases. The work load placed on the health services by screening can be very large, especially since most screening programmes also lead to incidental pathological findings unrelated to the disease at which the programme is aimed.

6.13. Combining screening for several diseases into a multiple screening procedure may seem to be convenient to the individual and economic to the programme, but such a 'package deal' may negatively influence the extent to which most of the criteria for screening including age limit and frequency would be met.

7. Research

7.1. Research into new, more effective, screening tests must be encouraged and the long-term effects of the various methods of treatment and provision for positive subjects studied. Research must be further developed to answer the numerous social, ethical, legal, medical, organisational and economic questions as well as psychological problems raised by screening, on which evidence is incomplete.

7.2. Quality assurance concerning research programmes should be conducted into the effectiveness of the various screening tests, the practical arrangements for screening, the measures to increase participation, the means of improving test efficiency, follow-up to and provisions for those screened positive, an assessment process and all the economic aspects.

7.3. Information gathered during screening should be available for the purpose of scientific research, for the improvement of health services, and for the benefit of future screening, taking into account full respect of autonomy and confidentiality and the protection of personal privacy.

8. General remarks

8.1. It is particularly important that political decision-makers and target groups should be kept informed of the current state of knowledge about the value of screening for particular diseases. Improved communication should be encouraged.

8.2. Governments should promote the research and evaluation necessary for assessing the value of both new and existing programmes. This form of research necessarily means large-scale research which, in some instances, may be designed as international collaborative studies. Scientific evaluation is the only way in which the positive and negative effects of screening can be assessed in order that a rational decision can be taken on whether a screening programme should be implemented and what resources should be allocated.

Quality assurance (as defined by World Health Organization):

'All those planned and systematic actions necessary to provide adequate confidence that a structure, system or component will perform satisfactorily in service (ISO 6215 1980). Satisfactory performance in service implies the optimum quality of the entire diagnostic process i.e., the consistent production of adequate diagnostic information with minimum exposure of both patients and personnel.'

Quality control (as defined by World Health Organization):

'The set of operations (programming, co-ordinating, carrying out) intended to maintain or to improve [...] (ISO 35341977). As applied to a diagnostic procedure, it covers monitoring, evaluation and maintenance at optimum levels of all characteristics of performance that can be defined, measured, and controlled.'

Council Directive 97/43/Euratom

of 30 June 1997 on health protection of individuals against the dangers of ionizing radiation in relation to medical exposure, and repealing Directive 84/466/Euratom

The Council of the European Union,

Having regard to the Treaty establishing the European Atomic Energy Community, and in particular Article 31 thereof,
Having regard to the proposal from the Commission, drawn up after obtaining the opinion of a group of persons appointed by the Scientific and Technical Committee,

Having regard to the opinion of the European Parliament (1),

Having regard to the opinion of the Economic and Social Committee (2),

(1)   Whereas the Council has adopted Directives laying down the basic safety standards for the protection of the health of workers and the general public against the dangers arising from ionizing radiation, as last amended by Directive 96/29/Euratom (3);

(2)   Whereas in accordance with Article 33 of the Treaty, each Member State is to lay down the appropriate provisions, whether by legislation, regulation or administrative action, to ensure compliance with the basic standards which have been established and take the necessary measures with regard to teaching, education and vocational training;

(3)   Whereas, on 3 September 1984 the Council adopted Directive 84/466/Euratom laying down the basic measures for the radiation protection of persons undergoing medical examination or treatment (4);

(4)   Whereas, as in 1984, medical exposure continues to constitute the major source of exposure to artificial sources of ionizing radiation of European Union citizens; whereas the use of ionizing radiation has enabled great progress to be made in many aspects of medicine; whereas practices causing medical exposure need to be carried out in optimized radiation protection conditions;

(5)   Whereas, recognizing the development of scientific knowledge in the field of radiation protection applied to medical exposure, the International Commission on Radiological Protection reviewed the subject in its 1990 and 1996 recommendations;

(6)   Whereas such developments make it necessary to repeal Directive 84/466/ Euratom;

(7)   Whereas Directive 96/29/Euratom lays down basic safety standards for the protection of the workers administering the medical exposure and of the members of the public; whereas the same Directive ensures that the total of contributions to the exposure of the population as a whole, is kept under review;

(8)   Whereas health and safety requirements, including radiation protection aspects, regarding the design, manufacture and placing on the market of the medical devices are dealt with by Council Directive 93/42/EEC of 14 June 1993 concerning medical devices (5); whereas pursuant to Article 1 (8) of that Directive, the relevant Directives adopted under the Euratom Treaty are not to be affected by its provisions; whereas it is necessary to set out radiation protection requirements for the medical use of radiological installations from the date of the commencement of their operation;

(9)   Whereas provisions need to be adapted for the protection as regards exposure incurred by volunteers and persons knowingly and willingly helping persons undergoing medical examination or treatment;

(10)   Whereas the Committee of Ministers of the Council of Europe adopted on 6 February

1990 Recommendation R(90)3 on medical research on human beings, concerning inter alia the setting up of an ethics committee;

(11) Whereas detailed requirements are needed for the correct application of the justification and optimization principles in relation to exposure within the scope of this Directive;

(12) Whereas responsibilities for administering medical exposure need to be set out;

(13) Whereas appropriate training for the staff involved, the establishment of quality assurance and audit programmes, and inspections by the competent authorities are necessary to ensure that medical exposure is delivered under good radiation protection conditions;

(14) Whereas specific provisions are necessary as regards special practice, pregnant and breastfeeding females, volunteers in research and helping persons;

(15) Whereas potential exposure needs to be taken into account,

Has adopted this directive:

Article 1 Purpose and scope

1. This Directive supplements Directive 96/29/Euratom and lays down the general principles of the radiation protection of individuals in relation to the exposure referred to in paragraphs 2 and 3.

2. This Directive shall apply to the following medical exposure:
   (a) the exposure of patients as part of their own medical diagnosis or treatment;
   (b) the exposure of individuals as part of occupational health surveillance;
   (c) the exposure of individuals as part of health screening programmes;
   (d) the exposure of healthy individuals or patients voluntarily participating in medical or biomedical, diagnostic or therapeutic, research programmes;
   (e) the exposure of individuals as part of medico-legal procedures.

3. This Directive shall also apply to exposure of individuals knowingly and willingly helping (other than as part of their occupation) in the support and comfort of individuals undergoing medical exposure.

Article 2 Definitions

For the purpose of this Directive, the following terms have the meaning hereby assigned them:

- Clinical audit: a systematic examination or review of medical radiological procedures which seeks to improve the quality and the outcome of patient care through structured review whereby radiological practices, procedures and results are examined against agreed standards for good medical radiological procedures, with modification of practices where indicated and the application of new standards if necessary.

- Clinical Responsibility: responsibility regarding individual medical exposures attributed to a practitioner, notably: justification; optimization; clinical evaluation of the outcome; cooperation with other specialists and the staff, as appropriate, regarding practical aspects; obtaining information, if appropriate, of previous examinations; providing existing radiological information and/or records to other practitioners and/or prescribers, as required; giving information on the risk of ionizing radiation to patients and other individuals involved, as appropriate.

- Competent Authorities: any authority designated by a Member State.

- Diagnostic Reference Levels: dose levels in medical radiodiagnostic practices or, in the case of radio-pharmaceuticals, levels of activity, for typical examinations for groups of standard-sized patients or standard phantoms for broadly defined types of equipment. These levels are expected not to be exceeded for standard procedures when good and normal practice regarding diagnostic and technical performance is applied.

- Dose Constraint: a restriction on the prospective doses to individuals which may result from a defined source, for use at the planning stage in radiation protection whenever optimization is involved.
- Exposure: the process of being exposed to ionizing radiation.
- Health screening: a procedure using radiological installations for early diagnosis in population groups at risk.
- Holder: any natural or legal person who has the legal responsibility under national law for a given radiological installation.
- Individual Detriment: clinically observable deleterious effects that are expressed in individuals or their descendants, the appearance of which is either immediate or delayed and, in the latter case, implies a probability rather than a certainty of appearance.
- Inspection: inspection is an investigation by any competent authority to verify compliance with national provisions on radiological protection for medical radiological procedures, equipment in use or radiological installations.
- Medical Physics Expert: an expert in radiation physics or radiation technology applied to exposure, within the scope of this Directive, whose training and competence to act is recognized by the competent authorities; and who, as appropriate, acts or gives advice on patient dosimetry, on the development and use of complex techniques and equipment, on optimization, on quality assurance, including quality control, and on other matters relating to radiation protection, concerning exposure within the scope of this Directive.
- Medical Radiological Procedure: any procedure concerning medical exposure.
- Medico-legal procedures: procedures performed for insurance or legal purposes without a medical indication.
- Occupational health surveillance: the medical surveillance for workers as specified by Member States or competent authorities.
- Patient dose: the dose, concerning patients or other individuals undergoing medical exposure.
- Patient dosimetry: the dosimetry concerning patients or other individuals undergoing medical exposure.
- Practical Aspects: the physical conduct of any of the exposure referred to in Article 1 (2) and any supporting aspects including handling and use of radiological equipment, and the assessment of technical and physical parameters including radiation doses, calibration and maintenance of equipment, preparation and administration of radio-pharmaceuticals and the development of films.
- Practitioner: a medical doctor, dentist or other health professional, who is entitled to take clinical responsibility for an individual medical exposure in accordance with national requirements.
- Prescriber: a medical doctor, dentist or other health professional, who is entitled to refer individuals for medical exposure to a practitioner, in accordance with national requirements.
- Quality Assurance: all those planned and systematic actions necessary to provide adequate confidence that a structure, system, component or procedure will perform satisfactorily complying with agreed standards.
- Quality control: is a part of quality assurance. The set of operations (programming, coordinating, implementing) intended to maintain or to improve quality. It covers monitoring, evaluation and maintenance at required levels of all characteristics of

performance of equipment that can be defined, measured, and controlled.
- Radiological: pertaining to radiodiagnostic and radiotherapeutic procedures, and interventional radiology or other planning and guiding radiology.
- Radiological installation: a facility containing radiological equipment.
- Radiodiagnostic: pertaining to in vivo diagnostic nuclear medicine, medical diagnostic radiology, and dental radiology.
- Radiotherapeutic: pertaining to radiotherapy including nuclear medicine for therapeutic purposes.

Article 3 Justification

1. Medical exposure referred to in Article 1 (2) shall show a sufficient net benefit, weighing the total potential diagnostic or therapeutic benefits it produces, including the direct health benefits to an individual and the benefits to society, against the individual detriment that the exposure might cause, taking into account the efficacy, benefits and risks of available alternative techniques having the same objective but involving no or less exposure to ionizing radiation.
   In particular:
   (a) - all new types of practices involving medical exposure shall be justified in advance before being generally adopted,
       - existing types of practices involving medical exposure may be reviewed whenever new, important evidence about their efficacy or consequences is acquired.
   (b) all individual medical exposures shall be justified in advance taking into account the specific objectives of the exposure and the characteristics of the individual involved.
   If a type of practice involving a medical exposure is not justified in general, a specific individual exposure of this type could be justified in special circumstances, to be evaluated on a case-by-case basis.
   The prescriber and the practitioner as specified by Member States, shall seek, where practicable, to obtain previous diagnostic information or medical records relevant to the planned exposure and consider these data to avoid unnecessary exposure.
   (c) medical exposure for biomedical and medical research shall be examined by an ethics committee, set up in accordance with national procedures and/or by the competent authorities.
   (d) special attention shall be given to the justification of those medical exposures where there is no direct health benefit for the person undergoing the exposure and especially for those exposures on medico-legal grounds.
2. Exposure referred to in Article 1 (3) shall show a sufficient net benefit, taking into account also the direct health benefits to a patient, the benefits to individuals referred to in Article 1 (3) and the detriment that the exposure might cause.
3. If an exposure can not be justified, it should be prohibited.

Article 4 Optimization

1. (a) All doses due to medical exposure for radiological purposes except radiotherapeutic procedures referred to in Article 1 (2) shall be kept as low as reasonably achievable consistent with obtaining the required diagnostic information, taking into account economic and social factors.
   (b) For all medical exposure of individuals for radiotherapeutic purposes, as mentioned

in Article 1 (2) (a), exposures of target volumes shall be individually planned; taking into account that doses of non-target volumes and tissues shall be as low as reasonably achievable and consistent with the intended radiotherapeutic purpose of the exposure.

2. Member States shall:

(a) promote the establishment and the use of diagnostic reference levels for radiodiagnostic examinations, as referred to in Article 1 (2) (a), (b), (c) and (e), and the availability of guidance for this purpose having regard to European diagnostic reference levels where available;

(b) ensure that for each biomedical and medical research project as mentioned in Article 1 (2) (d):

- the individuals concerned shall participate voluntarily,
- these individuals shall be informed about the risks of this exposure,
- a dose constraint is established for individuals for whom no direct medical benefit is expected from this exposure,
- in the case of patients, who voluntarily accept to undergo an experimental diagnostic or therapeutic practice and who are expected to receive a diagnostic or therapeutical benefit from this practice, the target levels of doses shall be planned on an individual basis by the practitioner and/or prescriber;

(c) ensure that special attention be given, to keep the dose arising from the medico-legal exposure referred to in Article 1 (2) (e) as low as reasonably achievable.

3. The optimization process shall include the selection of equipment, the consistent production of adequate diagnostic information or therapeutic outcome as well as the practical aspects, quality assurance including quality control and the assessment and evaluation of patient doses or administered activities, taking into account economic and social factors.

4. Member States shall ensure that:

(a) dose constraints are established for exposure, as referred to in Article 1 (3), of those individuals knowingly and willingly helping (other than as part of their occupation) in the support and comfort of patients undergoing medical diagnosis or treatment where appropriate;

(b) appropriate guidance is established for exposure as referred to in Article 1 (3);

(c) in the case of a patient undergoing a treatment or diagnosis with radionuclides, where appropriate the practitioner or the holder of the radiological installation provides the patient or legal guardian with written instructions, with a view to the restriction of doses to persons in contact with the patient as far as reasonably achievable and to provide information on the risks of ionizing radiation.

These instructions shall be handed out before leaving the hospital or clinic or a similar institution.

Article 5 Responsibilities

1. The prescriber as well as the practitioner shall be involved as specified by Member States in the justification process at the appropriate level.

2. Member States shall ensure that any medical exposure referred to in Article 1 (2) is effected under the clinical responsibility of a practitioner.

3. The practical aspects for the procedure or part of it may be delegated by the holder of the radiological installation or the practitioner, as appropriate, to one or more

individuals entitled to act in this respect in a recognized field of specialization.

4. Member States shall ensure the laying down of procedures to be observed in case of medico-legal examinations.

Article 6 Procedures

1. Written protocols for every type of standard radiological practice shall be established for each equipment.

2. Member States shall ensure that recommendations concerning referral criteria for medical exposure, including radiation doses, are available to the prescribers of medical exposure.

3. In radiotherapeutic practices, a medical physics expert shall be closely involved. In standardized therapeutical nuclear medicine practices and in diagnostic nuclear medicine practices, a medical physics expert shall be available. For other radiological practices, a medical physics expert shall be involved, as appropriate, for consultation on optimization including patient dosimetry and quality assurance including quality control, and also to give advice on matters relating to radiation protection concerning medical exposure, as required.

4. Clinical audits shall be carried out in accordance with national procedures.

5. Member States shall ensure that appropriate local reviews are undertaken whenever diagnostic reference levels are consistently exceeded and that corrective actions are taken where appropriate.

Article 7 Training

1. Member States shall ensure that practitioners and those individuals mentioned in Articles 5 (3) and 6 (3) have adequate theoretical and practical training for the purpose of radiological practices, as well as relevant competence in radiation protection. For this purpose Member States shall ensure that appropriate curricula are established and shall recognize the corresponding diplomas, certificates or formal qualifications.

2. Individuals undergoing relevant training programmes may participate in practical aspects for the procedures mentioned in Article 5 (3).

3. Member States shall ensure that continuing education and training after qualification is provided and, in the special case of the clinical use of new techniques, the organization of training related to these techniques and the relevant radiation protection requirements.

4. Member States shall encourage the introduction of a course on radiation protection in the basic curriculum of medical and dental schools.

Article 8 Equipment

1. Member States shall take such steps as they may consider necessary with a view to avoiding unnecessary proliferation of radiological equipment.

2. Member States shall ensure that:
    - all radiological equipment in use is kept under strict surveillance regarding radiation protection,
    - an up-to-date inventory of radiological equipment for each radiological installation is available to the competent authorities,
    - appropriate quality assurance programmes including quality control measures and

patient dose or administered activity assessments are implemented by the holder of the radiological installation, and
- acceptance testing is carried out before the first use of the equipment for clinical purposes, and thereafter performance testing on a regular basis, and after any major maintenance procedure.

3. Competent authorities shall take steps to ensure that necessary measures are taken by the holder of the radiological installation to improve inadequate or defective features of the equipment. They shall also adopt specific criteria of acceptability for equipment in order to indicate when appropriate remedial action is necessary, including, if appropriate, taking the equipment out of service.

4. In the case of fluoroscopy, examinations without an image intensification or equivalent techniques are not justified and shall therefore be prohibited.

5. Fluoroscopic examinations without devices to control the dose rate shall be limited to justified circumstances.

6. If new radiodiagnostical equipment is used, it shall have, where practicable, a device informing the practitioner of the quantity of radiation produced by the equipment during the radiological procedure.

Article 9 Special practices

1. Member States shall ensure that appropriate radiological equipment, practical techniques and ancillary equipment are used for the medical exposure
   - of children,
   - as part of a health screening programme,
   - involving high doses to the patient, such as interventional radiology, computed tomography or radiotherapy.
   Special attention shall be given to the quality assurance programmes, including quality control measures and patient dose or administered activity assessment, as mentioned in Article 8, for these practices.

2. Member States shall ensure that practitioners and those individuals referred to in Article 5 (3) performing the exposure referred to in the first paragraph obtain appropriate training on these radiological practices as required by Article 7 (1) and (2).

Article 10 Special protection during pregnancy and breastfeeding

1. (a) In the case of a female of childbearing age, the prescriber and the practitioner shall inquire as specified by Member States whether she is pregnant, or breastfeeding, if relevant; and
   (b) if pregnancy cannot be excluded, depending on the type of medical exposure, in particular if abdominal and pelvic regions are involved, special attention shall be given to the justification, particularly the urgency, and to the optimization of the medical exposure taking into account the exposure both of the expectant mother and the unborn child.

2. In the case of breastfeeding females, in nuclear medicine depending on the type of medical examination or treatment, special attention shall be given to the justification, particularly the urgency, and to the optimization of the medical exposure, taking into account the exposure both for the mother and the child.

3. Without prejudice to Article 10 (1) and (2), any measure contributing to increasing the awareness of women subject to this Article, such as public notices in appropriate places, could be helpful.

Article 11 Potential exposure

Member States shall ensure that all reasonable steps to reduce the probability and the magnitude of accidental or unintended doses of patients from radiological practices are taken, economic and social factors being taken into account.

The main emphasis in accident prevention should be on the equipment and procedures in radiotherapy, but some attention should be paid to accidents with diagnostic equipment. Working instructions and written protocols as referred to in Article 6 (1) and quality assurance programmes as referred to in Article 8 (2) and the criteria referred to in Article 8 (3) are of particular relevance for this purpose.

Article 12 Estimates of population doses

Member States shall ensure that the distribution of individual dose estimates from medical exposure referred to in Article 1 (2) is determined for the population and for relevant reference groups of the population as may be deemed necessary by the Member State.

Article 13 Inspection

Member States shall ensure that a system of inspection as defined in Article 2 enforces the provisions introduced in compliance with this Directive.

Article 14 Transposition into Member State law

1. Member States shall bring into force the laws, regulations and administrative provisions necessary to comply with this Directive before 13 May 2000. They shall forthwith inform the Commission thereof.

    When Member States adopt these measures, they shall contain a reference to this Directive or shall be accompanied by such reference on the occasion of their official publication. The methods of making such reference shall be adopted by Member States.

2. Member States shall communicate to the Commission the text of the main laws, regulations or administrative provisions which they adopt in the field covered by this Directive.

Article 15 Repeal

Directive 84/466/Euratom is hereby repealed with effect from 13 May 2000.

Article 16

This Directive is addressed to the Member States.

Done at Luxembourg, 30 June 1997.

For the Council | The President | A. NUIS

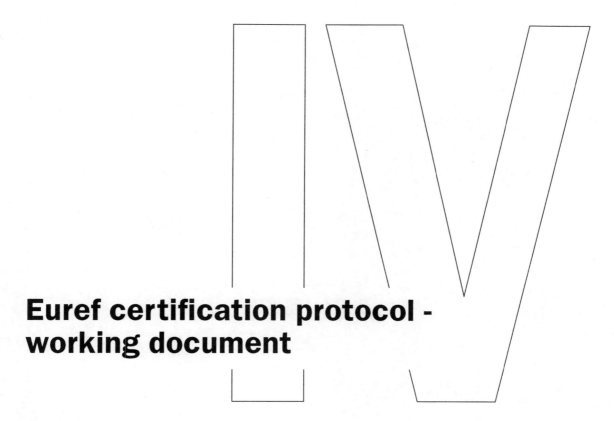

Euref certification protocol - working document

Authors
N. Perry
M. Broeders
J. Ennis
R. Holland
M. Rosselli del Turco
J. Schouten
C. de Wolf

The following should be regarded as a working document to be used for a feasibility study period which commenced in the year 2000 which we hope will lead towards the implementation of a formal programme for certification of mammography units in Europe. The basic elements necessary for the study period are set out below.

Executive summary

Mammography (X-ray examination of the breast) is a widely used imaging procedure - undergone by some 5 - 10 million women per year in the European Member States. The main benefits are those of reassurance of normality, early detection of breast cancer and reduction in mortality from breast cancer by mammography screening. The potential harm in terms of the creation of unnecessary anxiety and morbidity, untoward economic costs and the use of ionising radiation should not be underestimated.

Use of sub-optimal equipment by insufficiently trained and skilled professional staff will negate the major benefits of screening and result in poorly effective and cost-ineffective mammography services. We believe that positive steps are necessary to abolish such practice and that it is important to help consumers, health care professionals, government authorities and other interested parties to identify high quality mammography services appropriate to women's needs.

We therefore propose the development of a European programme for voluntary certification of high quality mammography services with continued efforts to promote quality improvement. Certification allows tangible and demonstrable recognition of adherence to a recognised quality system and will take into account the special requirements of both symptomatic and screening services. This voluntary certification programme will be developed for the European Commission by EUREF in cooperation with the European Network of Breast Screening programmes, competent departments of the European Commission, European agencies and other interested national authorities in Member States.

Methodology and criteria are described for four chosen categories of certification, two for the provision of diagnostic mammography services and two for the provision of mammography screening programmes. These categories range from the ability to produce an adequate quality mammogram up to a centre performing population screening to European Reference Centre level.

Introduction

Europe currently leads the world in implementation of organised population based breast cancer screening programmes using mammography of demonstrable high quality. Considerable progress has been made with effective population based screening in several Member States. The experience gained in these activities has demonstrated the complex technical, organisational and professional aspects of maintaining an appropriate balance between the beneficial and potentially harmful effects of mammography. This need for a high quality service in mammography and breast screening has become increasingly recognised over recent years. Attention to technical detail has been scientifically demonstrated to increase cancer detection rates and in particular to increase detection of small invasive cancers[1], a major prerequisite for maximising mortality reduction from breast cancer screening by mammography.

Training and adherence to audit have played a significant part in such advances. One of the lessons learnt is that effective mammography screening cannot be established in the framework of opportunistic screening within a symptomatic mammography service. It is essential to have in place high quality diagnostic mammography services which may or may not participate within a fully organised quality assured breast screening process. Benefits and advances gained by quality assured screening programmes working to recognised high standards should be introduced into programmes that are less experienced and also into the realms of diagnostic mammography.

In 1988 the European Commission funded Europe Against Cancer Programme initiated a Pilot Project Network in the Member States. This would examine and develop the methodologies of breast cancer screening in different health care environments, share knowledge and experience, provide a common logo under which the Network could move forward together, and provide reliable information for political decision making in each Member State as to the future of any national breast screening programmes. After the first few years, the pilot projects matured into a more quality based network for breast cancer screening, with funding only provided for quality improvement initiatives. EUREF - see annex VIII - was set up in order to facilitate and coordinate training in these screening centres. EUREF would provide epidemiological and physico-technical support and ultimately have the aim of bringing each of the network members to Reference Centre status within its own country. The breast screening network has received funding from The Europe Against Cancer programme and up until now the provision of such funding for quality assurance measures, the coordinating of training by EUREF and the site visits performed by consultants to the programme have been the major means by which a quality service has been documented and recognised.

We regard it as crucial that adherence to a quality system receives tangible and demonstrable recognition by way of certification. Certification of health care services is an endeavour receiving increasing attention from government agencies, professional bodies and health care purchasers and providers in Europe. There is an increasing awareness of the benefits of this process in improving the outcome and the cost-effectiveness of health care services through successful implementation of quality assurance systems. The inference from certification is two fold. Firstly that a certain level of performance has been achieved, secondly that a certificate may be withdrawn if standards are not maintained. In order to ensure that previous standards have not deteriorated, it is suggested that re-certification must be obtained every five years.

Certification in this instance may be defined as the granting of documentation in the form of a certificate bearing the EUREF logo and signed by a suitably senior executive within the EUREF organisation. The certificate will be time limited and will state that a recognised visiting team of professionals, approved by EUREF, has visited the unit/organisation concerned and has found it to have achieved satisfactory standards to the level of certification granted in accordance with the protocol and published guidelines.

Such requests for certification have been received by the EUREF office in Nijmegen from various centres within and outside the Breast Screening Network. We believe that it is important for EUREF to respond to these requests and to extend its activity in this manner. By so doing it will increase its commitment to quality assurance activities throughout Europe and will bring benefit from its extensive team of associated experts to those European areas not currently experienced in high quality mammography.

Some workers believe that the way forward in this matter is to undergo the process of obtaining the ISO 9000 Standard. Experience in the UK Breast Screening Programme has shown that this methodology is not optimal for the purpose required in breast cancer screening. The voluntary accreditation system for mammography in the United States organised initially by The American College of Radiology demonstrated most effectively how such a system rapidly takes hold and may become mandatory in the short to medium term. Ultimately, 'purchasing power' from general practitioners, women's groups or health insurance agencies is likely to be of great significance. Certification can act in support of this.

All requests for certification will be of a voluntary nature until such time in the future that the European Commission or other authorities consider this to be mandatory. These certification activities should not be detrimental to any worthwhile local quality initiatives taking place in units or programmes, and as far as possible should eventually become integrated with, and work alongside initiatives being taken at national level by recognised authorities in each Member State.

Screening versus diagnostic activity

It is important to distinguish clearly between the differing requirements for a diagnostic service (predominantly symptomatic) and a screening programme (predominantly asymptomatic). It is important to avoid confusion between the wider organisational and epidemiological support that will be necessary for a screening programme and to some extent the differing facilities and skills that may be required between both services.

We are committed to recognising and protecting the considerable skills and expertise acquired by numerous funded screening programmes as part of the Europe Against Cancer Breast Screening Network, and already quality assured by EUREF.

To this end we have separated the certification categories between screening and diagnostic activity. We intend to further clarify this issue by issuing certificates which will be marked as EUREF DIAGNOSTIC or EUREF SCREENING. The issuing of a EUREF DIAGNOSTIC Certificate will therefore make no judgement or reference to the ability to perform screening, likewise the possession of a EUREF DIAGNOSTIC certificate in no way implies that the EUREF organisation considers this unit as suitable to perform screening activities.

EUREF SCREENING Certificates will only be available to organised population based screening programmes, not to individual screening units.

Four certification categories are described:
1. Diagnostic Mammography Unit
2. Breast Assessment Centre
3. Loco-regional Screening Programme
4. European Reference Centre for Screening

It is quite possible that a Diagnostic Mammography Unit or a Breast Assessment Centre may individually form part of a Loco-regional programme or European Reference Centre. However in a decentralised screening programme it is acknowledged that the participating offices may not individually achieve complete Diagnostic Mammography Unit or Breast Assessment Centre standard. However all participating offices under these circumstances will be required to form part of the centralised physico-technical and professional quality control requirements as described, and comply with all relevant criteria.

Under these circumstances the mammographic image quality will be assured, as will the experience of the second radiologist performing centralised double reading.

Euref certification categories

Different categories of certification should be acknowledged from the ability to produce an adequate quality mammogram in an individual mammography unit, up to a facility that is capable of acting as a European Reference Centre for population screening activities. Reference will be made to whether the programme is working in a centralised or decentralised setting.

Volume requirements as stated in these sections are regarded as the absolute minimum required to allow the production of adequate diagnostic quality images. Greater numbers may not guarantee higher quality, but are much more likely to be associated with a significantly higher level of professional skill and physico-technical excellence. For this reason, higher volume throughputs are strongly recommended.

In all cases *a mammogram refers to a full set of mammograms performed on a woman*, and should not under any circumstances for the purposes of numerical advantage be counted in terms of individual mammographic exposures.

Euref diagnostic certification

Diagnostic Mammography Unit

This level reflects the ability of any office or clinic to provide mammographic image quality of satisfactory physico-technical and professional standards according to published criteria in the European guidelines.[2] EUREF will be satisfied as to the performance levels of equipment, radiographic staff, radiological staff and physics support services as laid out in the European guidelines. Adequate and regular quality control procedures will be followed.

The following basic criteria will be required from a Diagnostic Mammography Unit, which should:

a. Perform at least 1,000 mammograms per year.
b. Have dedicated equipment specifically designed for application in diagnostic mammography e.g. mammography system with magnification ability and dedicated processing, and be able to provide adequate viewing conditions for mammograms.
c. Comply with the physico-technical protocol in the European guidelines.
d. Ensure that the radiographer, technologist or other member of staff performing the mammographic examination must have had at least 40 hours of training specific to the radiographic aspects of mammography and regularly participate in external quality assessment schemes where available and radiographic update courses. This person must also take the lead in the radiographic aspects of quality control.
e. Employ a trained radiologist, i.e. a person who has had at least 60 hours of training specific to mammography and who in volume requirements reads at least 500 mammograms per year.
f. Keep a record of mammogram results and monitor numbers of women referred for further assessment.
g. Provide feedback of further assessment outcomes to the unit radiologists.

Breast Assessment Centre

In addition to the standards achieved by the Diagnostic Mammography Unit, a centralised system of diagnostic assessment for mammographically or clinically detected lesions must be available. There should be a full range of assessment facilities provided in order to allow complete and adequate work up by the Centre without necessarily having to refer the woman on for further investigation elsewhere. The Breast Assessment Centre should:

a. Perform at least 2,000 mammograms a year.
b. Be able to perform physical examinations and ultrasound examinations as well as the full range of radiographic procedures. Provide cytological examination and/or core biopsy sampling under radiological (including stereotactic) or sonographic guidance.
c. Employ a trained radiologist reading at least 1,000 mammograms a year.
d. Have organised and specialist cytological and histopathological support services.
e. Participate in multidisciplinary communication and review meetings with others responsible for diagnostic and treatment services.
f. Monitor data and feedback of results.
g. Keep a formal record of the assessment process and outcomes.

Euref screening certification

Loco-regional Screening Programme

In addition to the physico-technical and professional standards required for high quality mammography, it will be necessary to demonstrate a significant level of organisational success with regard to population based mammographic screening, and in addition to meet recognised performance standards and targets widely regarded as essential for successful screening. The Loco-regional Screening Programme should:

a. Perform at least 5,000 examinations a year (the minimum number in the European guidelines).

b. Operate a successful personalised invitation system and/or a promotional campaign as well as an organised system for re-inviting all previously screened women.

c. Serve an area and age defined target population of at least 20,000 eligible women.

d. Have a centralised physico-technical quality control service.

e. Have centralised reading or, in a case of a decentralised programme, centralised double reading by one or more fully trained and experienced radiologists each reading at least 5,000 mammograms per year.

f. Ensure that in a decentralised programme with multiple smaller screening offices participating, the central and experienced double reading radiologist judges the mammograms from both the diagnostic and an image quality point of view. This radiologist must take full responsibility for the image quality of the mammograms reported and ensure that where necessary images are repeated until they be of satisfactory standard.

g. Ensure that there is a nominated Programme Director with overall responsibility for the programme, having the authority to suspend unsatisfactory smaller units in a decentralised system, where repeated attempts at image quality improvement have failed.

h. Have adequate and satisfactory equipment dedicated to the use of mammography, and dedicated processing with all necessary facilities for full and complete assessment of women with screen-detected abnormalities.

i. Have an approved protocol for referral of women with screen-detected abnormalities within a decentralised screening programme to centres with adequate and full assessment facilities.

j. Observe all radiographic image quality criteria.

k. Have adequate viewing conditions including the use of roller viewers for multiple screen film reading by more than one reader if necessary in the most effective manner.

l. Comply with all physico-technical criteria set out in the European guidelines and ensure that adequate technical and professional quality assurance procedures are carried out in all units participating in the programme.

m. Receive satisfactory epidemiological support particularly with regard to the organisational, implementation and evaluation aspects as described in the European Guidelines - Quality Assurance in the Epidemiology of Breast Cancer Screening.[3]

n. Collect and monitor data according to the European guidelines.

o. Undergo multidisciplinary review meetings.

p. Process feedback of data and results to the professional staff involved in the programme.

q. Have a mechanism for identification and peer review of interval cancers. Interval cancer review will also form part of the certification visit.

r. Have undergone at least two full screening rounds.

European Reference Centre for Screening
In this context European refers to the performance of a centre according to the best European standards as opposed to its geographical connotations. In addition to the requirements listed above and the fulfilment of all published targets and conditions at organisational, professional and physico-technical levels, the Centre must be considered

capable of providing consultation services and training both internally and externally, being itself already certified as a screening programme. It will be expected to function on a more global level of furthering the processes of mammographic quality improvement regionally and nationally, both justifying and promoting the values of population screening by mammography for breast cancer. The European Reference Centre for Screening should:

a. Perform at least 10,000 mammograms a year.
b. Provide training by means of:
   - teaching files including interval cancers
   - training programmes with performance evaluation.
c. Comply with all required criteria of other levels of certification.
d. Employ a physicist and maintain regular contact with a reference pathologist, surgeon oncologist and epidemiologist.
e. Evaluate and report on the performance of the screening programme on a regular basis.

Sources and criteria

The major source for physico-technical and professional standards is the European guidelines for Quality Assurance in Mammography Screening.[2] Reference has been given to the American Mammography Quality Standards Act and in particular the Small Entity Compliance Guide - An Overview of the Final regulations Implementing the Mammography Quality Standards Act of 1992.[4] Reference is also made, and should be made by any office or programme wishing certification, to Council Directive 97/43/EURATOM[5], referring to the radiation protection of the exposure of individuals as part of health screening programmes.

Methodology

All requests for certification should be made to the organising offices of EUREF in Nijmegen by filing an application form with the Professional Coordinator. This form will include some preliminary questions, and the applicant should demonstrate that checklist criteria have been achieved. EUREF will then consider each request and on the basis of this checklist, the decision whether or not the site in question can be deemed viable for certification will be taken. In this case a site visit will be scheduled and a suitable team allocated. A protocol will be sent to the local unit laying out the time schedules involved and describing precisely the actions to be followed, the criteria which need to be achieved, and the documents and results that should be available for the visiting team to review. All visits will include a review of films, technical and patient facilities.

The visiting team for Diagnostic Mammography Unit and Breast Assessment Centre certification will consist of at least a radiologist, radiographer and physicist, with a team leader who may or may not be one of the professional representatives participating in the visit. Visiting teams for Loco-regional Screening Programme and European Reference Centre certification will include the above nominated members with the addition of a pathologist and epidemiologist. The membership will be stated prior to the visit and will be drawn from a pool of acknowledged experts from recognised centres.

The certification visit will take place at the offices of the unit or organisation requesting certification and it is expected that the relevant senior professionals involved in that programme will also be present. Following the visit and while still on site, the EUREF team will have an informal feedback session with each other. Provisional and brief comments on initial impressions will then be passed on confidentially by the leader of the EUREF team to the Senior Executive present at the local unit. Although the prime purpose of the visit will be to assess the suitability for certification, the visiting team will still make constructive suggestions as to any local improvements which could be made to further best practice.

The full written report in draft will be sent by EUREF to the nominated representative of the local unit within four weeks of the date of the visit. A formal reply must be made by the local unit within a further three weeks responding to issues of accuracy or interpretation. Following receipt of this response, EUREF will then issue a final report within two weeks and will state whether certification has been granted or withheld. There will be a mechanism for the right of appeal in cases of dispute.

When all procedures have been satisfactorily completed, full EUREF DIAGNOSTIC or EUREF SCREENING Certification will be issued. This signed certificate will bear the EUREF logo, and will state quite clearly the name of the unit or organisation concerned and the category of certification granted. Such a certificate may be displayed by the units or programmes concerned, and the relevant logo utilised on notepaper, reports etc as appropriate.

Frequency of certification
Re-certification should take place every five years with at least one data update in between full visits, so that the coordinating office may ensure that technical and professional standards are being adhered to.

Feasibility of project
A feasibility study of two years is to be carried out to estimate the viability of the certification programme in its present format.

30 March 2000

References
1. Young KC, Wallis MG, Ramsdale ML. Mammographic film density and detection of small breast cancers. Clinical Radiology 1994;49:461-465
2. De Wolf CJM, Perry NM (Eds). European Guidelines for Quality Assurance in Mammography Screening. Second Edition. European Commission. 1996.
3. Broeders MJM, Codd MB, Ascunce N, Linos A, Verbeek ALM. Quality Assurance in the Epidemiology of Breast Cancer Screening. In European Guidelines for Quality Assurance in Mammography Screening. European Commission. 1996.
4. Small Entity Compliance Guide - An Overview of the Final Regulations Implementing the Mammography Quality Standards Act of 1992.
Report to Mammography Facilities and the Public. United States Department of Health and Human Services. October 1997.
5. Health Protection of Individuals Against the Dangers of Ionising Radiation. Council Directive 97/43/EURATOM. European Commission. June 1997.

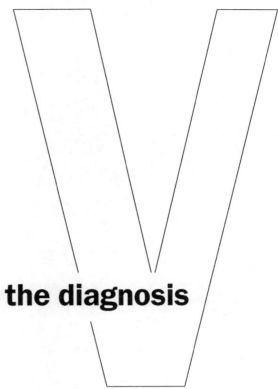

EUSOMA document

Quality Assurance in the diagnosis of breast disease

Nottingham Workshop
21st September 1999

This document has been accepted for publication in the European Journal of Cancer

Authors
N. Perry
L. Cataliotti
A. Wilson
I. Ellis
M. Blichert-Toft
J. Julien
R. Holland
C. Elston
M. Rosselli del Turco
R. Christiaens
I. Garas
Z. Pentek
M. Greco
C. van de Velde

Introduction

The diagnosis of breast disease has been subject to a sustained and widespread drive for quality control and quality improvement across Europe over the last ten years. Much of this has been confined to the provision of breast cancer screening services. Professionals working in the field have long since recognised that women using symptomatic breast services should be confident of receiving similar standards of diagnosis available in the screening sector.

Published guidelines for quality assurance in mammography screening already exist at European level and at a national level in several Member States. Guidelines for quality assurance in symptomatic breast diagnostic activity are not so well established. Their existence however is essential as they will potentially affect considerably more women than take part in screening programmes. This document attempts to lay out in a setting suitable for European usage, those aspects of quality assurance, quality objectives and outcome measures that are necessary to further these aims.

As far as possible we have tried to avoid screening or treatment issues unless of particular relevance to diagnostic activity. We have also chosen not to attempt to define clinical protocols.

Modern diagnosis of breast disease is a multidisciplinary activity requiring trained and experienced professionals using specialised equipment with up to date sampling and other diagnostic techniques. Screening is predominantly a radiological procedure with particular emphasis placed on the optimal balance of sensitivity and specificity. Many abnormalities are impalpable and priority is given to maximising the cancer detection rate while minimising anxiety and reducing the benign biopsy rate. The radiologist has the role of prime responsibility in screening. In symptomatic activity the clinician has the role of prime responsibility, this person is usually the referring General Practitioner or the surgeon that the patient is referred on to. The clinician may also be regarded as any medical professional who is trained and skilled specifically in clinical examination of the breast. In these circumstances however the role of imaging, interpretation and cytological/ histological sampling procedures will still be paramount as supportive diagnostic activities.

Practices are likely to vary across the Member States according to healthcare environments and availability of trained personnel, however these variations must not be allowed to interfere with the achievement of set targets and outcome measures.

If possible, all women requiring breast diagnosis should be referred to a specialist breast unit. However it is important to recognise that in a decentralised healthcare setting many women will not undergo more than basic imaging following a General Practitioner referral, and the benefits of full multidisciplinary assessment will not be available to them, or indeed necessary for many of them. These guidelines will therefore attempt to cover all pertinent aspects of basic diagnosis as well as assessment and underline the importance of ensuring that women who do require further assessment are not denied it. In order to ensure this, agreed protocols should be set up between diagnostic clinics and assessment centres, if the two are run as separate entities. Throughout this text the terms patients and women are referred to at various points as appropriate. It is recognised that on occasions, male patients will also require the services of a diagnostic breast clinic.

Asymptomatic women do not necessarily require initial clinical examination or other imaging investigation apart from mammography if taking part in a breast screening programme. However it is regarded as good practice that all women with breast symptoms undergo a clinical examination prior to any further investigation requested, and that this be performed by a suitably trained and experienced clinician.

Training and quality assurance

The key professional personnel involved in breast diagnosis are the surgeon (clinician), radiologist, radiographer, histo/cytopathologist, nurse counsellor and physicist. All such personnel must hold the requisite professional qualifications in their own country and have undergone specific training in the field of diagnosis/diagnostic imaging of the breast. They should regularly participate in Continuing Medical Education and update courses, also taking part in any existing external quality assessment schemes and being in possession of any necessary Certificate of Competence.

It is to be hoped that over the next few years there will be a move towards certification/accreditation for all professional staff and units participating in this activity.

A full and comprehensive quality assurance programme must be in place with clearly documented local quality control procedures and quality assurance manuals. As far as the imaging aspects of breast diagnosis are concerned – i.e. radiographic and radiological – these must comply with the technical and professional requirements laid out in the European Guidelines for Quality Assurance in Mammography Screening.

It is essential that there be a nominated person with responsibility for the physico-technical quality control aspects of every unit participating in breast diagnosis, at whatever level. Similarly, each service must have a Clinical Director or one member of the professional team acting as Lead Clinician with responsibility for overall performance and quality of the service, and with the requisite authority to make changes or suspend equipment if necessary.

Imaging procedures

Breast units, diagnostic clinics or assessment units must be in possession of local imaging protocols agreed by and made available to all clinic staff and forming part of the local QA manual.

Mammography and ultrasound either alone or in combination are the primary diagnostic imaging methods used for the breast. If mammography is required, a two view examination should be performed using the standard lateral oblique and cranio caudal projections. The use of mammography prior to the age of 35 is of limited diagnostic use and carries a higher theoretical risk from ionising radiation. Mammography in this age group should only be used in particular circumstances such as a strong clinical suspicion of malignancy and when specifically authorised by the radiologist in charge. If breast imaging is required below the age of 35, ultrasound is the method of choice. Other imaging techniques such as magnetic resonance imaging (MRI) of the breast have specific indications and do not form part of the initial diagnostic investigation at present.

Mammography is associated with a variable false negative rate in the order of 10% - 20%, but this may be as high as 50% if the image quality is compromised for any reason including the age of the patient and the density of the breast. If a woman complains of, or is found to have a discrete mass or other significant clinical sign in her breast which is not demonstrable mammographically, it is essential that she be referred for an ultrasound examination as part of standard triple assessment procedures. This will reduce the possibility of missed malignancy with negative mammography.

Women with breast implants should be advised that these may significantly reduce the efficacy of subsequent mammography and that mammographic imaging should be performed in clinics where ultrasound is available as it may frequently be required as an additional imaging technique. Magnetic resonance imaging is now recognised as the method of choice for investigating significant abnormalities in the breast in the presence of implants and for the assessment of possible intracapsular or extracapsular implant rupture.

Assessment of microcalcification is likely to require magnification views, and these should be performed in orthogonal projections i.e. true lateral and cranio caudal in order to maximise the diagnostic information available.

It is preferable to perform clinical examination prior to any image guided intervention sampling procedure so that subtle clinical signs are not disturbed by haematoma formation. For similar reasons it is preferable to perform any necessary basic imaging procedures such as mammography/ultrasound prior to any clinically guided sampling. If facilities and staffing allow, it may be logistically advantageous to perform sampling of clinically palpable lesions under image guided control

Communication at all times is an essential part of the process and this must exist between the members of the imaging team e.g. radiographer/radiologist, as well as with the patient and the referring clinician.

Diagnostic imaging clinic

In a decentralised healthcare setting there may be multiple clinics or offices present within a geographical area offering mammography and/or ultrasound examination of the breast. Some of these may be operating to significantly lower volume levels than that currently regarded as acceptable by specialist units. There are numerous problems with low volume throughput in breast imaging and a decentralised approach must not be allowed to jeopardise production of examinations having adequate image quality. The highest possible image quality is necessary to maximise diagnostic information and provide suitable levels of sensitivity and specificity. Inadequate quality of equipment, inadequate processing facilities, under used processing facilities, lack of a quality control programme and poorly trained and experienced radiological or radiographic staff will adversely affect optimum performance and interpretation of breast images. Minimum standards must be set in place so that this is not allowed to happen.

This section will describe certain requirements to be provided by any clinic offering diagnostic imaging services. This should be regarded as the most basic level of quality needed for adequate service provision. The next section will describe requirements for a fuller and more comprehensive breast assessment centre.

The end point of the diagnostic imaging clinic is to correctly identify and classify imaging characteristics, and should not include further formal assessment with tissue/cytology sampling, with the exception of simple cyst aspiration. Further investigations should be performed at or in conjunction with a breast assessment centre as laid out in the next section. This will ensure that cellular or tissue samples are analysed by a trained and recognised pathologist adhering to pathology quality assurance requirements.

Mammography equipment

Dedicated mammographic and film processing equipment must be available with the facility to produce low dose with high contrast and spatial resolution examinations. An adequately high optical density is required for satisfactory image interpretation due to the proven relationship between optical density and small cancer detection rates. Equipment should be up to date, of recognised manufacturer, suitable for its purpose, and subject to regular maintenance and quality control checks as laid out in the European Guidelines for Quality Assurance in Mammography Screening. For example it is not suitable to use a mammography machine without a foot operated compression system. All equipment in the clinic must be subject to regular radiographic quality control checks and performance tests by a medical physicist suitably trained and experienced in mammography. Consistent breaching of quality control levels should lead to suspension of the equipment from use by the nominated person charged with the overall responsibility for quality assurance of the unit.

Targets

The following are essential targets to be achieved, fuller requirements are laid out in the European Guidelines.
- High contrast/spatial resolution > 10 lp/mm
- Optical density 1.4 – 1.8
- Mean glandular dose per film ≤ 2mGy
- Daily processor control maintenance 100%

Ultrasound equipment

Breast ultrasound should only be carried out by members of medical staff specifically trained and experienced in this procedure. It should not be carried out by General Practitioners, gynaecologists, surgeons, radiologists, or radiographers who have not undergone such specific training and who do not participate in regular performance of this activity. The operating frequency of the ultrasound machine must be at least 7.5 MHz, and should preferably operate at 10 MHz or higher. Suitable recording facilities for sonographic images must be available.

Radiographic staff

Mammograms should be performed by suitably trained and experienced radiographic staff fulfilling all necessary training and working professional requirements and holding any relevant Certificate of Competence as previously described. In clinics where no mammographically trained radiographer is employed, the member of staff performing the mammograms must have undergone full training in the radiographic aspects of mammography, comply with all requirements as laid down for radiographic staff, including any necessary external quality assessment schemes and update courses and take the lead in regular radiographic quality control procedures. For the purpose of this document such a person will be referred to as the radiographer.

It is the radiographer's responsibility within the team to produce an optimum image with regard to positioning and technical aspects and in a manner acceptable to women. The radiographer must inform the woman about the procedure, how it is to be performed, how the woman will get her result, and in what time scale. The radiographer in charge of the unit is responsible for ensuring that a regular quality control programme is carried out and is responsible for reporting breaches of quality to the radiologist in charge of the clinic. Such a quality control programme will include both regular radiographic and physicist performed checks as listed in the European Guidelines.

In order to limit unnecessary exposure to ionising radiation and the creation of unnecessary anxiety, the technical retake level where repeat mammograms are necessary for positioning or technical faults must be kept to an absolute minimum, preferably below 1% but no more than 3%. All such retakes should be documented for audit purposes. Positioning performance requirements for adequate mammographic examinations are laid out in the European Guidelines and must be adhered to. The minimum requirements for positioning of the standard lateral oblique projection are that the pectoral muscle must be displayed down to nipple level, the inframammary fold should be visible and the nipple should be in profile. Skin folds, movement and other artefacts should be absent. An external quality assessment scheme should be in place so that peer review of adequate positioning is performed and satisfactory results obtained in at least 97% of images. All films must be appropriately named and marked correctly for side.

In order to maintain the skills and expertise required to carry out optimum mammography and be a useful member of the multidisciplinary team, the radiographer must be involved in performing at least 20 mammographic studies per week.

Targets

* Technical repeat rate minimum level < 3% - expected < 1%
* More than 97% of women will have an acceptable examination according to the positioning and exposure criteria given
* 100% of women will be informed by the radiographer of the method and timescale for receiving her results
* Minimum 20 mammographic studies per week to be performed by each radiographer

Basic quality control

The following is a basic summary of routine quality control tests to be performed by the radiographer, fuller details are available in the European Guidelines.

Daily
- Mechanical, safety and function checks
- Standard density consistency tests
- Reproducibility of mAs values
- Sensitometry
- Clean X-ray cross over rollers
- Screen inspection and cleaning
- Cassette inspection for wear and tear

Weekly
- Thickness variation
- Image quality

Quarterly
- Sensitivity and radiation absorption of cassettes
- Film screen contact
- Calibration of densitometer

Radiological staff

The radiologist must be specifically trained and experienced in breast imaging. This should include a knowledge of technical requirements of mammography equipment, processing, exposure factors and all those other factors of importance that are necessary in the production of good image quality. If possible, radiologists involved in symptomatic activity should also participate in local screening programmes.

A dedicated mammographic film viewer must be available and films should be read in a suitable room with control of background lighting. It is the responsibility of the radiologist to ensure that the mammograms are of adequate diagnostic standard, particularly with regard to positioning and film density. Where films are inadequate, they must be repeated. The radiologist must also ensure that feedback is provided to the radiographer on image quality. The report provided by the radiologist must state quite clearly the nature of any abnormality present, its side, site, size, description and extent. The radiologist should make clear the implication of the imaging findings and should recommend the most suitable necessary further investigation.

If a significant finding is present, carrying a high risk of malignancy, it is the responsibility of the reporting radiologist to ensure that the woman is aware that further investigation or management will be required. For this reason it is recommended that wherever possible the radiologist should be available within the clinic during the mammographic examination so that any necessary procedure such as an ultrasound can be performed while the woman is still present. This will avoid the need for a separate return visit, and allow the radiologist to pass on any necessary information to the woman, with due regard paid to the importance of not creating unnecessary anxiety.

Basic requirements of a Diagnostic Mammography Unit

Ultimately it is hoped that all clinics offering breast diagnostic services will be subject to accreditation/certification procedures. Until that time the following criteria are proposed in line with the EUREF Certification Protocols.

The following basic criteria will be required from a Diagnostic Mammography Unit, which should:

A   Perform at least 1,000 mammograms per year.

B   Have dedicated equipment specifically designed for application in diagnostic mammography e.g. mammography system with magnification ability and dedicated processing, and be able to provide adequate viewing conditions for mammograms.

C   Comply with the physico-technical protocol in the European Guidelines.

D   The radiographer, technologist or other member of staff performing the mammographic examination must have had at least 40 hours of training specific to the radiographic aspects of mammography and regularly participate in external quality assessment schemes where available and radiographic update courses. This person must also take the lead in the radiographic aspects of quality control.

E   Employ a trained radiologist, i.e. a person who has had at least 60 hours of training specific to mammography and who in volume requirements reads at least 500 mammograms per year.

F   Keep a record of mammogram results and monitor numbers of women referred for further assessment.

G   Provide feedback of further assessment outcomes to the unit radiologists.

NB
Volume requirements as stated in this section and the following section are regarded as the absolute minimum required to allow the production of adequate diagnostic quality images. Greater number may not guarantee higher quality, but are more likely to be associated with a significantly higher level of professional skill and physico-technical excellence. For this reason, higher volume throughputs are strongly recommended.

In all cases a mammogram refers to a full set of mammograms performed on a woman, and should not under any circumstances for the purposes of numerical advantage be counted in terms of individual mammographic exposures.

Breast Assessment Centre

While basic diagnostic imaging in the form of mammography/ultrasound may be sufficient for many women, those with significant symptoms, clinical findings, or mammographic findings need further workup which will require more specialist equipment and staff. A protocol should be in place with referring General Practitioners so that women with a clinical finding carrying a significant risk of malignancy should be referred directly to the breast assessment centre at a specialist breast unit. Such clinical findings will include a discrete new palpable mass, nipple discharge – particularly if single duct and unilateral, nipple retraction, nipple eczema, skin distortion such as tethering, dimpling or a change in breast shape, palpable axillary lymphadenopathy or inflammatory change. In this setting the woman will undergo a process of triple assessment i.e. clinical, imaging and cytological/histological investigation, performed by a specialist multidisciplinary team with access to more sophisticated imaging equipment and pre-operative diagnostic techniques.

Breast assessment centres which are not functioning as part of a specified breast unit must have written protocols available for triple assessment techniques. Additional mammographic techniques must include the ability to perform paddle compression and microfocus magnification views. Image guided sampling techniques must be available with the ability to perform these either under ultrasound or stereotactic control. Whether fine needle aspiration cytology procedures or core biopsy procedures are carried out will depend upon the local radiological and cytological expertise, and audit of results obtained. Immediate cytology reporting or checking for adequacy of cellularity can be performed. Core biopsy in expert hands can provide increased sensitivity and specificity compared to fine needle aspiration cytology. Radiographic, radiological and histo/cytopathological staff must be fully conversant with the accurate carrying out and interpretation of all these procedures. Specific standards of performance in sampling procedures must be adhered to, particularly with regard to insufficiency of results and pre-operative diagnosis (see Targets).

If abnormalities are visible sonographically, it is more suitable for sampling to be performed under ultrasound control. It is generally advisable for image guided sampling to be performed for any solid sonographically detected lesion. If required, microcalcification may occasionally be sampled under ultrasound control, but more usually stereotactic procedures will be required. Core biopsy is preferred for lesions of architectural distortion and microcalcifications, and may also allow definitive diagnosis of a benign lesion which will then not require surgical excision biopsy. If core biopsy is performed for microcalcification it is essential that specimen radiography of the cores be obtained to demonstrate the presence of calcification. Sampling techniques should be carried out with due regard to the imaging or clinical modality carrying the most suspicious features. Where there is a possibility of discordant clinical and imaging findings with regard to any lesion, it is advisable to carry out sampling under both imaging and clinical guidance. Very occasionally there may remain a significant discordance between suspicious radiological features and benign sampling where no reasonable pathological correlation can be made. Under these circumstances, open surgical excision is advisable.

It is regarded as good practice that lesions which are predominantly architectural distortion should be subject to excision biopsy following pre-operative diagnostic workup due to a significant risk of associated malignancy which may not be demonstrated even under ideal sampling conditions. Also lesions that are proven to contain atypical ductal hyperplasia should be subject to excision due to the risk of associated malignancy.

Where resources allow, mammotomy offers significant advantages for biopsy in a proportion of patients in achieving definitive pre-operative diagnosis and reducing the need for surgical intervention.

Diagnostic classification

A standard classification system is used as follows in addition to the normal descriptive methods.

Radiology

R1 Normal/benign
R2 A lesion having benign characteristics
R3 An abnormality present of indeterminate significance
R4 Features suspicious of malignancy
R5 Malignant features

Ultrasound

U1 Normal/benign
U2 A lesion having benign characteristics
U3 An abnormality present of indeterminate significance
U4 Features suspicious of malignancy
U5 Malignant features

A negative or benign clinical examination must not be allowed to downgrade the importance of suspicious imaging features unless the radiologist has been fully consulted.

Fine Needle Aspiration Cytology

C1 Inadequate
C2 Benign epithelial cells
C3 Atypia probably benign
C4 Suspicious of malignancy
C5 Malignant

Core Biopsy/Histology

B1 Unsatisfactory/normal
B2 Benign
B3 Benign but of uncertain malignant potential
B4 Suspicious of malignancy
B5 Malignant

Targets

• % of image guided FNAC procedures with an insufficient result
  Minimum standard < 25%   Expected < 15%
• % of image guided FNAC procedures from lesions subsequently proven to be malignant having an insufficient result
  Minimum standard < 10%

- % of women with breast cancer having a pre-operative diagnosis of malignancy (FNAC/CB reported as definitely malignant)
Minimum standard > 70%   Expected > 90%

Cytology/histology quality assurance
These figures are based on screening targets currently in use. Symptomatic requirements may well need to be reset higher in the light of experience.

- Absolute sensitivity > 60%
- Complete sensitivity > 80%
- Specificity > 60%
- Positive predictive value C5 > 95%
- False negative rate < 5%
- False positive rate < 1%

Audit
For audit purposes it is proposed that the standard assessment data set be used as recommended in the QT audit document approved by EUSOMA (see appendix 1).

Cytology/core biopsy reporting standards
These should be based upon examples given in appendices 2 and 3.

Basic requirements for a Breast Assessment Centre
In addition to the standards achieved by the Diagnostic Mammography Unit, a centralised system of diagnostic assessment for mammographically or clinically detected lesions must be available. There should be a full range of assessment facilities provided in order to allow complete and adequate work up by the centre without necessarily having to refer the woman on for further investigation elsewhere.

The Breast Assessment Centre should:

A   Perform at least 2,000 mammograms a year.

B   Be able to perform physical examinations and ultrasound examinations as well as the full range of radiographic procedures. Provide cytological examination and/or core biopsy sampling under radiological (including stereotactic) or sonographic guidance.

C   Employ a trained radiologist reading at least 1,000 mammograms a year.

D   Have organised and specialist cytological and histopathological support services.

E   Participate in multidisciplinary communication and review meetings with others responsible for diagnostic and treatment services.

F   Monitor data and feedback of results.

G   Keep a formal record of the assessment process and outcomes.

The requirements placed upon a breast assessment centre as part of a specialist breast unit may be even more rigorous than these.

Multidisciplinary activity

All breast assessment centres or breast units engaged in diagnostic excision biopsy must ensure the formation of proper multidisciplinary teamwork involving the following personnel:
Radiographer, radiologist, histo/cytopathologist, surgeon/clinician, nurse counsellor.

Ideally, before a woman is considered for surgical excision biopsy her case and results should have been discussed in the setting of a full multidisciplinary meeting. By so doing the surgeon will be best appraised of the likelihood of malignancy, the extent of abnormality on imaging and any discordant results which may have been obtained upon review of the case, which might lead to an alteration of surgical planning. Similarly all biopsy results should be discussed in a multidisciplinary audit setting to establish the nature of disease, its extent, completeness of excision and the appropriateness of the histology compared to the pre-operative diagnosis. Unexpected results should be discussed in this setting to establish their veracity, to confirm that the correct lesion has been excised and to provide a source of learning and experience.

Surgical aspects

The surgeon is a member of the multidisciplinary team and should participate in regular multidisciplinary review for case management and audit purposes. The surgeon should be fully involved in the assessment of women and should always see the patient before accepting her for surgery.

It should be agreed surgical policy that mammography is carried out prior to breast surgery providing the woman is in an appropriate age group. Firstly as a matter of good practice to demonstrate the nature and extent of any disease that is identifiable, secondly to ensure that full imaging information is available in the case of interval cancers arising in any local screening programme.

The surgeon should be discouraged from cutting specimens open after removal in theatre before sending them to pathology. All specimens should be marked and orientated according to recognised local protocols. The surgeon should ensure completeness of excision, which may be assisted by the use of two plane specimen radiography. At operation, the use of frozen sectioning is generally inappropriate, particularly in the assessment of clinically impalpable lesions. It may occasionally be justified to enable a firm diagnosis of invasive malignancy to be made in order to allow definitive surgery to be carried out in one operative procedure. In general terms surgeons should adhere to the

European Guidelines for Quality Assurance in the Surgical Management of Mammographically Detected Lesions, and in particular the monitoring of surgical outcome measures as defined in the European Guidelines on Quality Assurance in Mammography Screening (third edition).

Pre-operative localisation
Lesions that are either impalpable or difficult to locate with certainty on clinical examination will require some form of pre-operative localisation marking procedure provided by the radiologist. The most usual form is by wire placement either under X-ray or ultrasound guidance. The wire should be placed within 1 cm of the lesion if possible in at least 90% of cases, or a second wire should be inserted. It is acceptable under certain circumstances if the lesion is superficial for skin marking to be provided under ultrasound control. The surgeon must be provided with a full and accurate description of the procedure performed and a precise report of the relative placement of the wire compared to the lesion. Relevant images, correctly marked should also be provided.

Specimen radiographs must be available in, or in very close proximity to the operating theatre so that confirmation of excision of the lesion can be confirmed without delay and prior to skin closure. Successful excision of impalpable lesions is therefore a combination of surgical as well as radiological skill and the proportion of impalpable lesions successfully excised at the first operation should be in excess of 95%. Specimen radiographs must also be made available to the pathology department.

In order to limit the number of unnecessary biopsy procedures performed, it is recommended that the ratio of benign to malignant excision biopsies performed for diagnostic purposes should not exceed 0.5:1. Already diagnosed benign lesions and lesions removed due to patient choice are excluded. For cosmetic reasons it is important to minimise the extent of benign biopsy for impalpable lesions, and at present the most suitable discriminatory factor used is the weight of the specimen. Over 90% of diagnostic biopsies for impalpable lesions which subsequently prove benign should weigh less than 30 grams.

Targets
- Proportion of wires placed within 1 cm of an impalpable lesion prior to excision
  Minimum standard > 90%

- Proportion of impalpable lesions successfully excised at the first operation
  Minimum standard > 95%

- Proportion of benign diagnostic biopsies on impalpable lesions weighing less than 30 grams
  Minimum standard > 90%

- The rate of benign to malignant operations performed for diagnostic biopsy purposes (see text)
  Minimum standard 0.5:1

- No frozen section performed if tumour diameter < 10 mm
  Minimum standard 95%

Histopathology reporting forms

It is recommended that a minimum dataset for reporting be established by a form based on the example in appendix 4.

Anxiety and delays

Delays at any stage of the diagnostic process may result in anxiety for the woman, which sometimes may be considerable. Targets should be set in terms of working days (w.d.) at every stage where delay may arise.

- Delay between mammography and result
  Minimum standard < 5 w.d.

- Delay between result of imaging and offered assessment
  Minimum standard < 5 w.d.

- Delay between assessment and issuing of results
  Minimum standard < 5 w.d.

- Delay between decision to operate and date offered for surgery
  Minimum standard < 15 w.d.   Ideally < 10 w.d.

- 95% of women should receive full and adequate assessment in three appointments or less

- 80% of women with symptoms and signs strongly suggesting the presence of breast cancer should be seen within two weeks of referral

Unnecessary distress may be caused not only by delays as listed above but also by failure of efficient communication between the diagnostic team and the woman. Failure to reach a definitive diagnosis due to imprecise methods of assessment also results in anxiety.

If possible the radiologist should be present in the clinic at the time when a woman has her mammogram so that any necessary further investigation e.g. ultrasound examination, can be performed without delay. It is also important that full verbal information on the status of her investigations and diagnosis be given to the woman at suitably relevant stages throughout the diagnostic process. As far as possible the woman should be informed of the result of her examination before she leaves the clinic and of the need for any necessary further investigation to be performed.

The failure of the assessment process to make a definitive diagnosis of either a benign or a malignant condition is an undesirable outcome of assessment and further increases anxiety. For this reason the use of early recall for a repeat examination at a time shorter than that normally specified for a routine follow up is to be avoided. Women must be informed of when to expect results and should be provided with written information at appropriate stages in the diagnostic procedure. However women should not be informed by letter or telephone of the likelihood of malignancy being present. Such information should be given verbally to her in the presence of a nurse counsellor.

Rapid diagnostic/one stop clinics

There is considerable advantage to the formation of rapid diagnostic clinics, set up in breast units, where the diagnostic team may work together in a multidisciplinary setting. Women may receive a diagnosis and management plan in the quickest time possible, either during the same clinic, or having all necessary investigations at the same time and returning for results within 24 – 48 hours. The main advantages of this system are to reduce anxiety, and to provide a certain level of skill and teamwork not otherwise available. For this reason as previously recommended all women with discrete masses or significant signs or symptoms must be referred directly to a breast unit, and not to a basic diagnostic clinic.

Pathology QA aspects

Pathologists providing a breast histopathology and/or cytopathology service should have had specialist training and participate in a continuing education programme. They should follow recommended reporting guidelines and diagnostic protocols. They should participate in relevant external quality assessment schemes where available. Diagnostic cytology and needle core biopsy histology performance can be assessed using QA statistical methods. All pathology laboratories should be accredited according to national standards.

MRI and other diagnostic methods

As previously stated MRI is not yet part of the initial diagnostic workup. The full role and place of MRI in breast diagnosis is still being evaluated. However, when indicated, it already has an established role in the evaluation of breast implants and in the differentiation of recurrent disease from post surgical scarring, where it has a very high negative predictive value. There is however no evidence at present for its usefulness or cost effectiveness as routine follow up after breast cancer surgery. It is probably better than conventional techniques in assessing the full extent of malignant disease present within a breast, certainly in selected cases such as dense breasts. The technique is not sufficiently specific for routine use in younger women with dense breasts.

The precise place of sentinel node biopsy, scintimammography and P.E.T. is still under evaluation for breast diagnostic purposes.

Similarly, appraisal of the usefulness of invasive diagnostic procedures such as Mammotome and ABBI compared to FNAC/CB is underway. There is evidence that mammotomy has a better sensitivity and specificity than other biopsy methods. It appears to be well tolerated with a low complication rate and may hold significant advantages for patient management decisions.

Comparison will need to be made on the role, availability and cost effectiveness of all these techniques compared to more standard investigations

Reference documents

European Guidelines for Quality Assurance in Mammography Screening (third edition) 2001

Guidelines for Breast Pathology Services NHSBSP Publication No 2 1997

Minimum Dataset of Breast Cancer Histopathology Reports – Royal College of Pathologists 1998

Guidelines to Cytology Procedures and Reporting in Breast Cancer Screening NHSBSP Publication No 22 1993

Provision of Breast Services in the UK – British Breast Group

BASO Guidelines for Surgeons in the Management of Symptomatic Breast Disease in the UK 1998

Radiographic Quality Control Manual for Mammography NHSBSP Publication No 21 1999

Quality Assurance Guidelines for Radiologists NHSBSP Publication No 15 1997

European Guidelines for Quality Assurance in the Surgical Management of Mammographically Detected Lesions 1998

Report no. _____ Surname _____ Forename _____

Date of birth ___ / ___ / _____ Place of birth _____ Personal ID no. _____

Address _____

Town _____ District _____ Tel. _____ / _____

Trial _____

Assessment Section

Source of referral
1) Screening

_____

2) Other

_____

9) Unknown

Palpable lesion
0) No
1) Yes
9) Unknown

Other clinical findings

_____

Imaging/clinical size

_____ mm

Size-method (priority as follows)
1) Ultrasound
2) Mammographic
3) Clinical
9) Unknown

Breast side
R) Right
L) Left
U) Unknown

Lesion site
1) Superior-external
2) Central-external
3) Inferior-external
4) Inferior-central
5) Inferior-internal
6) Central-internal
7) Superior-internal
8) Superior-central
9) Areolar
88) Diffuse
99) Unknown

Ward stamp

Mammogram finding
0) Not done
R1 Negative/benign
R2 Benign lesion
R3 Abn., indetermined significance
R4 Suspicious of malignancy
R5 Malignant features
9) Unknown

Ultrasound finding
0) Not done
U1 Negative/benign
U2 Benign lesion
U3 Abn., indetermined significance
U4 Suspicious of malignancy
U5 Malignant features
9) Unknown

Disease extent
0) Localized
1) Multifocal (more foci in the same quadrant)
2) Multicentric (syncr. lesions in different quadrants: use 1 form per lesion)
9) Unknown

Mammogram pattern
0) No opacity or asymmetry
1) Well defined opacity
2) Poorly defined opacity
3) Spiculate opacity
4) Distortion/stellate opacity
5) Asymmetry
8) Other _____
9) Unknown

Microcalcifications
0) Absent
1) Predominantly punctate
2) Predom. pleomorphic / granular
3) Predom. linear branching
9) Unknown

Fine Needle Aspiration
0) Not done
C1 Inadequate
C2 Benign epithelial cells
C3 Atypia probably benign
C4 Suspicious of
   malignancy
C5 Malignant
9) Unknown

Core Biopsy
0) Not done
B1 Unsatisfactory / normal
B2 Benign
B3 Benign, uncertain
B4 Suspicious of malignancy
B5 Malignant
9) Unknown
If malignant
a) In situ
b) Invasive

Date of cytology or histology sample

_____ / _____ / _____

Department

_____

Nipple discharge
0) Absent
1) Present
9) Unknown

Nipple discharge cytology
0) Not done   4) Suspicious
1) Benign   5) Malignant
2) Papillary   8) Unsatisfactory
3) Dubious   9) Unknown

T N M by imaging or physical examination

T _____

N _____

M _____

Menstrual status
1) Fertile
2) Pregnancy
3) Post-menopause
4) Hormone replacement
   therapy
9) Unknown

This lesion with respect to any other lesions in the same patient
0) Single lesion   4) Metachronous, contralateral
1) Main lesion   5) Metachronous, ipsilateral
2) Double, contralateral 9) Unknown
3) Double, ipsilateral

First malignant lesion
0) No
1) Yes
9) Unknown

First treatment
1) Surgery   4) RT + CT
2) Radiotherapy 9) Unknown
3) Chemotherapy

Date of referral
_____ / _____ / _____

Notes

_____

_____

_____

Proposed cytology reporting form

Surname _____ Forenames _____

Date of birth _____ Screening no. _____

Hospital no. _____ Report no. _____

Side
☐ Right   ☐ Left

Specimen type
☐ FNA (solid lesion)   ☐ FNA (cyst)   ☐ Nipple discharge   ☐ Nipple or
                                                                       skin scrapings

Localisation technique
☐ Palpation   ☐ X-ray guided   ☐ Ultrasound guided   ☐ Stereotaxis

Opinion
☐ 1 Unsatisfactory
☐ 2 Benign
☐ 3 Atypia probably benign
☐ 4 Suspicious of malignancy
☐ 5 Malignant

☐ Case for review?

Pathologist _____ Name of aspirator _____

Date _____

Proposed wide bore needle biopsy form

Surname _____ Forenames _____

Date of birth _____

Screening no. _____ Hospital no. _____

Centre _____ Report no. _____

Side

☐ Right ☐ Left Number of cores _____

Calcification present on specimen X-ray?

☐ Yes ☐ No ☐ Radiograph not seen

Histological calcification

☐ Absent ☐ Benign ☐ Malignant ☐ Both

Localisation technique

☐ Palpation ☐ X-ray guided ☐ Ultrasound guided ☐ Stereotaxis

Opinion

☐ B1 Unsatisfactory/normal tissue only
☐ B2 Benign
☐ B3 Benign but of uncertain malignant potential
☐ B4 Suspicious of malignancy
☐ B5 Malignant ☐ a. In situ
☐ b. Invasive

Pathologist _____ Operator taking biopsy _____

Date _____

Comment _____

_____

_____

Pathology Section

Histopathology report no. _____

Date diagnostic report _____ / _____ / _____

Department _____

Pathologist _____

Date last report _____ / _____ / _____

Date lymph nodes report _____ / _____ / _____

Specimen cut
0) No
1) Yes
2) Unknown

Specimen orientation
0) No
1) Yes
2) Unknown

Weight of specimen _____ gm

Marker distance _____ mm

Main diagnosis
1) Benign
2) In situ
3) Microinvasive
4) Invasive
5) Non-epithelial
6) Other _____

9) Unknown

Benign (type)
1) Atypical ductal hyperplasia
2) Atypical lobular hyperplasia
3) Other _____
9) Unknown

In situ (type)
1) Ductal
2) Lobular
9) Unknown

Growth pattern (DCIS)
1) Solid
2) Comedo
3) Papillary
4) Micropapillary
5) Cribriform
6) Clinging
7) Other _____
9) Unknown

Histological grade (DCIS)
1) Low
2) Intermediate
3) High

0) Not done
9) Unknown

Classification

Invasive (type)
1) Ductal NST
2) Lobular
3) Medullary
4) Mucinous
5) Tubular, cribiform
6) Mixed ductal/lobular
7) Mixed ductal NST and other types
8) Mixed tubular/lobular
10) Metastatic
11) Other _____
88) Not assessable
99) Unknown

DCIS component
0) Absent
1) Present
9) Unknown

DCIS _____ %

Histological grade (invasive)
1) I
2) II
3) III

0) Not done
9) Unknown

Classification
1) WHO
2) Elston-Ellis
3) Other
9) Unknown

Vascular invasion
0) Not seen
1) Yes
8) Not evaluated
9) Unknown

Paget's disease

No   Yes   Unknown

Pathological size
_____ mm

Whole size (invasive+DCIS)
_____ mm

Disease extent
0) Localized
1) Multiple
9) Unknown

Specimen excision margins (at the definitive report)
1) T does not reach margin
2) Inv. T focally reaches margin
3) Inv. T reaches margin (extensive)
4) CIS focally reaches margin
5) CIS reaches margin (extensive)
9) Unknown

Margins
Minimum distance (invasive) _____ mm
Minimum distance (DCIS) _____ mm
Maximum distance _____ mm

pT

X	0	is	mic	1	1a	1b	1c	2	3	4	4a	4b	4c	4d	unknown

Lymph nodes
0) Negative
1) Positive
9) Unknown

Examined nodes (no.) _____

Positive nodes (no.) _____

pN

X	0	1	1a	1b	1bI	1bII	1bIII	1bIV	2	3	unknown

ER
0) Not done
1) Negative
2) Positive
9) Unknown

PR
0) Not done
1) Negative
2) Positive
9) Unknown

ER/PR method
1) Immunohistochemical
2) Biochemical
3) Other
9) Unknown

Antibody used _____
Antigen retrieval
0) No
1) Yes

Date of report _____ / _____ / _____

Other markers
0) No
1) Yes
9) Unknown

Notes
_____
_____
_____
_____
_____

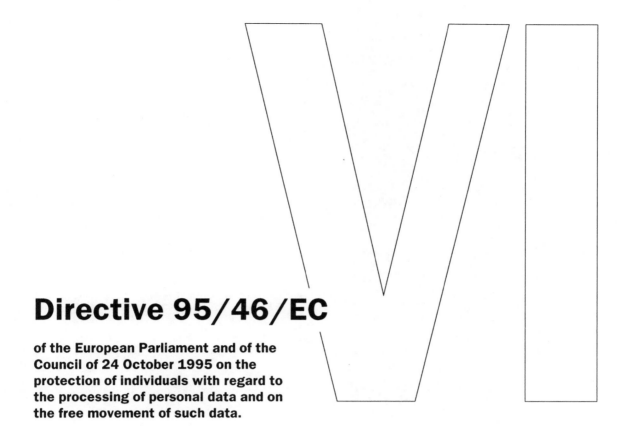

Directive 95/46/EC

of the European Parliament and of the Council of 24 October 1995 on the protection of individuals with regard to the processing of personal data and on the free movement of such data.

Introduction

The protection of individual data is a basic right of every citizen in the European Union. With this in mind, the European Union drafted directive 95/46/EC to control data collection and its usage in order to protect the individual rights of each person. This directive came into force in 1997, Member States being required to implement this as national law.

There are however occasions where rigorous data protection may interfere with the well being of the population concerned, in particular with regard to public health intervention. The organisation of an effective cancer screening programme requires accurate identification of the eligible target population. This information is available from population registers but protected by the above-mentioned directive. In certain circumstances therefore, exemptions may be made for public health reasons.

In the following paragraph, specific references are made to these exemptions. In case difficulties are encountered in any country with such data protection issues, reference should be made to this directive (article 8, paragraph 3).

This is an unofficial text. For the authoritative text of the Directive, reference should be made to the Official Journal of the European Communities of 23 November 1995 No L. 281 p. 31.

Contents

Recitals

Chapter I General provisions

Chapter II - General rules on the lawfulness

Chapter III - Judicial remedies, liability and sanctions
Article 22 Remedies
Article 23 Liability
Article 24 Sanctions

Chapter IV - Transfer of personal data to third countries
Article 25 Principles
Article 26 Derogations

Chapter V - Codes of conduct
Article 27

Chapter VI - Supervisory authority
Article 28 Supervisory authority
Article 29 Working Party on the Protection of Individuals
Article 30

Chapter VII - Community implementing measures
Article 31 The Committee

Final provisions
Article 32
Article 33
Article 34

Recitals

The European parliament and the council of the European Union,

Having regard to the Treaty establishing the European Community, and in particular Article 100a thereof,
Having regard to the proposal from the Commission 1,
Having regard to the opinion of the Economic and Social Committee 2,
Acting in accordance with the procedure referred to in Article 189b of the Treaty 3,

(1)   Whereas the objectives of the Community, as laid down in the Treaty, as amended by the Treaty on European Union, include creating an ever closer union among the peoples of Europe, fostering closer relations between the States belonging to the Community, ensuring economic and social progress by common action to eliminate the barriers which divide Europe, encouraging the constant improvement of the living conditions of its peoples, preserving and strengthening peace and liberty and promoting democracy on the basis of the fundamental rights recognized in the constitution and laws of the Member States and in the European Convention for the Protection of Human Rights and Fundamental Freedoms;

(2)   Whereas data-processing systems are designed to serve man; whereas they must, whatever the nationality or residence of natural persons, respect their fundamental rights and freedoms, notably the right to privacy, and contribute to economic and social progress, trade expansion and the well-being of individuals;

(3)   Whereas the establishment and functioning of an internal market in which, in accordance with Article 7a of the Treaty, the free movement of goods, persons, services and capital is ensured require not only that personal data should be able to flow freely from one Member State to another, but also that the fundamental rights of individuals should be safeguarded;

(4)   Whereas increasingly frequent recourse is being had in the Community to the processing of personal data in the various spheres of economic and social activity; whereas the progress made in information technology is making the processing and exchange of such data considerably easier;

(5)   Whereas the economic and social integration resulting from the establishment and functioning of the internal market within the meaning of Article 7a of the Treaty will necessarily lead to a substantial increase in cross-border flows of personal data between all those involved in a private or public capacity in economic and social activity in the Member States; whereas the exchange of personal data between undertakings in different Member States is set to increase; whereas the national authorities in the various Member States are being called upon by virtue of Community law to collaborate and exchange personal data so as to be able to perform their duties or carry out tasks on behalf of an authority in another Member State within the context of the area without internal frontiers as constituted by the internal market;

(6) Whereas, furthermore, the increase in scientific and technical cooperation and the coordinated introduction of new telecommunications networks in the Community necessitate and facilitate cross-border flows of personal data;

(7) Whereas the difference in levels of protection of the rights and freedoms of individuals, notably the right to privacy, with regard to the processing of personal data afforded in the Member States may prevent the transmission of such data from the territory of one Member State to that of another Member State; whereas this difference may therefore constitute an obstacle to the pursuit of a number of economic activities at Community level, distort competition and impede authorities in the discharge of their responsibilities under Community law; whereas this difference in levels of protection is due to the existence of a wide variety of national laws, regulations and administrative provisions;

(8) Whereas, in order to remove the obstacles to flows of personal data, the level of protection of the rights and freedoms of individuals with regard to the processing of such data must be equivalent in all Member States; whereas this objective is vital to the internal market but cannot be achieved by the Member States alone, especially in view of the scale of the divergences which currently exist between the relevant laws in the Member States and the need to coordinate the laws of the Member States so as to ensure that the cross-border flow of personal data is regulated in a consistent manner that is in keeping with the objective of the internal market as provided for in Article 7a of the Treaty; whereas Community action to approximate those laws is therefore needed;

(9) Whereas, given the equivalent protection resulting from the approximation of national laws, the Member States will no longer be able to inhibit the free movement between them of personal data on grounds relating to protection of the rights and freedoms of individuals, and in particular the right to privacy; whereas Member States will be left a margin for manoeuvre, which may, in the context of implementation of the Directive, also be exercised by the business and social partners; whereas Member States will therefore be able to specify in their national law the general conditions governing the lawfulness of data processing; whereas in doing so the Member States shall strive to improve the protection currently provided by their legislation; whereas, within the limits of this margin for manoeuvre and in accordance with Community law, disparities could arise in the implementation of the Directive, and this could have an effect on the movement of data within a Member State as well as within the Community;

(10) Whereas the object of the national laws on the processing of personal data is to protect fundamental rights and freedoms, notably the right to privacy, which is recognized both in Article 8 of the European Convention for the Protection of Human Rights and Fundamental Freedoms and in the general principles of Community law; whereas, for that reason, the approximation of those laws must not result in any lessening of the protection they afford but must, on the contrary, seek to ensure a high level of protection in the Community;

(11) Whereas the principles of the protection of the rights and freedoms of individuals, notably the right to privacy, which are contained in this Directive, give substance to

and amplify those contained in the Council of Europe Convention of 28 January 1981 for the Protection of Individuals with regard to Automatic Processing of Personal Data;

(12) Whereas the protection principles must apply to all processing of personal data by any person whose activities are governed by Community law; whereas there should be excluded the processing of data carried out by a natural person in the exercise of activities which are exclusively personal or domestic, such as correspondence and the holding of records of addresses;

(13) Whereas the activities referred to in Titles V and VI of the Treaty on European Union regarding public safety, defence, State security or the activities of the State in the area of criminal laws fall outside the scope of Community law, without prejudice to the obligations incumbent upon Member States under Article 56 (2), Article 57 or Article 100a of the Treaty establishing the European Community; whereas the processing of personal data that is necessary to safeguard the economic well-being of the State does not fall within the scope of this Directive where such processing relates to State security matters;

(14) Whereas, given the importance of the developments under way, in the framework of the information society, of the techniques used to capture, transmit, manipulate, record, store or communicate sound and image data relating to natural persons, this Directive should be applicable to processing involving such data;

(15) Whereas the processing of such data is covered by this Directive only if it is automated or if the data processed are contained or are intended to be contained in a filing system structured according to specific criteria relating to individuals, so as to permit easy access to the personal data in question;

(16) Whereas the processing of sound and image data, such as in cases of video surveillance, does not come within the scope of this Directive if it is carried out for the purposes of public security, defence, national security or in the course of State activities relating to the area of criminal law or of other activities which do not come within the scope of Community law;

(17) Whereas, as far as the processing of sound and image data carried out for purposes of journalism or the purposes of literary or artistic expression is concerned, in particular in the audiovisual field, the principles of the Directive are to apply in a restricted manner according to the provisions laid down in Article 9;

(18) Whereas, in order to ensure that individuals are not deprived of the protection to which they are entitled under this Directive, any processing of personal data in the Community must be carried out in accordance with the law of one of the Member States; whereas, in this connection, processing carried out under the responsibility of a controller who is established in a Member State should be governed by the law of that State;

(19) Whereas establishment on the territory of a Member State implies the effective and real exercise of activity through stable arrangements; whereas the legal form of such an establishment, whether simply branch or a subsidiary with a legal

personality, is not the determining factor in this respect; whereas, when a single controller is established on the territory of several Member States, particularly by means of subsidiaries, he must ensure, in order to avoid any circumvention of national rules, that each of the establishments fulfils the obligations imposed by the national law applicable to its activities;

(20) Whereas the fact that the processing of data is carried out by a person established in a third country must not stand in the way of the protection of individuals provided for in this Directive; whereas in these cases, the processing should be governed by the law of the Member State in which the means used are located, and there should be guarantees to ensure that the rights and obligations provided for in this Directive are respected in practice;

(21) Whereas this Directive is without prejudice to the rules of territoriality applicable in criminal matters;

(22) Whereas Member States shall more precisely define in the laws they enact or when bringing into force the measures taken under this Directive the general circumstances in which processing is lawful; whereas in particular Article 5, in conjunction with Articles 7 and 8, allows Member States, independently of general rules, to provide for special processing conditions for specific sectors and for the various categories of data covered by Article 8;

(23) Whereas Member States are empowered to ensure the implementation of the protection of individuals both by means of a general law on the protection of individuals as regards the processing of personal data and by sectorial laws such as those relating, for example, to statistical institutes;

(24) Whereas the legislation concerning the protection of legal persons with regard to the processing data which concerns them is not affected by this Directive;

(25) Whereas the principles of protection must be reflected, on the one hand, in the obligations imposed on persons, public authorities, enterprises, agencies or other bodies responsible for processing, in particular regarding data quality, technical security, notification to the supervisory authority, and the circumstances under which processing can be carried out, and, on the other hand, in the right conferred on individuals, the data on whom are the subject of processing, to be informed that processing is taking place, to consult the data, to request corrections and even to object to processing in certain circumstances;

(26) Whereas the principles of protection must apply to any information concerning an identified or identifiable person; whereas, to determine whether a person is identifiable, account should be taken of all the means likely reasonably to be used either by the controller or by any other person to identify the said person; whereas the principles of protection shall not apply to data rendered anonymous in such a way that the data subject is no longer identifiable; whereas codes of conduct within the meaning of Article 27 may be a useful instrument for providing guidance as to the ways in which data may be rendered anonymous and retained in a form in which identification of the data subject is no longer possible;

(27) Whereas the protection of individuals must apply as much to automatic processing of data as to manual processing; whereas the scope of this protection must not in effect depend on the techniques used, otherwise this would create a serious risk of circumvention; whereas, nonetheless, as regards manual processing, this Directive covers only filing systems, not unstructured files; whereas, in particular, the content of a filing system must be structured according to specific criteria relating to individuals allowing easy access to the personal data; whereas, in line with the definition in Article 2 (c) , the different criteria for determining the constituents of a structured set of personal data, and the different criteria governing access to such a set, may be laid down by each Member State; whereas files or sets of files as well as their cover pages, which are not structured according to specific criteria, shall under no circumstances fall within the scope of this Directive;

(28) Whereas any processing of personal data must be lawful and fair to the individuals concerned; whereas, in particular, the data must be adequate, relevant and not excessive in relation to the purposes for which they are processed; whereas such purposes must be explicit and legitimate and must be determined at the time of collection of the data; whereas the purposes of processing further to collection shall not be incompatible with the purposes as they were originally specified;

(29) Whereas the further processing of personal data for historical, statistical or scientific purposes is not generally to be considered incompatible with the purposes for which the data have previously been collected provided that Member States furnish suitable safeguards; whereas these safeguards must in particular rule out the use of the data in support of measures or decisions regarding any particular individual;

(30) Whereas, in order to be lawful, the processing of personal data must in addition be carried out with the consent of the data subject or be necessary for the conclusion or performance of a contract binding on the data subject, or as a legal requirement, or for the performance of a task carried out in the public interest or in the exercise of official authority, or in the legitimate interests of a natural or legal person, provided that the interests or the rights and freedoms of the data subject are not overriding; whereas, in particular, in order to maintain a balance between the interests involved while guaranteeing effective competition, Member States may determine the circumstances in which personal data may be used or disclosed to a third party in the context of the legitimate ordinary business activities of companies and other bodies; whereas Member States may similarly specify the conditions under which personal data may be disclosed to a third party for the purposes of marketing whether carried out commercially or by a charitable organization or by any other association or foundation, of a political nature for example, subject to the provisions allowing a data subject to object to the processing of data regarding him, at no cost and without having to state his reasons;

(31) Whereas the processing of personal data must equally be regarded as lawful where it is carried out in order to protect an interest which is essential for the data subject's life;

(32) Whereas it is for national legislation to determine whether the controller performing a task carried out in the public interest or in the exercise of official authority should be a public administration or another natural or legal person governed by public law, or by private law such as a professional association;

(33) Whereas data which are capable by their nature of infringing fundamental freedoms or privacy should not be processed unless the data subject gives his explicit consent; whereas, however, derogations from this prohibition must be explicitly provided for in respect of specific needs, in particular where the processing of these data is carried out for certain health-related purposes by persons subject to a legal obligation of professional secrecy or in the course of legitimate activities by certain associations or foundations the purpose of which is to permit the exercise of fundamental freedoms;

(34) Whereas Member States must also be authorized, when justified by grounds of important public interest, to derogate from the prohibition on processing sensitive categories of data where important reasons of public interest so justify in areas such as public health and social protection - especially in order to ensure the quality and cost-effectiveness of the procedures used for settling claims for benefits and services in the health insurance system - scientific research and government statistics; whereas it is incumbent on them, however, to provide specific and suitable safeguards so as to protect the fundamental rights and the privacy of individuals;

(35) Whereas, moreover, the processing of personal data by official authorities for achieving aims, laid down in constitutional law or international public law, of officially recognized religious associations is carried out on important grounds of public interest;

(36) Whereas where, in the course of electoral activities, the operation of the democratic system requires in certain Member States that political parties compile data on people's political opinion, the processing of such data may be permitted for reasons of important public interest, provided that appropriate safeguards are established;

(37) Whereas the processing of personal data for purposes of journalism or for purposes of literary of artistic expression, in particular in the audiovisual field, should qualify for exemption from the requirements of certain provisions of this Directive in so far as this is necessary to reconcile the fundamental rights of individuals with freedom of information and notably the right to receive and impart information, as guaranteed in particular in Article 10 of the European Convention for the Protection of Human Rights and Fundamental Freedoms; whereas Member States should therefore lay down exemptions and derogations necessary for the purpose of balance between fundamental rights as regards general measures on the legitimacy of data processing, measures on the transfer of data to third countries and the power of the supervisory authority; whereas this should not, however, lead Member States to lay down exemptions from the measures to ensure security of processing; whereas at least the supervisory authority responsible for this sector should also be provided with certain ex-post powers, e.g. to publish a regular report or to refer matters to the judicial authorities;

(38) Whereas, if the processing of data is to be fair, the data subject must be in a position to learn of the existence of a processing operation and, where data are collected from him, must be given accurate and full information, bearing in mind the circumstances of the collection;

(39) Whereas certain processing operations involve data which the controller has not collected directly from the data subject; whereas, furthermore, data can be legitimately disclosed to a third party, even if the disclosure was not anticipated at the time the data were collected from the data subject; whereas, in all these cases, the data subject should be informed when the data are recorded or at the latest when the data are first disclosed to a third party;

(40) Whereas, however, it is not necessary to impose this obligation of the data subject already has the information; whereas, moreover, there will be no such obligation if the recording or disclosure are expressly provided for by law or if the provision of information to the data subject proves impossible or would involve disproportionate efforts, which could be the case where processing is for historical, statistical or scientific purposes; whereas, in this regard, the number of data subjects, the age of the data, and any compensatory measures adopted may be taken into consideration;

(41) Whereas any person must be able to exercise the right of access to data relating to him which are being processed, in order to verify in particular the accuracy of the data and the lawfulness of the processing; whereas, for the same reasons, every data subject must also have the right to know the logic involved in the automatic processing of data concerning him, at least in the case of the automated decisions referred to in Article 15 (1); whereas this right must not adversely affect trade secrets or intellectual property and in particular the copyright protecting the software; whereas these considerations must not, however, result in the data subject being refused all information;

(42) Whereas Member States may, in the interest of the data subject or so as to protect the rights and freedoms of others, restrict rights of access and information; whereas they may, for example, specify that access to medical data may be obtained only through a health professional;

(43) Whereas restrictions on the rights of access and information and on certain obligations of the controller may similarly be imposed by Member States in so far as they are necessary to safeguard, for example, national security, defence, public safety, or important economic or financial interests of a Member State or the Union, as well as criminal investigations and prosecutions and action in respect of breaches of ethics in the regulated professions; whereas the list of exceptions and limitations should include the tasks of monitoring, inspection or regulation necessary in the three last-mentioned areas concerning public security, economic or financial interests and crime prevention; whereas the listing of tasks in these three areas does not affect the legitimacy of exceptions or restrictions for reasons of State security or defence;

(44) Whereas Member States may also be led, by virtue of the provisions of Community law, to derogate from the provisions of this Directive concerning the right of access, the obligation to inform individuals, and the quality of data, in order to secure certain of the purposes referred to above;

(45) Whereas, in cases where data might lawfully be processed on grounds of public interest, official authority or the legitimate interests of a natural or legal person, any data subject should nevertheless be entitled, on legitimate and compelling grounds relating to his particular situation, to object to the processing of any data relating to himself; whereas Member States may nevertheless lay down national provisions to the contrary;

(46) Whereas the protection of the rights and freedoms of data subjects with regard to the processing of personal data requires that appropriate technical and organizational measures be taken, both at the time of the design of the processing system and at the time of the processing itself, particularly in order to maintain security and thereby to prevent any unauthorized processing; whereas it is incumbent on the Member States to ensure that controllers comply with these measures; whereas these measures must ensure an appropriate level of security, taking into account the state of the art and the costs of their implementation in relation to the risks inherent in the processing and the nature of the data to be protected;

(47) Whereas where a message containing personal data is transmitted by means of a telecommunications or electronic mail service, the sole purpose of which is the transmission of such messages, the controller in respect of the personal data contained in the message will normally be considered to be the person from whom the message originates, rather than the person offering the transmission services; whereas, nevertheless, those offering such services will normally be considered controllers in respect of the processing of the additional personal data necessary for the operation of the service;

(48) Whereas the procedures for notifying the supervisory authority are designed to ensure disclosure of the purposes and main features of any processing operation for the purpose of verification that the operation is in accordance with the national measures taken under this Directive;

(49) Whereas, in order to avoid unsuitable administrative formalities, exemptions from the obligation to notify and simplification of the notification required may be provided for by Member States in cases where processing is unlikely adversely to affect the rights and freedoms of data subjects, provided that it is in accordance with a measure taken by a Member State specifying its limits; whereas exemption or simplification may similarly be provided for by Member States where a person appointed by the controller ensures that the processing carried out is not likely adversely to affect the rights and freedoms of data subjects; whereas such a data protection official, whether or not an employee of the controller, must be in a position to exercise his functions in complete independence;

(50) Whereas exemption or simplification could be provided for in cases of processing operations whose sole purpose is the keeping of a register intended, according to national law, to provide information to the public and open to consultation by the public or by any person demonstrating a legitimate interest;

(51) Whereas, nevertheless, simplification or exemption from the obligation to notify shall not release the controller from any of the other obligations resulting from this Directive;

(52) Whereas, in this context, ex post facto verification by the competent authorities must in general be considered a sufficient measure;

(53) Whereas, however, certain processing operation are likely to pose specific risks to the rights and freedoms of data subjects by virtue of their nature, their scope or their purposes, such as that of excluding individuals from a right, benefit or a contract, or by virtue of the specific use of new technologies; whereas it is for Member States, if they so wish, to specify such risks in their legislation;

(54) Whereas with regard to all the processing undertaken in society, the amount posing such specific risks should be very limited; whereas Member States must provide that the supervisory authority, or the data protection official in cooperation with the authority, check such processing prior to it being carried out; whereas following this prior check, the supervisory authority may, according to its national law, give an opinion or an authorization regarding the processing; whereas such checking may equally take place in the course of the preparation either of a measure of the national parliament or of a measure based on such a legislative measure, which defines the nature of the processing and lays down appropriate safeguards;

(55) Whereas, if the controller fails to respect the rights of data subjects, national legislation must provide for a judicial remedy; whereas any damage which a person may suffer as a result of unlawful processing must be compensated for by the controller, who may be exempted from liability if he proves that he is not responsible for the damage, in particular in cases where he establishes fault on the part of the data subject or in case of force majeure; whereas sanctions must be imposed on any person, whether governed by private of public law, who fails to comply with the national measures taken under this Directive;

(56) Whereas cross-border flows of personal data are necessary to the expansion of international trade; whereas the protection of individuals, guaranteed in the Community by this Directive does not stand in the way of transfers of personal data to third countries which ensure an adequate level of protection; whereas the adequacy of the level of protection afforded by a third country must be assessed in the light of all the circumstances surrounding the transfer operation or set of transfer operations;

(57) Whereas, on the other hand, the transfer of personal data to a third country which does not ensure an adequate level of protection must be prohibited;

(58) Whereas provisions should be made for exemptions from this prohibition in certain circumstances where the data subject has given his consent, where the transfer is necessary in relation to a contract or a legal claim, where protection of an important public interest so requires, for example in cases of international transfers of data between tax or customs administrations or between services competent for social security matters, or where the transfer is made from a register established by law and intended for consultation by the public or persons having a legitimate interest; whereas in this case such a transfer should not involve the entirety of the data or entire categories of the data contained in the register and, when the register is intended for consultation by persons having a legitimate interest, the transfer should be made only at the request of those persons or if they are to be the recipients;

(59) Whereas particular measures may be taken to compensate for the lack of protection in a third country in cases where the controller offers appropriate safeguards; whereas, moreover, provision must be made for procedures for negotiations between the Community and such third countries;

(60) Whereas, in any event, transfers to third countries may be effected only in full compliance with the provisions adopted by the Member States pursuant to this Directive, and in particular Article 8 thereof;

(61) Whereas Member States and the Commission, in their respective spheres of competence, must encourage the trade associations and other representative organizations concerned to draw up codes of conduct so as to facilitate the application of this Directive, taking account of the specific characteristics of the processing carried out in certain sectors, and respecting the national provisions adopted for its implementation;

(62) Whereas the establishment in Member States of supervisory authorities, exercising their functions with complete independence, is an essential component of the protection of individuals with regard to the processing of personal data;

(63) Whereas such authorities must have the necessary means to perform their duties, including powers of investigation and intervention, particularly in cases of complaints from individuals, and powers to engage in legal proceedings; whereas such authorities must help to ensure transparency of processing in the Member States within whose jurisdiction they fall;

(64) Whereas the authorities in the different Member States will need to assist one another in performing their duties so as to ensure that the rules of protection are properly respected throughout the European Union;

(65) Whereas, at Community level, a Working Party on the Protection of Individuals with regard to the Processing of Personal Data must be set up and be completely independent in the performance of its functions; whereas, having regard to its specific nature, it must advise the Commission and, in particular, contribute to the uniform application of the national rules adopted pursuant to this Directive;

(66) Whereas, with regard to the transfer of data to third countries, the application of this Directive calls for the conferment of powers of implementation on the Commission and the establishment of a procedure as laid down in Council Decision 87/373/EEC 4;

(67) Whereas an agreement on a modus vivendi between the European Parliament, the Council and the Commission concerning the implementing measures for acts adopted in accordance with the procedure laid down in Article 189b of the EC Treaty was reached on 20 December 1994;

(68) Whereas the principles set out in this Directive regarding the protection of the rights and freedoms of individuals, notably their right to privacy, with regard to the processing of personal data may be supplemented or clarified, in particular as far as certain sectors are concerned, by specific rules based on those principles;

(69) Whereas Member States should be allowed a period of not more than three years from the entry into force of the national measures transposing this Directive in which to apply such new national rules progressively to all processing operations already under way; whereas, in order to facilitate their cost-effective implementation, a further period expiring 12 years after the date on which this Directive is adopted will be allowed to Member States to ensure the conformity of existing manual filing systems with certain of the Directive's provisions; whereas, where data contained in such filing systems are manually processed during this extended transition period, those systems must be brought into conformity with these provisions at the time of such processing;

(70) Whereas it is not necessary for the data subject to give his consent again so as to allow the controller to continue to process, after the national provisions taken pursuant to this Directive enter into force, any sensitive data necessary for the performance of a contract concluded on the basis of free and informed consent before the entry into force of these provisions;

(71) Whereas this Directive does not stand in the way of a Member State's regulating marketing activities aimed at consumers residing in territory in so far as such regulation does not concern the protection of individuals with regard to the processing of personal data;

(72) Whereas this Directive allows the principle of public access to official documents to be taken into account when implementing the principles set out in this Directive,

Have adopted this directive:

Chapter I General provisions

Article 1 Object of the Directive

1. In accordance with this Directive, Member States shall protect the fundamental rights and freedoms of natural persons, and in particular their right to privacy with respect to the processing of personal data.

2. Member States shall neither restrict nor prohibit the free flow of personal data between Member States for reasons connected with the protection afforded under paragraph 1.

Article 2 Definitions

For the purposes of this Directive:

(a) 'personal data' shall mean any information relating to an identified or identifiable natural person ('data subject'); an identifiable person is one who can be identified, directly or indirectly, in particular by reference to an identification number or to one or more factors specific to his physical, physiological, mental, economic, cultural or social identity;

(b) 'processing of personal data' ('processing') shall mean any operation or set of operations which is performed upon personal data, whether or not by automatic means, such as collection, recording, organization, storage, adaptation or alteration, retrieval, consultation, use, disclosure by transmission, dissemination or otherwise making available, alignment or combination, blocking, erasure or destruction;

(c) 'personal data filing system' ('filing system') shall mean any structured set of personal data which are accessible according to specific criteria, whether centralized, decentralized or dispersed on a functional or geographical basis;

(d) 'controller' shall mean the natural or legal person, public authority, agency or any other body which alone or jointly with others determines the purposes and means of the processing of personal data; where the purposes and means of processing are determined by national or Community laws or regulations, the controller or the specific criteria for his nomination may be designated by national or Community law;

(e) 'processor' shall mean a natural or legal person, public authority, agency or any other body which processes personal data on behalf of the controller;

(f) 'third party' shall mean any natural or legal person, public authority, agency or any other body other than the data subject, the controller, the processor and the persons who, under the direct authority of the controller or the processor, are authorized to process the data;

(g) 'recipient' shall mean a natural or legal person, public authority, agency or any other body to whom data are disclosed, whether a third party or not; however, authorities which may receive data in the framework of a particular inquiry shall not be regarded as recipients;

(h) 'the data subject's consent' shall mean any freely given specific and informed indication of his wishes by which the data subject signifies his agreement to personal data relating to him being processed.

Article 3 Scope

1. This Directive shall apply to the processing of personal data wholly or partly by automatic means, and to the processing otherwise than by automatic means of personal data which form part of a filing system or are intended to form part of a filing system.

2. This Directive shall not apply to the processing of personal data:
   - in the course of an activity which falls outside the scope of Community law, such as those provided for by Titles V and VI of the Treaty on European Union and in any case to processing operations concerning public security, defence, State security (including the economic well-being of the State when the processing operation relates to State security matters) and the activities of the State in areas of criminal law,
   - by a natural person in the course of a purely personal or household activity.

Article 4 National law applicable

1. Each Member State shall apply the national provisions it adopts pursuant to this Directive to the processing of personal data where:
   (a) the processing is carried out in the context of the activities of an establishment of the controller on the territory of the Member State; when the same controller is established on the territory of several Member States, he must take the necessary measures to ensure that each of these establishments complies with the obligations laid down by the national law applicable;
   (b) the controller is not established on the Member State's territory, but in a place where its national law applies by virtue of international public law;
   (c) the controller is not established on Community territory and, for purposes of processing personal data makes use of equipment, automated or otherwise, situated on the territory of the said Member State, unless such equipment is used only for purposes of transit through the territory of the Community.

2. In the circumstances referred to in paragraph 1 (c), the controller must designate a representative established in the territory of that Member State, without prejudice to legal actions which could be initiated against the controller himself.

Chapter II General rules on the lawfulness of the processing of personal data

Article 5

Member States shall, within the limits of the provisions of this Chapter, determine more precisely the conditions under which the processing of personal data is lawful.

SECTION I - PRINCIPLES RELATING TO DATA QUALITY

Article 6

1. Member States shall provide that personal data must be:
   (a) processed fairly and lawfully;
   (b) collected for specified, explicit and legitimate purposes and not further processed in a way incompatible with those purposes. Further processing of data for historical, statistical or scientific purposes shall not be considered as incompatible provided that Member States provide appropriate safeguards;
   (c) adequate, relevant and not excessive in relation to the purposes for which they are collected and/or further processed;
   (d) accurate and, where necessary, kept up to date; every reasonable step must be taken to ensure that data which are inaccurate or incomplete, having regard to the purposes for which they were collected or for which they are further processed, are erased or rectified;
   (e) kept in a form which permits identification of data subjects for no longer than is necessary for the purposes for which the data were collected or for which they are further processed. Member States shall lay down appropriate safeguards for personal data stored for longer periods for historical, statistical or scientific use.

2. It shall be for the controller to ensure that paragraph 1 is complied with.

SECTION II - CRITERIA FOR MAKING DATA PROCESSING LEGITIMATE

Article 7

Member States shall provide that personal data may be processed only if:

(a) the data subject has unambiguously given his consent; or

(b) processing is necessary for the performance of a contract to which the data subject is party or in order to take steps at the request of the data subject prior to entering into a contract; or

(c) processing is necessary for compliance with a legal obligation to which the controller is subject; or

(d) processing is necessary in order to protect the vital interests of the data subject; or

(e) processing is necessary for the performance of a task carried out in the public interest or in the exercise of official authority vested in the controller or in a third party to whom the data are disclosed; or

(f) processing is necessary for the purposes of the legitimate interests pursued by the controller or by the third party or parties to whom the data are disclosed, except where such interests are overridden by the interests for fundamental rights and freedoms of the data subject which require protection under Article 1 (1).

SECTION III - SPECIAL CATEGORIES OF PROCESSING

Article 8 The processing of special categories of data
1. Member States shall prohibit the processing of personal data revealing racial or ethnic origin, political opinions, religious or philosophical beliefs, trade-union membership, and the processing of data concerning health or sex life.

2. Paragraph 1 shall not apply where:
    (a) the data subject has given his explicit consent to the processing of those data, except where the laws of the Member State provide that the prohibition referred to in paragraph 1 may not be lifted by the data subject's giving his consent; or
    (b) processing is necessary for the purposes of carrying out the obligations and specific rights of the controller in the field of employment law in so far as it is authorized by national law providing for adequate safeguards; or
    (c) processing is necessary to protect the vital interests of the data subject or of another person where the data subject is physically or legally incapable of giving his consent; or
    (d) processing is carried out in the course of its legitimate activities with appropriate guarantees by a foundation, association or any other non-profit-seeking body with a political, philosophical, religious or trade-union aim and on condition that the processing relates solely to the members of the body or to persons who have regular contact with it in connection with its purposes and that the data are not disclosed to a third party without the consent of the data subjects; or
    (e) the processing relates to data which are manifestly made public by the data subject or is necessary for the establishment, exercise or defence of legal claims.

3. Paragraph 1 shall not apply where processing of the data is required for the purposes of preventive medicine, medical diagnosis, the provision of care or treatment or the management of health-care services, and where those data are processed by a health professional subject under national law or rules established by national competent bodies to the obligation of professional secrecy or by another person also subject to an equivalent obligation of secrecy.

4. Subject to the provision of suitable safeguards, Member States may, for reasons of substantial public interest, lay down exemptions in addition to those laid down in paragraph 2 either by national law or by decision of the supervisory authority.

5. Processing of data relating to offences, criminal convictions or security measures may be carried out only under the control of official authority, or if suitable specific safeguards are provided under national law, subject to derogations which may be granted by the Member State under national provisions providing suitable specific safeguards. However, a complete register of criminal convictions may be kept only under the control of official authority.
    Member States may provide that data relating to administrative sanctions or judgements in civil cases shall also be processed under the control of official authority.

6. Derogations from paragraph 1 provided for in paragraphs 4 and 5 shall be notified to the Commission

7. Member States shall determine the conditions under which a national identification number or any other identifier of general application may be processed.

Article 9 Processing of personal data and freedom of expression

Member States shall provide for exemptions or derogations from the provisions of this Chapter, Chapter IV and Chapter VI for the processing of personal data carried out solely for journalistic purposes or the purpose of artistic or literary expression only if they are necessary to reconcile the right to privacy with the rules governing freedom of expression.

SECTION IV - INFORMATION TO BE GIVEN TO THE DATA SUBJECT

Article 10 Information in cases of collection of data from the data subject

Member States shall provide that the controller or his representative must provide a data subject from whom data relating to himself are collected with at least the following information, except where he already has it:

(a) the identity of the controller and of his representative, if any;

(b) the purposes of the processing for which the data are intended;

(c) any further information such as
   - the recipients or categories of recipients of the data,
   - whether replies to the questions are obligatory or voluntary, as well as the possible consequences of failure to reply,
   - the existence of the right of access to and the right to rectify the data concerning him in so far as such further information is necessary, having regard to the specific circumstances in which the data are collected, to guarantee fair processing in respect of the data subject.

Article 11 Information where the data have not been obtained from the data subject

1. Where the data have not been obtained from the data subject, Member States shall provide that the controller or his representative must at the time of undertaking the recording of personal data or if a disclosure to a third party is envisaged, no later than the time when the data are first disclosed provide the data subject with at least the following information, except where he already has it:
    (a) the identity of the controller and of his representative, if any;
    (b) the purposes of the processing;
    (c) any further information such as
       - the categories of data concerned,
       - the recipients or categories of recipients,
       - the existence of the right of access to and the right to rectify the data concerning him in so far as such further information is necessary, having regard to the specific circumstances in which the data are processed, to guarantee fair processing in respect of the data subject.

2. Paragraph 1 shall not apply where, in particular for processing for statistical purposes or for the purposes of historical or scientific research, the provision of such information proves impossible or would involve a disproportionate effort or if recording or disclosure is expressly laid down by law. In these cases Member States shall provide appropriate safeguards.

SECTION V - THE DATA SUBJECT'S RIGHT OF ACCESS TO DATA

Article 12 Right of access

Member States shall guarantee every data right to obtain from the controller:

(a) without constraint at reasonable intervals and without excessive delay or expense:
- confirmation as to whether or not data relating to him are being processed and information at least as to the purposes of the processing, the categories of data concerned, and the recipients or categories of recipients to whom the data are disclosed,
- communication to him in an intelligible form of the data undergoing processing and of any available information as to their source,
- knowledge of the logic involved in any automatic processing of data concerning him at least in the case of the automated decisions referred to in Article 15 (1);

(b) as appropriate the rectification, erasure or blocking of data the processing of which does not comply with the provisions of this Directive, in particular because of the incomplete or inaccurate nature of the data;

(c) notification to third parties to whom the data have been disclosed of any rectification, erasure or blocking carried out in compliance with (b), unless this proves impossible or involves a disproportionate effort.

SECTION VI - EXEMPTIONS AND RESTRICTIONS

Article 13

1. Member States may adopt legislative measures to restrict the scope of the obligations and rights provided for in Articles 6 (1), 10, 11 (1), 12 and 21 when such a restriction constitutes a necessary measures to safeguard:
    (a) national security;
    (b) defence;
    (c) public security;
    (d) the prevention, investigation, detection and prosecution of criminal offences, or of breaches of ethics for regulated professions;
    (e) an important economic or financial interest of a Member State or of the European Union, including monetary, budgetary and taxation matters;
    (f) a monitoring, inspection or regulatory function connected, even occasionally, with the exercise of official authority in cases referred to in (c), (d) and (e);
    (g) the protection of the data subject or of the rights and freedoms of others.

2. Subject to adequate legal safeguards, in particular that the data are not used for taking measures or decisions regarding any particular individual, Member States may, where there is clearly no risk of breaching the privacy of the data subject, restrict by a legislative measure the rights provided for in Article 12 when data are processed solely for purposes of scientific research or are kept in personal form for a period which does not exceed the period necessary for the sole purpose of creating statistics.

SECTION VII - THE DATA SUBJECT'S RIGHT TO OBJECT

Article 14 The data subject's right to object
Member States shall grant the data subject the right:

(a) at least in the cases referred to in Article 7 (e) and (f), to object at any time on compelling legitimate grounds relating to his particular situation to the processing of data relating to him, save where otherwise provided by national legislation. Where there is a justified objection, the processing instigated by the controller may no longer involve those data;

(b) to object, on request and free of charge, to the processing of personal data relating to him which the controller anticipates being processed for the purposes of direct marketing, or to be informed before personal data are disclosed for the first time to third parties or used on their behalf for the purposes of direct marketing, and to be expressly offered the right to object free of charge to such disclosures or uses.
Member States shall take the necessary measures to ensure that data subjects are aware of the existence of the right referred to in the first subparagraph of (b).

Article 15 Automated individual decisions
1. Member States shall grant the right to every person not to be subject to a decision which produces legal effects concerning him or significantly affects him and which is based solely on automated processing of data intended to evaluate certain personal aspects relating to him, such as his performance at work, creditworthiness, reliability, conduct, etc.

2. Subject to the other Articles of this Directive, Member States shall provide that a person may be subjected to a decision of the kind referred to in paragraph 1 if that decision:
   (a) is taken in the course of the entering into or performance of a contract, provided the request for the entering into or the performance of the contract, lodged by the data subject, has been satisfied or that there are suitable measures to safeguard his legitimate interests, such as arrangements allowing him to put his point of view; or
   (b) is authorized by a law which also lays down measures to safeguard the data subject's legitimate interests.

SECTION VIII - CONFIDENTIALITY AND SECURITY OF PROCESSING

Article 16 Confidentiality of processing
Any person acting under the authority of the controller or of the processor, including the processor himself, who has access to personal data must not process them except on instructions from the controller, unless he is required to do so by law.

Article 17 Security of processing
1. Member States shall provide that the controller must implement appropriate technical and organizational measures to protect personal data against accidental or unlawful destruction or accidental loss, alteration, unauthorized disclosure or access, in particular where the processing involves the transmission of data over a network, and against all other unlawful forms of processing.

   Having regard to the state of the art and the cost of their implementation, such measures shall ensure a level of security appropriate to the risks represented by the processing and the nature of the data to be protected.

2. The Member States shall provide that the controller must, where processing is carried out on his behalf, choose a processor providing sufficient guarantees in respect of the technical security measures and organizational measures governing the processing to be carried out, and must ensure compliance with those measures.

3. The carrying out of processing by way of a processor must be governed by a contract or legal act binding the processor to the controller and stipulating in particular that:
   - the processor shall act only on instructions from the controller,
   - the obligations set out in paragraph 1, as defined by the law of the Member State in which the processor is established, shall also be incumbent on the processor.

4. For the purposes of keeping proof, the parts of the contract or the legal act relating to data protection and the requirements relating to the measures referred to in paragraph 1 shall be in writing or in another equivalent form.

SECTION IX - NOTIFICATION

Article 18 - Obligation to notify the supervisory authority
1. Member States shall provide that the controller or his representative, if any, must notify the supervisory authority referred to in Article 28 before carrying out any wholly or partly automatic processing operation or set of such operations intended to serve a single purpose or several related purposes.

2. Member States may provide for the simplification of or exemption from notification only in the following cases and under the following conditions:
   - where, for categories of processing operations which are unlikely, taking account of the data to be processed, to affect adversely the rights and freedoms of data subjects, they specify the purposes of the processing, the data or categories of data undergoing processing, the category or categories of data subject, the recipients or categories of recipient to whom the data are to be disclosed and the length of time

the data are to be stored, and/or
- where the controller, in compliance with the national law which governs him, appoints a personal data protection official, responsible in particular:
- for ensuring in an independent manner the internal application of the national provisions taken pursuant to this Directive
- for keeping the register of processing operations carried out by the controller, containing the items of information referred to in Article 21 (2),
thereby ensuring that the rights and freedoms of the data subjects are unlikely to be adversely affected by the processing operations.

3. Member States may provide that paragraph 1 does not apply to processing whose sole purpose is the keeping of a register which according to laws or regulations is intended to provide information to the public and which is open to consultation either by the public in general or by any person demonstrating a legitimate interest.

4. Member States may provide for an exemption from the obligation to notify or a simplification of the notification in the case of processing operations referred to in Article 8 (2) (d).

5. Member States may stipulate that certain or all non-automatic processing operations involving personal data shall be notified, or provide for these processing operations to be subject to simplified notification.

Article 19 - Contents of notification
1. Member States shall specify the information to be given in the notification. It shall include at least:
   (a) the name and address of the controller and of his representative, if any;
   (b) the purpose or purposes of the processing;
   (c) a description of the category or categories of data subject and of the data or categories of data relating to them;
   (d) the recipients or categories of recipient to whom the data might be disclosed;
   (e) proposed transfers of data to third countries;
   (f) a general description allowing a preliminary assessment to be made of the appropriateness of the measures taken pursuant to Article 17 to ensure security of processing.

2. Member States shall specify the procedures under which any change affecting the information referred to in paragraph I must be notified to the supervisory authority.

Article 20 Prior checking
1. Member States shall determine the processing operations likely to present specific risks to the rights and freedoms of data subjects and shall check that these processing operations are examined prior to the start thereof.

2. Such prior checks shall be carried out by the supervisory authority following receipt of a notification from the controller or by the data protection official, who, in cases of doubt, must consult the supervisory authority.

---

3. Member States may also carry out such checks in the context of preparation either of a measure of the national parliament or of a measure based on such a legislative measure, which define the nature of the processing and lay down appropriate safeguards.

Article 21 Publicizing of processing operations

1. Member States shall take measures to ensure that processing operations are publicized.

2. Member States shall provide that a register of processing operations notified in accordance with Article 18 shall be kept by the supervisory authority.

   The register shall contain at least the information listed in Article 19 (1) (a) to (e). The register may be inspected by any person.

3. Member States shall provide, in relation to processing operations not subject to notification, that controllers or another body appointed by the Member States make available at least the information referred to in Article 19 (1) (a) to (e) in an appropriate form to any person on request.
   Member States may provide that this provision does not apply to processing whose sole purpose is the keeping of a register which according to laws or regulations is intended to provide information to the public and which is open to consultation either by the public in general or by any person who can provide provide of a legitimate interest.

Chapter III - Judicial remedies, liability and sanctions

Article 22 Remedies

Without prejudice to any administrative remedy for which provision may be made, inter alia before the supervisory authority referred to in Article 28 , prior to referral to the judicial authority, Member States shall provide for the right of every person to a judicial remedy for any breach of the rights guaranteed him by the national law applicable to the processing in question.

Article 23 Liability

1. Member States shall provide that any person who has suffered damage as a result of an unlawful processing operation or of any act incompatible with the national provisions adopted pursuant to this Directive is entitled to receive compensation from the controller for the damage suffered.

2. The controller may be exempted from this liability, in whole or in part, if he proves that he is not responsible for the event giving rise to the damage.

Article 24 Sanctions

The Member States shall adopt suitable measures to ensure the full implementation of the provisions of this Directive and shall in particular lay down the sanctions to be imposed in case of infringement of the provisions adopted pursuant to this Directive.

Chapter IV - Transfer of personal data to third countries

Article 25 Principles

1. The Member States shall provide that the transfer to a third country of personal data which are undergoing processing or are intended for processing after transfer may take place only if, without prejudice to compliance with the national provisions adopted pursuant to the other provisions of this Directive, the third country in question ensures an adequate level of protection.

2. The adequacy of the level of protection afforded by a third country shall be assessed in the light of all the circumstances surrounding a data transfer operation or set of data transfer operations; particular consideration shall be given to the nature of the data, the purpose and duration of the proposed processing operation or operations, the country of origin and country of final destination, the rules of law, both general and sectoral, in force in the third country in question and the professional rules and security measures which are complied with in that country.

3. The Member States and the Commission shall inform each other of cases where they consider that a third country does not ensure an adequate level of protection within the meaning of paragraph 2.

4. Where the Commission finds, under the procedure provided for in Article 31 (2), that a third country does not ensure an adequate level of protection within the meaning of paragraph 2 of this Article, Member States shall take the measures necessary to prevent any transfer of data of the same type to the third country in question.

5. At the appropriate time, the Commission shall enter into negotiations with a view to remedying the situation resulting from the finding made pursuant to paragraph 4.

6. The Commission may find, in accordance with the procedure referred to in Article 31 (2), that a third country ensures an adequate level of protection within the meaning of paragraph 2 of this Article, by reason of its domestic law or of the international commitments it has entered into, particularly upon conclusion of the negotiations referred to in paragraph 5, for the protection of the private lives and basic freedoms and rights of individuals.
Member States shall take the measures necessary to comply with the Commission's decision.

Article 26 Derogations

1. By way of derogation from Article 25 and save where otherwise provided by domestic law governing particular cases, Member States shall provide that a transfer or a set of transfers of personal data to a third country which does not ensure an adequate level of protection within the meaning of Article 25 (2) may take place on condition that:

   (a) the data subject has given his consent unambiguously to the proposed transfer; or

   (b) the transfer is necessary for the performance of a contract between the data subject and the controller or the implementation of precontractual measures taken in response to the data subject's request; or

   (c) the transfer is necessary for the conclusion or performance of a contract concluded in the interest of the data subject between the controller and a third party; or

   (d) the transfer is necessary or legally required on important public interest grounds, or for the establishment, exercise or defence of legal claims; or

   (e) the transfer is necessary in order to protect the vital interests of the data subject; or

   (f) the transfer is made from a register which according to laws or regulations is intended to provide information to the public and which is open to consultation either by the public in general or by any person who can demonstrate legitimate interest, to the extent that the conditions laid down in law for consultation are fulfilled in the particular case.

2. Without prejudice to paragraph 1, a Member State may authorize a transfer or a set of transfers of personal data to a third country which does not ensure an adequate level of protection within the meaning of Article 25 (2), where the controller adduces adequate safeguards with respect to the protection of the privacy and fundamental rights and freedoms of individuals and as regards the exercise of the corresponding rights; such safeguards may in particular result from appropriate contractual clauses.

3. The Member State shall inform the Commission and the other Member States of the authorizations it grants pursuant to paragraph 2.

   If a Member State or the Commission objects on justified grounds involving the protection of the privacy and fundamental rights and freedoms of individuals, the Commission shall take appropriate measures in accordance with the procedure laid down in Article 31 (2).
   Member States shall take the necessary to comply with the Commission's decision.

4. Where the Commission decides, in accordance with the procedure referred to in Article 31 (2), that certain standard contractual clauses offer sufficient safeguards as required by paragraph 2, Member States shall take the necessary measures to comply with the Commission's decision.

Chapter V - Codes of conduct

Article 27

1. The Member States and the Commission shall encourage the drawing up of codes of conduct intended to contribute to the proper implementation of the national provisions adopted by the Member States pursuant to this Directive, taking account of the specific features of the various sectors.

2. Member States shall make provision for trade associations and other bodies representing other categories of controllers which have drawn up draft national codes or which have the intention of amending or extending existing national codes to be able to submit them to the opinion of the national authority.
   Member States shall make provision for this authority to ascertain, among other things, whether the drafts submitted to it are in accordance with the national provisions adopted pursuant to this Directive. If it sees fit, the authority shall seek the views of data subjects or their representatives.

3. Draft Community codes, and amendments or extensions to existing Community codes, may be submitted to the Working Party referred to in Article 29 . This Working Party shall determine, among other things, whether the drafts submitted to it are in accordance with the national provisions adopted pursuant to this Directive. If it sees fit, the authority shall seek the views of data subjects or their representatives. The Commission may ensure appropriate publicity for the codes which have been approved by the Working Party.

Chapter VI Supervisory authority and working party on the protection of individuals with regard to the processing of personal data

Article 28 Supervisory authority

1. Each Member State shall provide that one or more public authorities are responsible for monitoring the application within its territory of the provisions adopted by the Member States pursuant to this Directive.
   These authorities shall act with complete independence in exercising the functions entrusted to them.

2. Each Member State shall provide that the supervisory authorities are consulted when drawing up administrative measures or regulations relating to the protection of individuals' rights and freedoms with regard to the processing of personal data.

3. Each authority shall in particular be endowed with:
   - investigative powers, such as powers of access to data forming the subject-matter of processing operations and powers to collect all the information necessary for the performance of its supervisory duties,

- effective powers of intervention, such as, for example, that of delivering opinions before processing operations are carried out, in accordance with Article 20 , and ensuring appropriate publication of such opinions, of ordering the blocking, erasure or destruction of data, of imposing a temporary or definitive ban on processing, of warning or admonishing the controller, or that of referring the matter to national parliaments or other political Institutions,
- the power to engage in legal proceedings where the national provisions adopted pursuant to this Directive have been violated or to bring these violations to the attention of the judicial authorities.

Decisions by the supervisory authority which give rise to complaints may be appealed against through the courts.

4. Each supervisory authority shall hear claims lodged by any person, or by an association representing that person, concerning the protection of his rights and freedoms in regard to the processing of personal data. The person concerned shall be informed of the outcome of the claim.

    Each supervisory authority shall, in particular, hear claims for checks on the lawfulness of data processing lodged by any person when the national provisions adopted pursuant to Article 13 of this Directive apply. The person shall at any rate be informed that a check has taken place.

5. Each supervisory authority shall draw up a report on its activities at regular intervals. The report shall be made public.

6. Each supervisory authority is competent, whatever the national law applicable to the processing in question, to exercise, on the territory of its own Member State, the powers conferred on it in accordance with paragraph 3. Each authority may be requested to exercise its powers by an authority of another Member State.

    The supervisory authorities shall cooperate with one another to the extent necessary for the performance of their duties, in particular by exchanging all useful information.

7. Member States shall provide that the members and staff of the supervisory authority, even after their employment has ended, are to be subject to a duty of professional secrecy with regard to confidential information to which they have access.

Article 29 Working Party on the Protection of Individuals with regard to the Processing of Personal Data

1. A Working Party on the Protection of Individuals with regard to the Processing of Personal Data, hereinafter referred to as 'the Working Party', is hereby set up.
    It shall have advisory status and act independently.

2. The Working Party shall be composed of a representative of the supervisory authority or authorities designated by each Member State and of a representative of the authority or authorities established for the Community institutions and bodies, and of a representative of the Commission.

Each member of the Working Party shall be designated by the institution, authority or authorities which he represents. Where a Member State has designated more than one supervisory authority, they shall nominate a joint representative. The same shall apply to the authorities established for Community institutions and bodies.

3. The Working Party shall take decisions by a simple majority of the representatives of the supervisory authorities.

4. The Working Party shall elect its chairman. The chairman's term of office shall be two years. His appointment shall be renewable.

5. The Working Party's secretariat shall be provided by the Commission.

6. The Working Party shall adopt its own rules of procedure.

7. The Working Party shall consider items placed on its agenda by its chairman, either on his own initiative or at the request of a representative of the supervisory authorities or at the Commission's request.

Article 30

1. The Working Party shall:
   (a) examine any question covering the application of the national measures adopted under this Directive in order to contribute to the uniform application of such measures;
   (b) give the Commission an opinion on the level of protection in the Community and in third countries;
   (c) advise the Commission on any proposed amendment of this Directive, on any additional or specific measures to safeguard the rights and freedoms of natural persons with regard to the processing of personal data and on any other proposed Community measures affecting such rights and freedoms;
   (d) give an opinion on codes Community level.

2. If the Working Party finds that divergences likely to affect the equivalence of protection for persons with regard to the processing of personal data in the Community are arising between the laws or practices of Member States, it shall inform the Commission accordingly.

3. The Working Party may, on its own initiative, make recommendations on all matters relating to the protection of persons with regard to the processing of personal data in the Community.

4. The Working Party's opinions and recommendations shall be forwarded to the Commission and to the committee referred to in Article 31 .

5. The Commission shall inform the Working Party of the action it has taken in response to its opinions and recommendations. It shall do so in a report which shall also be forwarded to the European Parliament and the Council. The report shall be made public.

6. The Working Party shall draw up an annual report on the situation regarding the protection of natural persons with regard to the processing of personal data in the Community and in third countries, which it shall transmit to the Commission, the European Parliament and the Council. The report shall be made public.

Chapter VII - Community implementing measures

Article 31 The Committee

1. The Commission shall be assisted by a committee composed of the representatives of the Member States and chaired by the representative of the Commission.

2. The representative of the Commission shall submit to the committee a draft of the measures to be taken. The committee shall deliver its opinion on the draft within a time limit which the chairman may lay down according to the urgency of the matter.

    The opinion shall be delivered by the majority laid down in Article 148 (2) of the Treaty. The votes of the representatives of the Member States within the committee shall be weighted in the manner set out in that Article. The chairman shall not vote.

    The Commission shall adopt measures which shall apply immediately. However, if these measures are not in accordance with the opinion of the committee, they shall be communicated by the Commission to the Council forthwith. In that event:
    - the Commission shall defer application of the measures which it has decided for a period of three months from the date of communication,
    - the Council, acting by a qualified majority, may take a different decision within the time limit referred to in the first indent.

Final provisions

Article 32

1. Member States shall bring into force the laws, regulations and administrative provisions necessary to comply with this Directive at the latest at the end of a period of three years from the date of its adoption.

    When Member States adopt these measures, they shall contain a reference to this Directive or be accompanied by such reference on the occasion of their official publication. The methods of making such reference shall be laid down by the Member States.

2. Member States shall ensure that processing already under way on the date the national provisions adopted pursuant to this Directive enter into force, is brought into conformity with these provisions within three years of this date.

By way of derogation from the preceding subparagraph, Member States may provide that the processing of data already held in manual filing systems on the date of entry into force of the national provisions adopted in implementation of this Directive shall be brought into conformity with Articles 6 , 7 and 8 of this Directive within 12 years of the date on which it is adopted. Member States shall, however, grant the data subject the right to obtain, at his request and in particular at the time of exercising his right of access, the rectification, erasure or blocking of data which are incomplete, inaccurate or stored in a way incompatible with the legitimate purposes pursued by the controller.

3. By way of derogation from paragraph 2, Member States may provide, subject to suitable safeguards, that data kept for the sole purpose of historical research need not be brought into conformity with Articles 6 , 7 and 8 of this Directive.

4. Member States shall communicate to the Commission the text of the provisions of domestic law which they adopt in the field covered by this Directive.

Article 33
The Commission shall report to the Council and the European Parliament at regular intervals, starting not later than three years after the date referred to in Article 32 (1), on the implementation of this Directive, attaching to its report, if necessary, suitable proposals for amendments. The report shall be made public.

The Commission shall examine, in particular, the application of this Directive to the data processing of sound and image data relating to natural persons and shall submit any appropriate proposals which prove to be necessary, taking account of developments in information technology and in the light of the state of progress in the information society.

Article 34
This Directive is addressed to the Member States.

Done at Luxembourg, 24 October 1995.

Footnotes
1 OJ No C 277, 5. 11. 1990, p. 3 and OJ No C 311, 27.11.1992, p. 30.
2 OJ No C 159, 17. 6. 1991, p. 38.
3 Opinion of the European Parliament of 11 March 1992 (OJ No C 94, 13. 4. 1992, p. 198), confirmed on 2 December 1993 (OJ No C 342, 20. 12. 1993, p. 30); Council common position of 20 February 1995 (OJ No C 93, 13. 4. 1995, p. 1) and Decision of the European Parliament of 15 June 1995 (OJ No C 166, 3. 7. 1995).
4 OJ No L 197, 18. 7. 1987, p. 33.

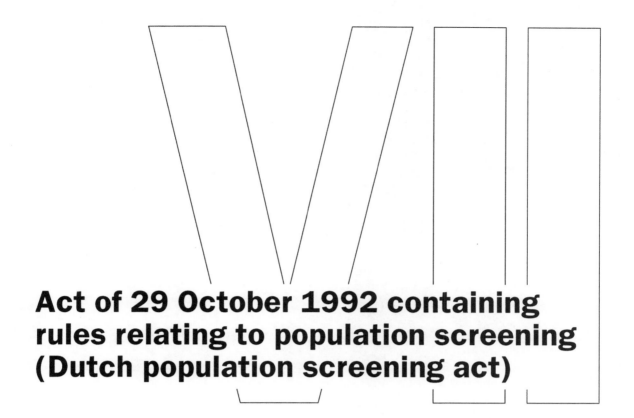

Act of 29 October 1992 containing rules relating to population screening (Dutch population screening act)

We, Beatrix, by the grace of God, Queen of the Netherlands, Princess of Orange-Nassau, etc.

Whereas it is desirable for the purpose of protecting the population to institute a system of authorisation for population screening programmes which may endanger the health of the persons to be examined, and whereas separate provisions concerning chest radiography to detect tuberculosis, as laid down in the Tuberculosis Screening Act (Bulletin of Acts, Orders and Decrees[*Staatsblad*] 1951, 288), are no longer required;

On the advice of the Council of State and in consultation with the Dutch Parliament, have approved and decreed the following:

Chapter I Definitions

Article 1
In this Act and in the provisions issued under it, the following definitions shall apply:
a) Our Minister: the Minister for Welfare, Health and Cultural Affairs;
b) the Health Council: the Health Council referred to in Article 21 of the Health Act (Bulletin of Acts, Orders and Decrees 1956, 51);
c) population screening: medical examination of persons performed under a programme covering the whole population or a section thereof and aimed at detecting specific diseases or risk indicators for the benefit, or in part for the benefit, of the persons examined.

Chapter II Population screening for which an authorisation is required

Article 2
1. Population screening programmes involving the use of ionising radiation, population screening for cancer and population screening for serious diseases or disorders which cannot be treated or prevented shall be subject to the safeguards referred to in Article 3.

2. If, on account of the nature of the screening method to be used or on account of the disease or risk indicator to be detected, Our Minister considers that provisions to protect public health are required immediately, he may designate the screening programmes that are to be subject to the safeguards referred to in Article 3.

3. A bill regulating the matters covered by a decree issued under 2 shall be introduced in the Lower House of the Dutch Parliament within 12 months of the entry into force of such a decree. If the bill is withdrawn or rejected by one of the Houses of the Dutch Parliament, the decree shall be immediately revoked.

Article 3
1. It is forbidden to carry out screening programmes as referred to in Article 2(1) or designated under Article 2(2) without the authorisation of Our Minister.

2. Rules designed to protect the persons to be examined against the risks associated with the screening programmes referred to in Article 2(1) or with the screening programmes designated under Article 2(2) may be laid down in regulations. Such rules may differ according to the various types of screening programme involved.

3. In the case of the screening programmes referred to in Article 2(1) and screening programmes designated under Article 2(2) that are partly carried out for medical research purposes, a regulation may be issued laying down rules concerning the manner in which permission is to be given and in which the individuals involved are to be informed about the purpose, nature and consequences of the examination and about protection of privacy for the persons to be examined.

4. An authorisation may be granted subject to restrictions or with requirements attached, solely insofar as is necessary having regard to the nature of the screening programme for which authorisation is granted, the purpose in either case being to protect the persons to be examined against the risks or to ensure adequate benefit from the screening programme in question.

5. In the case of a designation as referred to in Article 2(2), Our Minister may impose rules as referred to in Article 3(2) and (3); these rules, if not revoked earlier, shall lapse 12 months after they enter into force.

Article 4
1. An application for authorisation as referred to in Article 3(1) shall contain a detailed description of:
   a) the methods of examination to be used;
   b) the diseases or risk indicators to be detected;
   c) the population category to be examined;
   d) the organisation of the screening programme;
   e) the quality assurance measures to be taken in respect of the screening programme.

2. Rules concerning other information to be submitted with an application may be laid down in regulations. Such rules may differ according to the various types of screening programme involved.

Article 5
Repealed.

Article 6
Our Minister shall consult the Health Council before taking a decision on an application.

Article 7
1. An application shall be rejected if:
   a) the screening programme is scientifically unsound;

b) the screening programme does not conform to statutory provisions governing medical practice;

c) the anticipated benefits of the screening programme are outweighed by the attendant risks to the health of the persons examined.

2. In the case of the screening programmes referred to in Article 3(3), an application may be rejected if such an examination is not required for public health purposes.

3. In the case of population screening for serious diseases or disorders that cannot be treated or prevented, an authorisation shall be issued only in special circumstances.

Article 8

1. The inspectors referred to in Article 9[1] shall be informed of the decision on the application insofar as they exercise authority in the locality concerned.

2. The decision shall also be announced in the Netherlands Government Gazette (*Staatscourant*).

Article 9

1. An authorisation may be withdrawn only if:
   a) the information submitted in order to obtain the said authorisation proves to be incorrect or inadequate to the extent that a different decision on the application would have been taken if the true circumstances had been fully known when the application was assessed;
   b) a restriction subject to which the authorisation has been granted is contravened;
   c) a requirement attached to the authorisation is not complied with;
   d) a different decision on the application would have been taken if subsequent scientific knowledge concerning the screening programme for which authorisation has been granted had been known when the application was assessed;
   e) a medical research study is added to the screening programme after authorisation has been granted and a different decision on the application would have been taken if this had been known when the application was assessed.

2. In cases where an authorisation may be withdrawn, restrictions or requirements may be added to it or the restrictions or requirements attached to it may be amended instead.

3. Our Minister shall consult the Health Council before giving effect to paragraphs 1 or 2.

Chapter III Further provisions

Article 10

The public health inspectors designated for the purpose by Our Minister and the officials of the Public Health Supervisory Service acting on their instructions shall be responsible for monitoring compliance with the provisions of this Act and those issued pursuant to it.

Article 11
1. The persons referred to in Article 10 shall be authorised to request information and to demand access to documents and take copies thereof insofar as such actions can reasonably be deemed necessary for the performance of their duties.

2. All persons shall be obliged to lend the persons referred to in Article 10 any assistance that may reasonably be deemed necessary for the performance of their duties.

Article 12
Repealed.

Article 13
1. Persons contravening
   a) the provisions of Article 3(1),
   b) provisions issued pursuant to Article 3(2), (3) or (5),
   c) a requirement attached to an authorisation pursuant to Article 3(4),
   d) the provisions of Article 11(2),
   shall be liable to a class four fine.

2. The punishable actions referred to in (1) constitute offences.

Article 14
1. Persons who on the date on which this Act or a decree issued under Article 2(2) enters into force are already carrying out a screening programme for which an authorisation is required under Article 3(1) shall not be required to comply with the said provision[2] and the provisions issued under Article 3(2), (3) or (5) for 13 weeks following the above date, provided that an application for the necessary authorisation has been submitted within that period, or for four weeks after the order containing the decision on that application enters into force.

2. If in his judgment immediate steps have to be taken in the interests of public health, Our Minister may stipulate that the time limits set out in paragraph 1 shall not apply to the persons referred to in the said paragraph who are already carrying out a screening programme.

Article 15
Within five years of the entry into force of this Act, Our Minister shall submit a report on its implementation to both Houses of the Dutch Parliament.

Article 16
The Tuberculosis Screening Act (Bulletin of Acts, Orders and Decrees 1951, 288) is repealed.

Article 17
This Act shall enter into force on a date to be determined by Royal Decree.

Article 18
This Act may be cited as the Population Screening Act.

We order and command that this Act shall be published in the Bulletin of Acts, Orders and Decrees (*Staatsblad*), and that all ministerial departments, authorities, bodies and officials whom it may concern shall diligently implement it.

Done at The Hague, 29 October 1992

Beatrix

The State Secretary for Welfare, Health and Cultural Affairs | H.J. Simons

Published on 1 December 1992

The Minister for Justice | E.M.H. Hirsch Ballin

Decree of 1 August 1995 laying down regulations pursuant to Articles 3(3) and 4(2) of the Population Screening Act (Population Screening Decree)

We, Beatrix, by the grace of God, Queen of the Netherlands, Princess of Orange Nassau, etc.

On the recommendation issued by the Minister for Health, Welfare and Sport on 11 April 1995 (PAO/GZ-952378);
Taking account of Articles 3(3) and 4(2) of the Population Screening Act;
Having obtained the opinion of the Health Council (opinion of 7 September 1994);
Having consulted the Council of State (opinion of 27 June 1995, No W13.95.0195);
Having seen the more detailed report of the Minister for Health, Welfare and Sport, dated 14 July 1995 (No PAO/GZ/95-6771);

Have approved and decreed the following:

Article 1
In this Decree 'the Act' means 'the Population Screening Act'.

Article 2
1. The examination of a person as part of a screening programme as referred to in Article 3(3) of the Act may only be carried out:
a) where the person to be examined has come of age and subsection c) does not apply: with the written consent of the person concerned;
b) where the person to be examined is a minor who is at least 12 years old and subsection c) does not apply: with the written consent of the person concerned together with the written consent of the parents who are effectively responsible for him or of his guardian;
c) where the person to be examined is at least 12 years old and is unable to exercise reasonable judgment in the matter: with the written consent of the parents who are effectively responsible for him or of his guardian, or if he is of age, of his legal representative, spouse or other partner;
d) where the person to be examined has not yet reached the age of 12: with the written consent of the parents who are effectively responsible for him or of his guardian.

2. If the person referred to in paragraph 1(c) and (d) clearly objects to a procedure being performed on him, it shall be deemed that the consent referred to in paragraph 1(c) has not been given.

3. Persons who have given their consent may withdraw it at any time without indicating the reasons. Such a withdrawal shall not entail the payment of any compensation.

Article 3
1. Before any consent is requested, the persons carrying out the examination[3] shall ensure that the person whose consent is required is informed in writing of the following:

---

a) the purpose, type and duration of the examination;
b) the risks associated with the examination in respect of the health of the person undergoing the examination;
c) the risks to the person who is to be examined arising from failure to complete the examination[4];
d) the inconvenience or other adverse effects associated with undergoing the examination.

2. The information referred to in 1 shall be provided in such a way that it may reasonably be assumed that the person concerned has understood its contents. The latter shall be given sufficient time to enable him, on the basis of this information, to reach a carefully considered decision concerning the consent that has been requested.

3. If the person to be examined is not yet 12 years old or is unable to exercise reasonable judgment in the matter, the person carrying out the examination shall ensure that the individual concerned is given information in a manner appropriate to his ability to understand.

Article 4

Without prejudice to the provisions of Article 4(1) of the Act, applications for an authorisation as referred to in Article 3(1) of the Act shall include:
a) the dates on which the screening programme will commence and end;
b) a detailed description of the purpose of the programme;
c) a detailed description of the potentially detrimental effects of the examinations involved;
d) a description of the type and layout of the areas or rooms where the screening is to take place.

Article 5

1. Where application is made for an authorisation concerning a screening programme in which X-ray equipment is used and where the use of such equipment requires an authorisation under the Nuclear Energy Act, a copy of the latter authorisation or of the application for such an authorisation shall be submitted.

2. Where application is made for an authorisation concerning a screening programme for a serious disease or disorder which cannot be treated or prevented, the said application shall contain a description of the special circumstances justifying the programme in question.

Article 6

This Decree shall enter into force on a date to be determined by Royal Decree.

Article 7

This Decree may be cited as the Population Screening Decree.

We order and command that this Decree together with the relevant explanatory memorandum shall be published in the Bulletin of Acts, Orders and Decrees (*Staatsblad*).

The Hague, 1 August 1995

Beatrix

The Minister for Public Health, Welfare and Sport I E. Borst-Eilers

Published on 5 September 1995

The Minister for Justice I W. Sorgdrager

---

[1] Translator's note: this is wrong - the correct reference is to Article 10.

[2] Translator's note: it is not clear from the original what provision is being referred to.

[3] Translator's note: here, as in the rest of Article 3 and elsewhere, it is not clear whether 'onderzoek' means the whole programme or a single examination.

[4] Translator's note: the exact meaning of 'tussentijds beëindigen' is unclear.

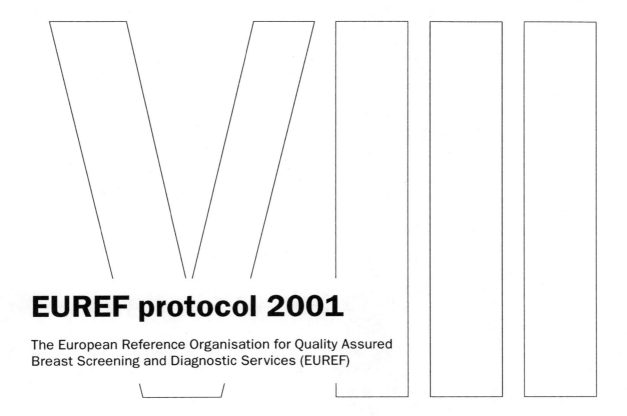

EUREF protocol 2001

The European Reference Organisation for Quality Assured
Breast Screening and Diagnostic Services (EUREF)

The European Reference Organisation for Quality Assured Breast Screening and Diagnostic Services (EUREF)

Breast screening and diagnostic services have expanded rapidly throughout Western Europe. This growth will accelerate as activity increases in certain Member States of the European Community and is also taken up by Eastern European nations.

The primary benefits of such services include reduction of mortality from breast cancer and better overall management and care of women with breast problems. However, poor quality of service provision may cause harm and can lead to significant negative outcomes in term of morbidity, anxiety, efficiency and cost-effectiveness.

Current European experience is that breast services vary considerably in the quality of organisation, delivery and professional support. Concepts of specialist training, professional guidelines and standards, audit and quality assurance are not widely recognized nor implemented.

EUREF believes it is neither appropriate nor desirable for women in Europe to be subject to such haphazard standards of care when breast cancer is so prevalent and causes such concern. Furthermore, knowledge gained through successful breast screening programmes must be disseminated widely throughout screening and diagnostic services for the benefit of all women.

Experience of national screening programmes and the European Network for Breast Cancer Screening has demonstrated the need for three key activities:

1 **Certification** of breast services,
2 **Guidelines** – the production and regular updating of technical and professional quality assurance guidelines,
3 **Training** – the promotion and organisation of mandatory training programmes for staff in all professional and administrative disciplines related to breast screening and diagnosis.

EUREF commits itself to the furtherance of these activities at a local, regional and national level and will provide support and advice on such issues upon request.

The structure of the EUREF organization will be as follows:

a Council,
b Management Board,
c Affiliated experts,
d Administrative office.

The Council will consist of nationally recognized professionals, prominent in the fields of health politics or breast care services. They will provide high level and high profile support for the aims of the organisation both politically and professionally. They will also provide advice to the management board on key issues as required.

The Management Board will be drawn from recognized and experienced staff actively involved in the professional or administrative aspect of breast screening and diagnostic services. They will drive and steer the activities of EUREF, communicate with the Council where necessary and either as a whole or in nominated subgroups receive reports from and oversee the activities of those experts affiliated to EUREF. A designated member of the Management Board will attend Council meetings in order to report activities and to provide a liaison function.

A panel of affiliated experts to EUREF will be drawn up, consisting of at least two recognized and experienced persons from all of the disciplines associated with breast screening and diagnostic services. They will participate in the practical activities carried out by the EUREF organization, whether they be related to certification, guideline production or training. They and the EUREF organization will pay due respect to confidentiality issues with regard to the findings and reports arising from any such activity.

EUREF is a pan European organization, widely drawn from different Member States and is operated on a non-profit making basis. Its name and logo have been registered at a European level. At the present time the administrative office will be located in Nijmegen where facilities and administrative staff are available, although it may be necessary in the future to have subsidiary offices based in other European centres as certification activities expand. EUREF already has considerable experience in the planning and practical performance of certification activities as part of a European Commission funded study.

Amsterdam, January 11, 2001

European Commission

European guidelines for quality assurance in mammography screening — Third edition

Luxembourg: Office for Official Publications of the European Communities

2001 — 366 pp. — 21 x 29.7 cm

ISBN 92-894-1145-7

Price (excluding VAT) in Luxembourg: EUR 15